The Behavioural and Emotional Complications of Traumatic Brain Injury

Studies on Neuropsychology, Neurology and Cognition

Series Editor:
Linas Bieliauskas, University of Michigan

The Studies on Neuropsychology, Neurology and Cognition series provides state-of-the-art overviews of key areas of interest to a range of clinicians, professionals, researchers, instructors, and students working in clinical neuropsychology, neurology, and related fields.

Topics cover a broad spectrum of core issues related to theory and practice in the field of brain injury, including:

- Practical and professional issues (e.g. diagnosis, treatment, rehabilitation)
- Lifespan (e.g. child, geriatric)
- Domain-specific (e.g. sport, toxicology)
- Methodology (e.g. functional brain imaging, statistics and research methods)
- Essential related issues (e.g. ethics, minorities and culture, forensics)

The authors, editors, and contributors to each title are internationally recognized professionals and scholars in their field. Each volume provides an essential resource for clinicians and researchers wanting to update and advance their knowledge in their specific field of interest.

Many news titles are currently in development, so please return often to this website for continually updated information on new and forthcoming publications.

PUBLISHED TITLES

Neuropsychology & Substance Misuse / Kalechstein, Van Gorp
Cognitive Reserve / Stern
Perspectives in Mild Cognitive Impairment / Tuokko, Hultsch
Quantified Process Approach to Neuropsychological Assessment / Poreh
Neurobehavioral Toxicology: Vol I. Foundations and Methods / Albers, Berent
Neurobehavioral Toxicology: Vol II. Peripheral Nervous System / Albers, Berent
Geriatric Neuropsychology / Bush, Martin
A Casebook of Ethical Challenges in Neuropsychology / Bush
Ethical Issues in Clinical Neuropsychology / Bush, Drexler
Methodological and Biostatistical Foundations of Clinical Neuropsychology and Medical and Health Disciplines, 2nd Edition / Cicchetti, Rourke
Minority and Cross-Cultural Aspects of Neuropsychological Assessment / Ferraro
The Practice of Clinical Neuropsychology / Lamberty, Courtney, Heilbronner
Traumatic Brain Injury in Sports / Lovell, Barth, Collins, Echemendia
Practice of Child-clinical Neuropsychology / Rourke, Rourke, van der Vlugt
Forensic Neuropsychology / Sweet
Neuropsychological Rehabilitation / Wilson

FORTHCOMING TITLES

Brain Injury Treatment / Leon-Carrion, von Wild, Zitnay
Geriatric Neuropsychology Casebook / Dunkin
Neuropsychology of Malingering / Morgan, Sweet

For continually updated information about the *Studies on Neuropsychology, Neurology and Cognition* series, please visit: www.psypress.co.uk/nnc/

The Behavioural and Emotional Complications of Traumatic Brain Injury

Simon F. Crowe

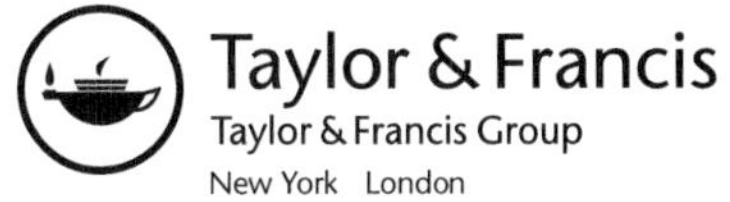

Psychology Press
Taylor & Francis Group
711 Third Avenue
New York, NY 10017

Psychology Press
Taylor & Francis Group
27 Church Road
Hove, East Sussex BN3 2FA, UK

First issued in paperback 2014

Psychology Press is an imprint of the Taylor and Francis Group, an informa business

International Standard Book Number-13: 978-1-84169-441-2 (Hardcover)
International Standard Book Number-13: 978-1-138-00620-1 (pbk)

Library of Congress Cataloging-in-Publication Data

Crowe, Simon F.
The behavioural and emotional complications of traumatic brain injury / Simon F. Crowe.
p. ; cm. -- (Studies on neuropsychology, neurology, and cognition)
Includes bibliographical references.
ISBN 978-1-84169-441-2 (alk. paper)
1. Brain--Wounds and injuries--Complications. 2. Mental illness--Etiology. I. Title. II. Series.
[DNLM: 1. Mental Disorders--etiology. 2. Behavioral Symptoms. 3. Brain Injuries--complications. 4. Brain Injuries--psychology. WM 140 C953b 2007]

RD594.C76 2007
617.4'81044--dc22 2007041885

Visit the Taylor & Francis Web site at
http://www.taylorandfrancis.com

and the Psychology Press Web site at
http://www.psypress.com

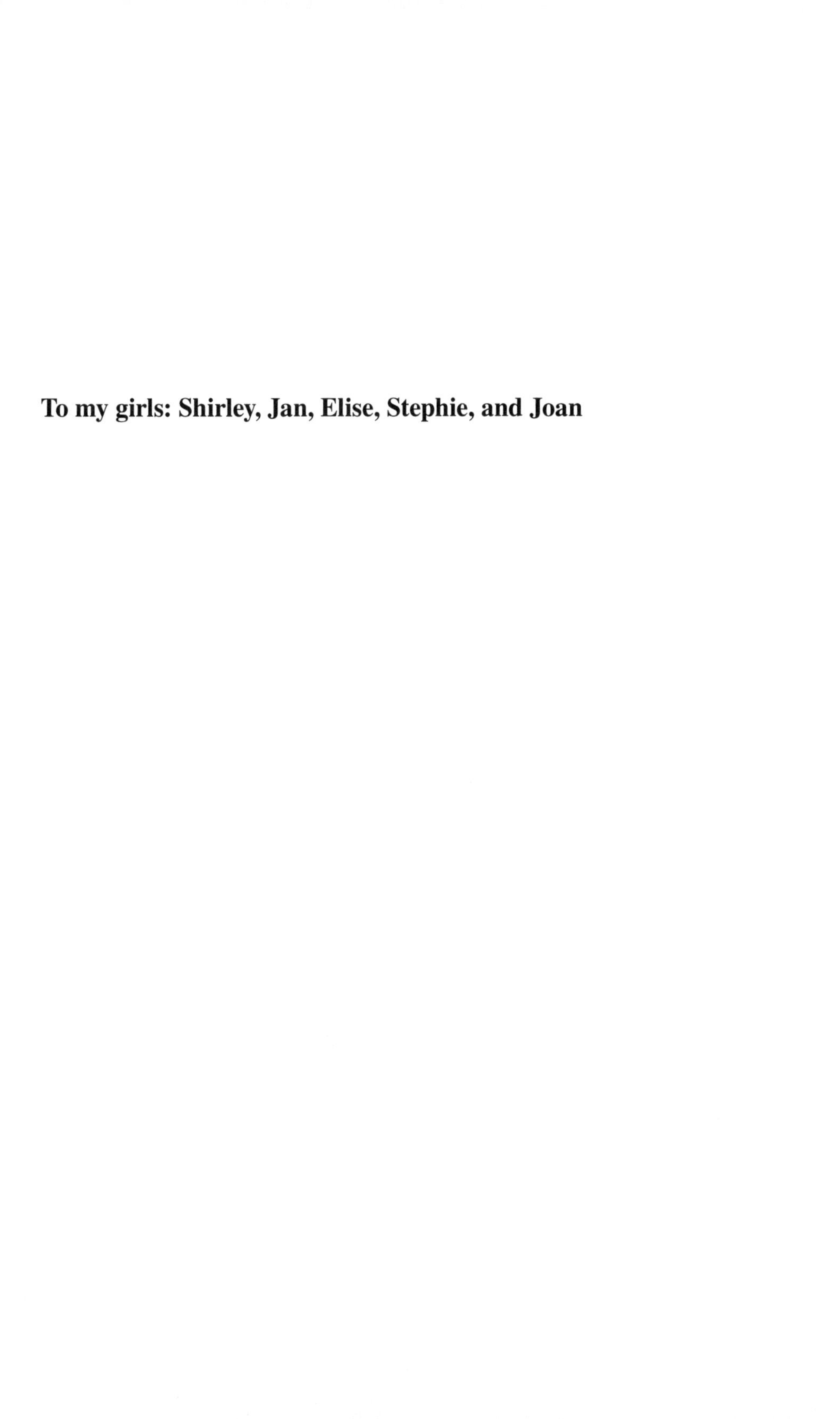

To my girls: Shirley, Jan, Elise, Stephie, and Joan

Men ought to know that from the brain, and from the brain only, arise our pleasures, joys, laughter, and jests, as well as our sorrows, pains, griefs and tears. Through it, in particular, we think, see, hear, and distinguish the ugly from the beautiful, the bad from the good, the pleasant from the unpleasant….It is the same thing which makes us mad or delirious, inspires us with dread and fear, whether by night or by day, brings sleeplessness, inopportune mistakes, aimless anxieties, absent mindedness and acts that are contrary to habit

(Hippocrates 4th Century, B.C.)

Contents

About the author

Simon Crowe, Ph.D., is the Professor and Head of the School of Psychological Science at La Trobe University in Bundoora, Australia. He has a Ph.D. in the neurobiological basis of memory formation and has also completed a training program in clinical neuropsychology at the University of Melbourne. He is the past Chair of the Department and Schools of Psychology Association, Vice President of the Australian Psychological Society (APS), and Cochair of the Science and Research Advisory Group of the APS.

Dr. Crowe maintains strong research programs in the biological basis of memory formation as well as conducting studies into the neuropsychology of neuropsychiatric disorders and a variety of neuropsychological assessment issues. He has published one previous monograph, *The Neuropsychological Effects of the Psychiatric Disorders*, and has authored more than 80 refereed journal articles and numerous book chapters, conference presentations, notes, and commentaries. He is the past editor of the journal *Australian Psychologist* (2000–2005). He has supervised 40 doctoral degree candidates (Ph.D. and D.Psych.) as well as numerous Masters and fourth year theses.

He is a member of the Expert Reference Group of beyond blue and a grant evaluator for the ARC, NH&MRC, beyond blue, Smoking and Health Research Foundation, and the Neurological Foundations of New Zealand and Israel.

Dr. Crowe continues to conduct and extensively practice largely in the area of medicolegal disputation and is an independent neuropsychological examiner for the Workcover Authority and the Transport Accident Commission in Victoria, Australia, from which his extensive experience of the behavioural and emotional effects of TBI has been drawn.

About the authors

1 Introduction

It is hard to imagine what it must be like for an individual following the personal crisis and catastrophe that ensues as a result of a serious traumatic brain injury (TBI). The individual is confronted with a huge range of alterations in his or her normal functioning operating at the biological, psychological, and social levels. A range of primary and secondary neurological events can occur culminating in pain, seizures, compromise in movement, sensation, perception, orthopaedic and other injuries, neuropsychological compromise including disorientation, confusion, retrograde and anterograde memory deficits, decrease in attention and concentration, slowed speed of information processing, executive deficits including concreteness in idea generation, disinhibition and impulsivity, psychosocial deficits including diminished self-esteem, loneliness, a renewed dependency on parents or spouse, infantilization by the wider community, diminution of sexual functioning and interest, depression, anxiety, social isolation, and economic deficits including loss of income, loss of one's employment as a defining feature of one's social persona, prohibitive medical costs, loss of treasured interests or hobbies, and the unenviable role of the plaintiff in any medico-legal proceeding surrounding the claim. All of these changes are also occurring to an individual who has just had a near death experience possibly also having lost, or feeling that they have caused the loss or injury of the other individuals in the vehicle, culminating in heightened levels of guilt, shame, and the not too surprising focus upon "Who am I?" and "Why am I here?"

The long-term outcome arising as a consequence of a brain injury and its behavioural and emotional consequences will be directly dependent upon the severity of the initial injury sustained. However, each individual case will result in a different structural and behavioural pathology depending upon the nature of the injury and the physical forces of the impact, as well as the age, sex, genetic endowment, and experience of the individual at the time of injury (Bigler, 2001). Thus, while TBI can be treated as if it were a common diagnostic entity, the nature of the individual component in terms of the blow, the neural substrate, and the unique psychology of the individual who sustains the injury each vary the explanation of the postinjury outcome.

Individuals can develop a wide range of psychiatric conditions following traumatic brain injuries. These can include: depression, bipolar disorder, secondary mania, psychotic states, posttraumatic stress disorder (PTSD), obsessive compulsive disorder, phobic disorders, and generalised anxiety disorders. These individuals can also be subject to a number of neuropsychiatric syndromes including disorders of drive and motivation and disorders of impulse control.

The aim of this book is to try to tame this maelstrom of contributing factors and attempt to predict which patients will suffer from the various conditions discussed in the ensuing chapters and how it is that they have come to suffer condition X rather than condition Y or, in fact, to suffer no long-term consequences at all.

The discussion begins with a focus upon the nature of the injury, looking at this from a range of perspectives including measurement of the injury, epidemiology, neuropathology, and the mechanics of the blow. I then consider the various classification schemes for the severity of the injury and focus particularly on the issue of the postconcussion syndrome. The discussion then moves to a consideration of organic personality change as a result of injury, then focuses on affective disorder, the most commonly reported behavioural and emotional disruption that occurs following TBI (van Reekum, Cohen, & Wong, 2000). I discuss anxiety and affective disorders including posttraumatic stress associated with the injury and then move on to describe abnormal illness behaviour, psychotic states, and denial of illness following injury. The discussion will then address the effects of the injury on neurovegetative functioning including eating, sleeping, pain, and substance abuse and, as a corollary of these, disruptions of sexual functioning. In the final chapter, with a view to the predicting the behavioural and emotional outcome in individuals who sustain TBI, I attempt to synthesize the various aspects of the injury, the individual who sustains it, and his or her experience both preceding and in the wake of the injury.

Defining traumatic brain injury (TBI)

Let's begin with a few definitions surrounding this complex area. As head injuries can range from a mild bump on the head to serious trauma leading to coma or death, the need to classify patients for both treatment and to predict outcome has led to the classification of patients based on the severity of the initial injury.

Cerebral concussion is the most mild form of TBI and is defined as

> a short-lasting disturbance of neural function typically induced by a sudden acceleration or deceleration of the head usually without skull fracture....The most dramatic aspect of concussion is an abrupt loss of consciousness with the patient dropping motionless to the ground and possibly appearing to be dead. This is usually quite brief, typically lasting just 1–3 min, and is followed by spontaneous recovery of awareness....There appears to be an intimate link between amnesia and concussion so much so that if a patient claims no memory loss, it is unlikely that concussion has occurred. (Shaw, 2002, p. 283)

In association with the loss of consciousness, other commonly observed features of a cerebral concussion include respiratory arrest, generalised vasoconstriction, loss of corneal reflexes, and paralysis of swallowing (Lishman, 1997).

Posttraumatic amnesia (PTA) is the acute, temporary phase of recovery from TBI characterised by impaired orientation, attention, and memory. It is a transient state, which typically includes a period of coma, with a broad spread between individuals in time to resolution, ranging from seconds to months. PTA duration is a useful, although not definitive, indicator of the severity of brain injury (Forrester, Encel, & Geffen, 1994; McMillan, Jongen, & Greenwood, 1996; Russell & Smith, 1961; Wilson, Teasdale, Hadley, Wiedmann, & Lang, 1993), a good predictor of recovery of cognitive function (Boake et al., 2001; Brooks, Aughton, Bond, Jones, & Rizvi, 1980; Dikmen, Temkin, McLean, Wyler, & Machamer, 1987; Geffen, Encel, & Forrester,

1991; Haslam et al., 1994; Mandleberg, 1976), and a relatively good predictor of functional outcome (Bishara, Partridge, Godfrey, & Knight, 1992; Ellenberg, Levin, & Saydjari, 1996; Fleming, Tooth, Hassel, & Chan, 1999; Levin, O'Donnell, & Grossman, 1979; Russell & Smith, 1961).

Patients in PTA are typically disorientated for time, place, and person and suffer from anterograde amnesia (i.e., they cannot lay down new memories) and in association with this they often feature a relatively brief (although not always so) period of loss of memory for the period preceding the injury referred to as retrograde amnesia. Patients also feature diminished alertness and attentional functioning and are usually easily fatigued. They may also be more susceptible to environmental stimulation including heightened sensitivity to light and sound. Their disorientation and confusion often lead to high levels of agitation (Corrigan, 1989). Individuals are deemed to have emerged from PTA when their orientation for person, place, and time has returned, along with the resumption of continuous memory (Fortuny, Briggs, Newcombe, Ratcliffe, & Thomas, 1980; Russell & Smith, 1961).

The definition of delirium, a sometimes noted complication of TBI, is

> A disturbance of consciousness with reduced ability to focus, sustain or shift attention; a change in cognition; or the development of a perceptual disturbance that occurs over a short period of time and tends to fluctuate over the course of the day....Historically, delirium also has been referred to as acute confusional state, acute brain syndrome and toxic psychosis. Although the symptoms of delirium typically resolve within 10–12 days and the majority of patients have full recovery, delirium is associated with increased morbidity and mortality. (Weber, Coverdale, & Kunik, 2004, p. 115)

Considerable overlap between PTA and posttraumatic confusion does exist (Nakase-Thompson, Sherer, Yablon, Nick, & Trzepacz, 2004). Nakase et al. found that of 69% (59/85) of patients admitted to a neurorehabilitation unit featuring the *Diagnostic and Statistical Manual of Mental Disorders–Text Revision* (*DSM-IV-TR*); (American Psychological Association [APA], 2000) criteria for delirium, 71% (42/59) resolved during their inpatient rehabilitation stay.

Whiplash is a term first used in 1928 (Crowe, 1964a, 1964b) that describes the typical hyperextension followed by flexion of the neck that occurs when the occupant of a motor vehicle is struck from behind by another vehicle (Evans, Evans, & Sharp, 1994). Although neck injuries do occur following side or head-on collisions, approximately 85% of "whiplash" injuries occur as a result of rear-end impacts (Deans, McGalliard, & Rutherford, 1986).

There are a variety of scales and methods used to classify the effects of TBI. The two most commonly employed methods are estimation of the duration of PTA (usually as determined by self- or eyewitness report) and the Glasgow Coma Scale (GCS). More formal estimation of duration of PTA is made by using the Galveston Orientation and Amnesia Test (GOAT) (Levin, O'Donnell, & Grossman, 1979) or the Westmead PTA Scale (Shores, Marosszeky, Sandanam, & Batchelor, 1986) in addition to other instruments.

Other measures such as the Ranchos Los Amigos Scale (Hagen, 1984) and the Glasgow Outcome Scale (GOS) (Jennett & Bond, 1975) are also used to predict outcomes following TBI.

Duration of posttraumatic amnesia (PTA)

PTA has been defined as the period of loss of memory following a traumatic event. Specifically, ongoing experience is not registered or the registration of that experience is not continuous (Russell & Smith, 1961). PTA duration is measured from the time of the injury and includes the disorientation, confusion, and coma periods and continues up to the point when the patient resumes continuous registration of experience (Schacter & Crovitz, 1977). Table 1.1 provides estimates of injury severity based on PTA duration.

During the period of PTA, "islands of memory" may occur. These are described as brief periods during the ongoing PTA during which normal periods of encoding and retrieval of episodic memories may transpire despite the return to the amnesic state. Glenys Forrester and colleagues (Forrester et al., 1994) have indicated that these islands of memory occur in about one third of mild and moderate TBI patients.

In a more recent study Williams, Evans, Wilson, and Needham (2002) noted that of their 66 TBI survivors, 18 (27%) had islands of memory for the events. Interestingly, they noted that the recall of these islands was not necessarily associated with the later emergence of PTSD.

From a purely mechanistic point of view, it is difficult to determine how it is possible for a blow sufficient to cause PTA and to disrupt the mechanisms of laying down memory, might transiently resolve for a sufficient period of time to permit memory formation to resume, only to revert to the former state and again disrupt memory formation without further insult to the system. However, as noted above, there are consistent reports in the literature that such a process does occur in as many as one third of patients, although how or why such a process might occur remains obscure.

The end of PTA is defined as the point from which ongoing accurate recall of events takes place (Symonds & Russell, 1943). Researchers must be careful to ensure that the endpoint of PTA is not defined as the first recalled event (McMillan, 1997), which may merely be an "island of memory," but the time from which ongoing recall is restored. Duration of PTA is most reliably assessed over an extended period of

Table 1.1 Estimates of Injury Severity Based on PTA Duration

PTA Duration	*Severity*
<5 minutes	Very mild
5–60 minutes	Mild
1–24 hours	Moderate
1–7 days	Severe
1–4 weeks	Very severe
>4 weeks	Extremely severe

From Jennett & Teasdale, 1981, p. 90. Adapted from Russell & Smith, 1961.

time (i.e., three or more days) using psychometrically validated measures of ongoing recall (see a discussion of these instruments below).

When a formal assessment of this type is not available, the less reliable retrospective account provided by questioning the patient regarding the sequence and detail of events in chronological order until the time of continuous record of events is established (Gronwall & Wrightson, 1980; McMillan et al., 1996) and can be used as a substitute.

Difficulties can arise in using PTA duration as a measure of injury severity due to the intrinsic problems associated with the use of self-reports as data. This is made more difficult in determining when continuous registration occurs in confused or aphasic patients, patients who have been intubated or have significant facial or jaw injuries, or patients who have been administered drugs including analgesics, barbiturates, or paralytic drugs used to lower intracranial pressure (Levin, Benton, & Grossman, 1982).

These difficulties are compounded by the possibility that the patient's first reaction to an accident may be to attempt to make sense of the sudden unexpected impact and to focus upon any imminent threat. These initial seconds and minutes may manifest as an unawareness of surrounding events or a dissociative state, and thus misinterpreted as a state of unconsciousness or PTA. In addition, patients are often emotionally stunned and depersonalised by the sudden trauma, a state sometimes misinterpreted as PTA (Margulies, 2000).

PTA duration has also failed to discriminate reliably between moderately and severely impaired patients in the longer-term, suggesting that the measure may not be sensitive enough in classifying subjects for research purposes. While PTA duration and final functional outcome have been demonstrated to be significantly related, and more strongly so than any other individual variable, in most studies this relationship explains little more than one third of the variance in outcome (Ponsford, Sloan, & Snow, 1995). Clearly, many factors beyond the duration of PTA are at work in the long-term sequelae of the injury.

Glasgow Coma Scale (GCS)

The GCS devised by Teasdale and Jennett in 1974 and revised in 1976 (see Table 1.2) (Teasdale & Jennett, 1974, 1976) is the most commonly used method of classification of injury severity and prognosis. The major purpose of the GCS is the early prediction of mortality and morbidity (Hagen, 1984). It is based on the presence, degree, and duration of coma. The GCS is divided into three dimensions from which the patient's best response is rated. The scores are awarded in each dimension: eye opening (score 1–4), best verbal response (score 1–5), and best motor response (score 1–6). These scores are added together to indicate a total coma score. In calculating severity, a total score range of 3–5 is considered very severe, 6–8 severe, 9–12 moderate, and a score in the range from 13–15 is considered mild. The notion of the "complicated mild" TBI situation involves an individual with a GCS of 13–15, but with positive CT findings or other evidence of neurological injury, which would inevitably predict a worse prognosis than the uncomplicated situation (Williams, Levin, & Eisenberg, 1990). A score of less than or equal to 8 is defined as coma.

Table 1.2 The Glasgow Coma Scale from Teasdale and Jennett (1974)

Response Dimension	*Patient's Response*	*Score*[a]
Eye opening	Opens eyes spontaneously	4
	Opens eyes in response to speech	3
	Opens eyes in response to pain	2
	Does not open eyes	1
Best verbal response	Oriented	5
	Confused	4
	Inappropriate	3
	Incomprehensible	2
	None	1
Best motor response	Obeys commands	6
	A localising response—pulls examiner's hand away on painful stimuli	5
	A localising response—pulls a part of body away on painful stimulus	4
	Flexor response	3
	Extensor posturing	2
	No response	1

[a] In Teasdale and Jennett's original article scores were not assigned. The assigned scores in the table are taken from Lezak (1995).

[b] In Teasdale and Jennett's original article there were only four types of motor response. The division of a localizing response into two discrete response types is taken from Lezak (1995).

In a small percentage of cases, the individual may pass from coma into the "persistent vegetative state," a state characterised by eye opening, preservation of sleep and wake cycles, some rudimentary visual tracking, minor reflex and postural adjustments and primitive reflexes, but no evidence of ongoing responsivity to the environment (Jennett & Teasdale, 1981).

The GCS continues to be the most commonly employed and reliable measure of injury severity in use today because it can be used by each of the disciplines involved in the early assessment of patients following injury including neurosurgeons, neurologists, psychiatrists, and neuropsychologists, and has successfully been implemented internationally to determine initial injury severity. It has been extensively researched in its prediction of global outcome (e.g., the GOS), best predicts both important early outcomes such as death and later outcomes such as employment, and can be obtained within 24 hours of injury (Sherer & Struchen, 2004). Nonetheless, there are some disadvantages.

A key limitation of the GCS is that it is a time-dependent assessment tool (Ruff & Jurica, 1999). If a clinician were to administer the GCS two weeks after the injury there is no sense that this would provide an accurate assessment of the acute injury and, by extension, its implication to long-term outcome. The scale is also difficult to apply in cases where injury or medical intervention prevents initial assessment of any of the three sections of the scale or where intubation, alcohol intoxication, or medication effects (such as opiates applied for pain relief) are present, as these can spuriously reduce the score. Also, when the scale is applied within the first few hours or day following injury as intended, there is a risk of wrongly classifying those patients who later deteriorate in functioning due to secondary injury such as haematoma or herniation of the brain (the so-called "talk and die" syndrome originally described by Reilly and colleagues; Reilly, Adams, Graham, & Jennett, 1975). Implicit within the notion of the patient who has "talked and deteriorated" after a TBI is the concept that this patient has not sustained overwhelming or lethal impact damage to the brain as evidenced by his or her ability to talk after the injury (Ratanalert, Chompikul, & Hirunpat, 2002).

The more recent literature indicates that a subcomponent of the GCS—the time to follow commands (TFC)—may also be a useful indicator of injury severity. TFC is defined as the interval in days from the time of the injury until the individual is able to follow instructions on two consecutive assessments within a 24-hour period (Dikmen, McLean, Temkin, & Wyler, 1986; Dikmen et al., 1994; Katz & Alexander, 1994; Sherer et al., 2003).

Rimel and colleagues (Rimel, Giordani, Barth, Boll, & Jane, 1981; Rimel, Giordani, Barth, & Jane, 1982) have proposed that a TFC of less than or equal to 20 minutes indicates a mild injury, less than or equal to 6 hours after admission to the emergency department indicates a moderate injury, and greater than 6 hours after admission to the emergency department indicates a severe injury. While there is substantial overlap between TFC, PTA, and the TFC and PTA intervals between the various severity clusters of the GCS, TFC provides the best separation between the clusters of severity (Sherer & Struchen, 2004).

The advantages of TFC include its ability to predict both intermediate and long-term outcomes in both trauma and rehabilitation series, it can be obtained early, and it takes into account early complications. Its disadvantages include the fact that TFC is not immediately available, is affected by sedation, requires the close monitoring of the patient over an extended period of time, can be difficult to interpret, fluctuates, and lacks a commonly used scheme for characterizing severity (Sherer & Struchen, 2004).

The neuropsychological profile of PTA continues to be relatively poorly understood. Beyond the use of the common PTA assessment tools, there has been little systematic investigation to determine the exact nature of the cognitive impairments that occur during PTA, most notably in memory functioning. The retrograde component of the amnesia temporally shrinks during PTA, with older memories returning before more recent ones in line with Ribot's Law, suggesting interference with retrieval processes (Baddeley, 1990; High, Levin, & Gary, 1990; Levin, High, & Eisenberg, 1985; Ribot, 1882).

The early work carried out by Yarnell and Lynch (1970) with concussed American football players clearly indicates that the retrograde amnesia is not related to encoding deficits. After a blow to the head, players were able to remember events from immediately before the injury. However, a few minutes later they could not recall these events, which suggests that the information was encoded at the time. Whether the subsequent recall deficits were due to impaired consolidation or to impaired retrieval is unclear. The fact that the memories from immediately preceding the event rarely return in TBI tends to support the notion that the initial consolidation of the information may have been compromised.

Schwartz and Sisler (1971) found that after additional trials were given to allow the concussed sample to adequately learn a list of paired associates, PTA patients displayed recall comparable to the controls at 8 minutes but not at 1 hour following the learning. Similarly, after normal recognition of pictures following a 10-minute delay, patients in PTA display reduced retention over a 32-hour period compared to individuals with resolved PTA and controls (Levin, High, & Eisenberg, 1988).

Some researchers have also argued that in patients with PTA, recognition for newly learned information resolves before free recall of the same material (Geffen, Encel, & Forrester, 1991; Stuss et al., 1999). These results suggest that while encoding and consolidation impairments are likely during PTA, retrieval deficits are the last to resolve.

Due to the problems noted above with regard to specifying the exact nature and duration of PTA, a number of psychometric approaches to the measurement of duration of PTA have been developed. These techniques rely upon the restitution of the continuous ability to recall as the hallmark sign of emergence from PTA and thus usually involves serial assessment to determine ongoing continuity of recall from one day to the next.

A number of tools have been developed and these prospective measures of PTA are as important, if not more important, than retrospective measures since clinical observations—even those of very experienced clinicians—often misdiagnose patients (Tate et al., 2005). The two most commonly used such instruments are the GOAT and the Westmead PTA Scale.

Galveston Orientation and Amnesia Test (GOAT)

The first standardised scale for measuring PTA was the GOAT (Levin et al., 1979), which primarily assesses orientation, but also assesses memory of the last event before the injury and the first postinjury recollection (Levin et al., 1979). This instrument gathers biographical information (name, address, and birth date), and assesses orientation for time, place, and recollection of events surrounding the injury and admission to the hospital as well as eliciting description of the first recall of events following the injury. The total number of points scored for these items are deducted from 100, and scores below 65 are considered to be in the defective range, from 66–75 borderline, and those above 75, normal. The test was designed for daily administration, and Levin et al. (1982) reported significant associations between the score and length of PTA, acute neurological impairment as measured by the GCS, and social and vocational recovery as rated by the Glasgow Outcome Scale (GOS) (Jennett & Bond, 1975).

Westmead PTA Scale

The Westmead PTA scale (Shores et al., 1986) is a structured set of questions used to assess orientation and the ability to demonstrate ongoing recall from one day to the next. The patient is asked a number of orientation questions and asked to recall the examiner's name and face, and asked to recognize pictures of common objects that he or she had been presented with the day before. The procedure is repeated until a perfect score of 12 is obtained on three consecutive days and the period of PTA is deemed to have ended on the first of these three days. The Westmead PTA scale is a more comprehensive assessment tool than the GOAT as it measures new learning, in addition to orientation (Shores et al., 1986). Modifications of these tests and other similar scales have also been devised (Forrester et al., 1994; Fortuny et al., 1980; Mysiw, Bogner, Arnett, Clinchot, & Corrigan, 1996; Ponsford et al., 2004). There is variable agreement between these scales regarding when the exact end point of PTA occurs (Mysiw, Corrigan, Carpenter, & Chock, 1990; Schwartz et al., 1998; Tate, Pfaff, & Jurjevic, 2000), indicating that there are differences in the conception of PTA by researchers and certainly no agreed upon gold standard measure of it at this time (Ahmed, Bierley, Sheikh, & Date, 2000; Tate & Pfaff, 2000).

Ranchos Los Amigos Scale

Unlike the GCS (Teasdale & Jennett, 1974), which is particularly useful during the acute phase of treatment, the Ranchos Los Amigos scale (Hagen, 1984) is helpful in identifying a patient's level of cognitive functioning throughout recovery (see Table 1.3). This scale consists of eight levels of functioning and has mostly been used to track recovery after injury. The main criticism of the Ranchos Los Amigos Scale is that while it provides an indication of the patient's general cognitive status, the actual details of the patient's functioning cannot clearly be deduced from the patient's level (Lezak, 1995).

Glasgow Outcome Scale (GOS)

The GOS (Jennett & Bond, 1975) is a complementary instrument to the GCS (Teasdale & Jennett, 1974, 1976) providing criteria by which to evaluate injury outcome. The scale consists of five levels: (1) death, (2) persistent vegetative state, (3) severe disability, (4) moderate disability, and (5) good recovery. The scale has been criticised due to its insensitivity, particularly with the classification of patients who are semi-dependent or independent, but is useful as a broad range estimate of the trajectory of functioning in the injured individual.

Epidemiology

TBI is the most common form of brain injury (McDonald, Togher, & Code, 1999) and occurs as a result of external forces hitting the skull, such as when the head strikes the windshield of a vehicle or when a blunt object strikes the head. In these circumstances the brain is damaged when the force of impact causes it to smash against the bony surfaces on the base of the skull. Neurological damage may also occur as a result of "whiplash" injury, which causes the head to snap forward and backward rapidly, resulting in acceleration/deceleration forces causing shearing or stretching of the nerve fibres (Bigler & Snyder, 1995). The brain may also be injured as a result of a penetrating force such as when a bullet enters the skull or when the skull is hit with such power as to cause fracturing. In most instances the former type of injury is referred to as a "closed head injury" while the latter is referred to as a "penetrating brain injury" or an "open head injury," and both types of injury may result in localised and diffuse damage (de Kruijk, Twijnstra, & Leffers, 2001).

Table 1.3 The Ranchos Los Amigos Scale: Levels of Cognitive Functioning*

I	No Response: The patient is in a coma and is completely unresponsive to stimuli.
II	Generalized Response: Patient reacts inconsistently and nonpurposefully to stimuli in a nonspecific manner. Responses are limited and often the same regardless of stimulus presented.
III	Localised Response: Patient reacts specifically, but inconsistently, to discrete stimuli. Responses are directly related to the type of stimulus presented.
IV	Confused–Agitated: Behaviour is bizarre and nonpurposeful relative to immediate environment. Does not discriminate among persons or objects, is unable to cooperate directly with treatment efforts, verbalizations are frequently incoherent and/or inappropriate to the environment, confabulation may be present. Gross attention to environment is brief, and selective attention is often nonexistent. Patient lacks short-term recall.
V	Confused–Inappropriate: Nonagitated: patient is able to respond to simple commands fairly consistently. However, with increased complexity of commands, or lack of any external structure, responses are nonpurposeful, random, or fragmented. Has gross attention to the environment, but is highly distractible and lacks ability to focus attention on a specific task; with structure may be able to converse on a social-automatic level for short periods of time; verbalization is often inappropriate and confabulatory; memory is severely impaired, often shows inappropriate use of objects; may perform previously learned tasks with structure, but is unable to learn new information.
VI	Confused–Appropriate: Patient shows goal-directed behaviour, but is dependent on external input for direction; follows simple directions consistently and shows carry-over for relearned tasks with little or no carry-over for new tasks; responses may be incorrect due to memory problems, but appropriate to the situation; past memories show more depth and detail than recent memory.
VII	Automatic–Appropriate: Patient appears appropriate and oriented within hospital and home settings, goes through daily routine automatically, but is frequently robot-like, with minimal-to-absent confusion; has shallow recall of activities; shows carry-over for new learning, but at a decreased rate; with structure, is able to initiate social or recreational activities; judgement remains impaired.
VIII	Purposeful and Appropriate: Patient is able to recall and integrate past and recent events, and is aware of and responsive to the environment, shows carry-over for new learning and needs no supervision once activities are learned; may continue to show a decreased ability, relative to premorbid abilities in language, abstract reasoning, tolerance for stress and judgment in emergencies or unusual circumstances.

Source: Hagen, 1984, pp. 257–258.

The number of persons sustaining a TBI cannot be understated. It is estimated that in America one person every 15 seconds sustains some form of TBI, with approximately 50,000 people losing their lives each year as a result of TBI (Thurman et al., 1999). The annual incidence of head trauma in United States is approximately 1.5 million per year (Thurman et al., 1999). Of these, 500,000 will require hospitalisation and approximately 80,000 to 90,000 will suffer from some level of chronic disability (Frankowski, 1986; Thurman et al., 1999).

In their comprehensive review of 16 studies, Kraus and Chu (2005) noted that the incidence of TBI ranges from a low of 92 per 100,000 to a high of 618 per 100,000 across the United States. Their estimate of the current average rate of fatal plus nonfatal TBI reported in all of the U.S. studies is approximately 150 per 100,000 population per year. They further note that the fatality rate varies from 14 to 30 per 100,000 population per year. They also note that only 16% of all head injuries result in hospital admission (i.e., 1 in 6) and that approximately 80% of TBIs are mild, with a further 10% moderate and 10% severe.

Approximately 395,000 individuals are hospitalised annually for the condition (Bernstein, 1999; Gerberding & Binder, 2003). The vast majority of all TBI (i.e., 75–80% are in the mild TBI range with approximately 25% of those hospitalized, 35% treated and then released from emergency rooms, 14% treated as outpatients only, and about 25% receiving no medical care at all (Gerberding & Binder, 2003).

The average prevalence rate for what could be termed "mild" TBI is approximately 618 per 100,000. It is estimated that between 80,000 and 90,000 people experience long-term disability as a result of brain trauma (Kraus & MacArthur, 1996), and altogether 5.3 million men, women, and children live with a permanent disability as a result of TBI (Thurman et al., 1999).

In the United States, motor vehicle accidents are the most common cause of head injury accounting for more than 45–50% of those injuries suffered. Other causes include falls (21–30%), occupational accidents (10%), violence (5–12%), and injuries from sporting and recreational activities (10%: McAllister, 1992). In Australia, road accidents cause 70% of all traumatic brain injuries followed by falls and assaults (McCarthy, 2001). From July 2000 to June 2001, 350,000 cases were treated in emergency departments for sports- or recreation-related head injuries, and 200,000 of these were diagnosed with a brain injury (Gotsch, Annest, Holmgreen, & Gilchrist, 2002; Kraus & Chu, 2005).

In the United Kingdom, in the mid-1980s it was estimated that 1 million patients per year were entering emergency rooms with TBI, with nearly 5000 dead on arrival, and 1500 with permanent brain impairment (Jennett, 1996).

Recent estimates by the Australian Institute of Health and Welfare give a range of 57 to 377 injuries per 100,000 population per year with a mean of about 150 per 100,000 population per year (i.e., 149 per 100,000 between July 1996 and June 1997: Fortune & Wren, 1999; 154 per 100,000 between July 1995 and June 1996: O'Connor & Cripps, 1999). Adverse outcomes range from 3% with moderate disability or worse to 40% with some residual difficulties on discharge from hospital (Fortune & Wren, 1999). In the early 1990s, health costs arising from TBI were estimated to be $37.8 billion per year (Max, McKenzie, & Rice, 1991) up from the estimated figure of the early 1980s of $4 billion per year (Kalsbeek, McLaurin, Harris, & Miller, 1980). Today's figure would surely be more still.

There is a clear pattern of age specificity with respect to the incidence of TBI. Rates for people under age 10, and most particularly for those under age 5, are high across all studies that report age-specific data (Kraus & Chu, 2005; Kraus & Sorenson, 1994). These figures feature a peak in incidence after age 15 and then a decline after age 24 (Kraus & Chu, 2005; Kraus & Sorenson, 1994; Rapoport & Feinstein, 2000). More than 60% of those suffering brain injury are aged from 16 to 29 (Rosenthal,

Griffith, Bond, & Miller, 1990). Figures tend to decline through middle age but rise again for ages over 60 (Kraus & Sorenson, 1994; Rapoport & Feinstein, 2000). In persons under the age of 45, TBI is the leading cause of death and disability, with an overall mortality rate of 25 per 100,000.

Younger TBI individuals also tend to be more commonly studied than older individuals (i.e., those over 65: Goldstein, Levin, Goldman, Clark, & Altonen, 2001), and the nature of the injuries sustained by these individuals tends to differ with the younger groups characterised by high-velocity motor vehicle accidents while the older group are more likely to be affected by low-velocity falls, possibly as a result of sensory changes (e.g., vision, vestibular, auditory) as well as due to slower speeds of information processing and diminution in the speed of motor responses necessary for righting reflexes.

Before the crash

Beyond the effects of age on TBI incidence, the data clearly indicate that people with head injuries are *not* a random sample of those in their age group (Jennett, 1990). Rather, they include "...an undue proportion of people with some kind of social deviancy. Some are risk-takers in cars and on motorcycles, and some are drinkers or declared alcoholics" (p. 5). For example, 31–58% of those injured in road accidents have blood alcohol levels in excess of 100ml/dl (Corrigan, 1995), while 50–66% had premorbid evidence of substance dependency. In the TBI group studies conducted by Brooks (1988) and Kreutzer, Marwitz, and Wittol (1995), 15–20% had prior convictions for criminal offences preceding the injury.

Men sustain TBI far more commonly than do women, and studies in the United States (Kraus & Chu, 2005) have noted a ratio of 1.6–2.8 men injured to every woman. The incidence rates of TBI are also highest for those groups with the lowest socioeconomic status (Kraus & Chu, 2005).

Rimel, Jane, and Bond (1990) summarised the cross-cultural research findings with TBI sufferers and note that someone sustaining a TBI is more likely to be male than female (two to three times more likely), between 15 and 29 years of age, single rather than married, unemployed, of lower socioeconomic status, living in a congested urban area, and more likely than the general population to have a previous history of alcohol and/or drug abuse, marital discord, and learning disability (Kraus & Chu, 2005). Inevitably, this demographic picture has important implications for the focus of this discussion on the effects of TBI on emotional and behavioural functioning.

An alternative perspective on this issue pertains to the degree to which a variety of demographic and intra-individual features may protect against the ravages of TBI. Ommaya, Goldsmith, and Thibault (2001) indicate that greater brain mass is protective with respect to brain injury. In contrast, smaller brain size may represent a risk factor for the cognitive and emotional effects of TBI. Similarly, Bigler, Johnson, and Blatter (1999) noted that a TBI group with lower IQ (i.e., less than 90) had significantly more enlarged third ventricles and temporal horn compartments than did similarly injured individuals with IQs greater than 90. Bigler et al. (1999) noted that lower psychometric intelligence may be related to more atrophy of the temporal horn and the subcortex and that smaller premorbid brain size may be a risk factor for poorer outcome post TBI.

This observation has received further support from Kesler, Adams, Blasey, and Bigler (2003). In their study of 25 TBI patients, they observed that the participants with lower IQ and lower educational achievement had significantly lower total intracranial volume, irrespective of injury severity, and also suffered greater decline in IQ from the pre- to postinjury assessments. Kesler et al. (2003) noted that "individuals with smaller brain volumes and lower education may be more vulnerable to the functional impact of TBI on IQ outcome, regardless of injury severity and degree of structural brain damage" (p. 160).

It is interesting to speculate on this point about the implications for the sex differences noted in brain weight, with women generally noted to have a brain weight some 10–15% lower than the more heavily brain-weighted male of our species!

Biomechanics of traumatic brain injury

The long-term outcome arising as a consequence of brain injury and its behavioural and emotional consequences will be directly dependent upon the severity of the injury sustained. The final effects of the blow will be an additive or interactive total of a number of forces set in train by the blow. These will include the nature of the blow itself, the nature of the head that is hit, the physical forces of the impact, as well as the age, sex, genetic endowment, and experience of the individual at the time of injury (Bigler, 2001). These issues are further compounded by individual differences related to the requirements of daily life, the environment in which he or she lives, his or her past experiences, and other factors, such as the degree of family of financial support. It is crucial to understand the interplay between these individual or environmental factors and the neuropsychological and psychological deficits, including the circumstances in which the deficits appear, to understand how these various environmental factors may define the way the specific deficits interact (Ponsford et al., 1995).

Despite the various manners in which a blow to the head can be delivered, all concussive injuries have one thing in common: they involve a virtually instantaneous transfer of kinetic energy to the skull that will require either absorption (acceleration) or release (deceleration) of the energy that has been applied to the brain (Shaw, 2002).

For example, neither a slow crushing impact to the brain nor a bullet fired into the brain will induce concussion. The first will not do so because the kinetic energy must be transferred and expended rapidly, thus it would only result in damage to the skull. Equally, the second would not cause loss of consciousness, because the mass of the bullet is insufficient to impart the necessary kinetic energy to the head to cause loss of consciousness (Shaw, 2002). This also explains why it is difficult to produce a concussion when the head is fixed. A beating victim who maintains his head in contact with a wall or with the ground during the attack (by no means an easy feat I am sure) is unlikely to lose consciousness (Shaw, 2002).

The nature of the skull that is struck also has a significant bearing upon the final outcome. The variables of relevance here include skull shape, density and mass of neural tissue, thickness of the scalp and skull, extent, nature and direction of the blow, head–body relationships and mobility of the head and neck at the time of the blow (Shaw, 2002).

The effects of closed head injury can be further subdivided on the basis of the mechanics of the initial injury: those where the body is moving and then strikes a stationary object (as in a fall or motor vehicle accident) and those where the head and body is stationary and the head receives a blow from an object (as in an assault). Of these two injury types the former (i.e., the acceleration–deceleration injury where the head is moving and hits a stationary object) is both more common and causes more extensive brain injury than the latter type (Morse & Montgomery, 1992). Gennarelli and colleagues (Gennarelli et al., 1982; Gennarelli, Thibault, & Graham, 1998) have similarly contended that the brain is most vulnerable to diffuse axonal injury (DAI) when it is moved laterally and is least affected by sagittal movement.

A number of early studies conducted into the mechanics of blows to the crania of monkeys indicate that rotational acceleration consistently produced macroscopically visible lesions exclusively in concussed animals (Ommaya, Faas, & Yarnell, 1968). These authors note that "at equivalent levels of input, acceleration rotation of the head appears to be necessary for loss of consciousness as well as productive of diffuse and focal lesions in the brain" (Ommaya & Gennarelli, 1974, p. 635). They further noted that "paralytic coma (traumatic unconsciousness) is not developed until the magnitude of shear strain is large enough to reach the well-protected mesencephalic part of the brain stem and thus complete the disconnexion (sic) of the alerting system of the brain" (Ommaya & Gennarelli, 1974, p. 637).

It should be noted that a number of possible mechanisms for the cause of loss of consciousness have been proposed including a vascular hypothesis, a reticular hypothesis, a centripetal hypothesis, a pontine cholinergic hypothesis, and a convulsive hypothesis. (See Shaw, 2002, for a comprehensive review and argument in support of the convulsive theory.)

Plum and Posner (1972) have observed that consciousness may be impaired by widespread damage to the cerebral hemispheres and/or by suppression of brain stem activating mechanisms. The two essential elements of consciousness then are arousal and awareness. These processes rely respectively on the subcortical and cortical regions of the brain. Whereas arousal reflects a primitive brain stem function in response to internal or external stimuli, awareness reflects higher level integration of cognitive processes via cortical activity.

Ommaya and Gennarelli (1974) compared the effects of nonimpact acceleration in monkeys when the head was fixed by the application of a stiff collar or when allowed to rotate. They noted that all of the rotated group exhibited concussion and diffuse, widespread, symmetrical lesions throughout the brain. However, there was a total absence of concussion in the monkeys whose heads were fixed at the time of impact. Rotational movement of the brain is less likely to occur when the head is fixed (Pudenz & Shelden, 1946).

Ommaya et al., (1968) noted that if they applied a cervical collar to the monkeys, it raised the threshold for concussion in 50% of the monkeys studied. Interestingly, despite the fact that these monkeys featured no loss of consciousness, brain injury still did occur. The extent of the brain damage was considerably less in the fixed than in the rotated group, with the fixed group featuring a neuropathological lesion distribution that was focal and asymmetric only involving the outer cortical layers. Ommaya and Gennarelli (1974) proposed a

> graded set of clinical syndromes following head injury wherein increasing severity of disturbance in level of consciousness is caused by mechanically induced strains affecting the brain in a centripetal sequence of disruptive effect on function and structure. The effect of this sequence always begins at the surface of the brain in the mild cases and extends inwards to affect the diencephalic-mesencephalic core at the most severe levels of trauma. (p. 637)

Thus from first principles it should be possible to determine a threshold of force applied to the skull below which the brain is never injured, a threshold at which the brain is only temporarily injured, and a threshold above which the brain is always permanently injured. It should be stressed that loss of consciousness will only occur in those situations in which the force of the blow has been sufficient to cause disruption of the activity of the mesencephalic core of the brain (cf. discussion of alternative views provided by Shaw, 2002 above).

The transfer of kinetic energy associated with the traumatic blow sets in train a series of vectors of force each of which may have a distinct effect on the final injury outcome. In a high-velocity side impact to the skull, the brain is set in rotation along its long axis causing a twisting action consistent with the angular rotation of the blow. A similar process of twisting is set in train along the superior inferior axis causing sliding of the bottom half of the brain beneath the top half. A third physical distortion caused by twisting and stretching of the lateral surface of the brain also occurs, possibly culminating in stretching and fracture of the axons (Bigler, 2001).

Translational injuries in which the head remains fixed relative to the shoulders, are not thought to cause diffuse axonal damage (Crowe, 2000). The effect of maintaining the head in a rigid posture may explain why the famous X-15 test pilot Scott Crossfield suffered only retinal damage after a 100-plus g deceleration, why "Indy" race car drivers have survived crashes of 50 to 80 g (Margulies, 2000), and why woodpeckers can decelerate their brains up to 1200 g (May, Fuster, Haber, & Hirschman, 1979) without TBI.

Neuropathological effects of the blow

A TBI can be defined as an insult to the brain caused by an external force that may produce diminished or altered states of consciousness, which may result in impaired cognitive abilities or physical functioning (National Head Injury Foundation [NHIF], 1989). The events that might cause such injuries include road traffic accidents, falls, assaults, penetrating missile wounds, or blunt trauma. The injury arising as a consequence of these blows can be classified as either open or closed head injuries.

An open head injury is an injury in which the skull is penetrated, the dura is breached, and the brain is exposed. Open head injuries differ from closed head injuries in that there is frequently no disruption of consciousness as a consequence of the blow due to the lesser level of kinetic energy imparted to the skull. The deficits arising as a result of open head injuries tend to be localised and the cognitive deficits that occur tend to be relatively predictable depending on the location of the lesion produced. Individuals who suffer open head injuries may undergo rapid, spontaneous recovery. However, as the skull has been opened, they may show later signs of deterioration as a result of contamination and infection, including the development of meningitis and the formation of cerebral abscesses.

These individuals may also show cerebrospinal fluid (CSF) leakage as a result of basilar skull fracture either due to damage to the cribriform plate in association with laceration of the dura producing CSF leakage from the nose (rhinorrhea), or as a result of fracture of the squamous portion of temporal bone leading to deformity of the external ear canal or rupture of the tympanic membrane or both. If this latter injury occurs in association with a dural tear, leakage of the CSF from the ear canal (otorrhea) can occur (Friedman, 1983).

Closed head injury, in contrast, occurs as a result of nonpenetrating injury where the skull remains intact, the dura is not breached, and the brain is not exposed. Deficits as a result of a closed head injury are thus more diffuse.

Subsequent to the blow, these individuals often feature disruption of consciousness and impairment in their continuity of recall of events. Three processes are begun as a consequence of the injury: (1) loss of consciousness probably as a consequence of disruption of the alerting and orienting centres in the brain stem, (2) a variable period of PTA, and (3) often a somewhat unpredictable and variable period of retrograde amnesia (loss of recall of events for the period preceding the blow).

Lishman (1997) has contended that an acute posttraumatic psychosis may also ensue in the early development of the condition. He notes

> Some patients pass through an excitable and overactive phase with florid disturbance of behaviour which can be long continued and pose serious problems of management. Sometimes this is attributable to the abnormal experiences and delusional misinterpretations of a posttraumatic delirium, but sometimes it proves to foreshadow enduring changes of temperament and behaviour occasioned by the injury. The patient may be abusive, aggressive and markedly uncooperative. Very occasionally crimes of violence are committed at the height of such disturbance, and afterwards the patient has no knowledge of their occurrence….the period of acute traumatic psychosis comes to be incorporated within the posttraumatic amnesic gap. (p. 168)

Damage as a result of a traumatic event is the result of a two-stage process, primary injury followed by secondary injury, although some investigators (e.g., Reilly, 2001) further divided this process into a series of four phases: (1) primary injury, (2) evolution of the primary injury, (3) secondary or additional injury, and (4) recovery. Although the issues of evolution and recovery are crucial to the effects of the final injury, these stages are difficult to disentangle from each other, and this discussion will persevere with the former categorization for the purposes of simplicity.

Primary injury

The skull contains three relatively incompressible substances: bone, neural material, and fluids including blood, CSF, and the interstitial fluid, all of which are contained within the relatively fixed volume of the skull. The dynamics of the blow that results in the closed head injury causes a series of physical reactions within the brain substance in response to the applied force. It is also useful to recall that the consistency of the brain within the skull (due to its high concentration [60%] of lipids in the myelin sheaths) is equivalent to that of butter at room temperature.

Primary damage from a traumatic blow occurs through two paths: focal injury and diffuse injury. At the site of impact bruising (contusion) develops. As the bones of the base of skull and in the anterior temporal fossa are relatively inflexible while the brain tissue is soft and fragile, the collision of the brain substance with bone, including the knife-like projection of the sphenoid bones and their anterior clinoid projections, produces marked contusion to the base of the brain (like a knife through butter so to speak!) and its vasculature as it compresses against these bony processes and rebounds. Rotation of the brain also may lead to avulsion of the veins leaving the upper borders of the cerebral hemispheres, causing further vascular compromise.

Contusions can also develop at the opposite side of the brain to the point of impact, a process referred to as *coup-contrecoup* injury. *Contrecoup* damage is the result of the translation of the force and direction of impact to the brain, which sits on a flexible brain stem in a liquid medium. In effect, the brain is "bounced" off the skull on the side opposite of the site of impact causing contusion. In some instances the damage at the site of the *contrecoup* lesion may be greater than that sustained at the site of impact (Morse & Montgomery, 1992), and some investigators (e.g., Russell, 1932) consider that the *contrecoup* effect is likely to cause more severe damage than that at the site of the impact itself.

The specific and localisable changes in functioning that occur in TBI can be accounted for by the site of the *coup* and *contrecoup* lesions (Courville, 1942, 1952), which invariably occur to the frontal (typically inferiorly or posterolaterally) and temporal (typically inferior–anterior and/or medial) lobes (Bigler, 2001), culminating in clinical syndromes featuring executive, memory, attention, and emotional compromise (e.g., Bigler & Clement, 1997).

Bigler (2001) noted that the use of the term "lesion" in association with TBI can be misleading. Despite what may be visualised on any contemporary neuroimaging analysis of the brain lesions as a result of TBI, be they single or multiple lesions, damage to the brain will always be beyond the visually identified lesion represented on the scan (Bigler, 2001).

More recently, data arising from the diffusion tensor imaging and magnetic resonance relaxometry techniques have emerged as techniques for detecting axonal disruption *in vivo*. The former measure focuses on the direction of the diffusion of water molecules (fractional anisotropy), a measure of the intactness of the myelin sheaths. Regions of reduced anisotropy are noted in white matter in the first 24 hours following TBI (Jones et al., 2000) indicating that these techniques may be a powerful means of further characterising the injury following TBI.

The second pathway of insult in a closed head injury is diffuse injury, the result of focal shear injury, contusion, vascular compromise, oedema, diffuse axonal injury (DAI) or the more recently employed terminology: traumatic axonal injury (TAI) (Gennarelli & Graham, 2005), excitotoxic reactions, and diffuse brain injuries (Bigler, 2001).

Oedema or brain swelling comes about as a result of accumulation of excess water within the brain tissue. This usually occurs as a consequence of leakage from the cerebral blood vessels (i.e., vasogenic oedema) at least in the initial stages following injury. This can, however, spread to the underlying white matter by passing between the myelin sheaths (Levin et al., 1982).

TAI, also known as white matter shearing, occurs from the combination of the translated force of the impact onto the brain and the rotational acceleration of the brain within the skull. Nerve axons and blood vessels are rotated and stretched causing: (1) changes to the permeability of the axonal membranes rendering electrical transmission of impulses dysfunctional or (2) shearing. Iverson (2005) notes that contrary to popular misconception, brain injuries do not result in the "shearing" of axons. The process actually occurs as a consequence of the neurons stretching, swelling, and finally separating, but this process only occurs in a small proportion of neurons with most affected neurons recovering over time.

The biochemical changes set in motion as a consequence of TAI include: (1) physical disruption of the cell membrane and the cytoskeleton and (2) increased membrane permeability resulting in major ionic fluxes into and out of the cell (Graham & Gennarelli, 1997). Ca^{2+} is the primary cause of the damaging cascades that follow as a result of trauma and which ultimately leads to cell death (Obrenovich & Urenjak, 1997; Vespa et al., 1998; Xiong, Gu, Petersen, Muizelaar, & Lee, 1997). These processes include: mechanical disruption of the membrane permeability, opening of postsynaptic calcium channels, and depletion of Mg^{2+}. The ionic changes of themselves cause activation of calpains, enzymes that break down the cytoskeleton, mitochondrial uptake of Ca^{2+} leading to disruption of ATP production, production of free radicals, and lipid peroxidation (Reilly, 2001). Excitotoxic insult due to glutamate release has also been extensively discussed in the literature (Lishman, 1997).

The damage caused to the nerve axons as a result of these various processes causes slowed speed of neuronal processing, which is postulated to be the primary cause of cognitive impairment in TBI (Morse & Montgomery, 1992). Bigler (2001) prefers the term diffuse brain injury (DBI) to DAI, as this term includes DAI but also incorporates damage secondary to vascular injury, oedema, and ischaemic injury. As noted above, Gennarelli (Gennarelli & Graham, 2005) prefers the term TAI.

Focal shear injury (FSI) occurs as a consequence of the intense shear, strain, and/or rotational forces that occur at the point of rapid acceleration/deceleration that accompany high-speed impact injuries such as motor vehicle accidents (Bigler, 2001). Shear is most likely to occur at the boundary between the grey and the white matter and may result in a disproportionate reduction in white matter, particularly of the corpus callosum (Levin et al., 2000; Thatcher et al., 1997), following TBI.

Other changes such as elevation in the expression of beta amyloid precursor protein, a protein strongly implicated in the development of Alzheimer's disease, has been immunohistochemically identified at points of axonal injury as early as 1.75 hours after injury (Blumbergs et al., 1995).

Gennarelli and colleagues (1998) have proposed three grades or levels of TAI: level 1 in which diffuse nonspecific axonal damage is present without focal abnormalities; level 2 in which the deficits associated with level 1 are accompanied by focal abnormalities particularly in the corpus callosum and often associated with small tissue tear haemorrhages; and level 3 in which the injury associated with levels 1 and 2 is observed with the addition of damage to the anterior parts of the brain stem often with multiple tissue tears.

The microscopic signature of TAI are axon retraction balls and microglial clusters that are located primarily in the corpus callosum, adjacent deep white matter, and upper brain stem (Strich, 1956). The distribution of retraction balls can also vary as a function of the mechanics of the blow. Bundles of fibres running in one direction may be specifically damaged, while others running in a different direction may be spared (Levin et al., 1982; Strich, 1956).

While the pathological changes associated with the injury obviously are set in motion as soon as the injury occurs, the earliest stage at which these changes can be identified by electron microscopy is at about one hour following the injury. The full force of the injury is then revealed over the ensuing several days. Delayed axonal death can also occur between 6 to 72 hours following the initial injury. The axonal process seems to be particularly sensitive to the changes associated with TAI with the nodes of Ranvier being the weakest point and the site at which the morphological changes associated with TAI appear as early as 10 minutes following the injury (Gennarelli et al., 1998).

Over the next 4 to 24 hours following the injury, the stretched axons undergo transection with death of the distal axonal segments and sealing off at the proximal axonal stump. The distal axon is phagocytosed by microglial cells, hence the microglial clusters noted on histological examination. Once axonal transport starts again, the products being transported from the cell body accumulate against the sealed axonal stump, causing it balloon up into an axon retraction ball (Margulies, 2000).

Secondary injury

Following a blow to the head, the primary injury can be further complicated by the development of secondary injuries including hemorrhages and their sequelae, laceration of the brain due to depressed skull fracture, oedema, and systemic processes including anaemia (a decrease of haemoglobin in the blood), hypoxia (inadequate oxygenation of the tissue), and hypercapnea (greater than normal amounts of carbon dioxide in the blood) (Harris Nagy, & Vardaxis, 2006; Morse & Montgomery, 1992; Reilly et al., 1975).

The development of haemorrhage following a TBI can occur both extradurally or intradurally. Extradural (epidural) haematomas are formed by bleeding from the meningeal blood vessels (particularly the middle meningeal artery), which pool and strip the dura away from the overlying skull. These generally occur in an oval pattern and cause compression of the brain beneath them (Graham, 1996; McIntosh et al., 1996), and constitute an urgent and life-threatening medical emergency.

Intradural haematomas tend to occur as a result of the friction between the meninges and the bony structures of the skull (Povlishock & Christman, 1995) and are classified as subarachnoid, intracerebral, and intercerebellar. The subdural haematomas are more widespread that intracerebral bleeds as they can diffuse throughout the subdural space covering the entire hemisphere (Graham & McIntosh, 1996). Intracerebral bleeding tends to be found deep in the parenchyma often within the frontal and temporal lobes (Graham & McIntosh, 1996; Povlishock & Christman, 1995), and is thought to be caused by rotational and shear forces stretching small blood vessels and causing them to rupture.

Bigler (2001) believes that the effects of vascular compromise in the wake of TBI have been an "overlooked source of pathology as part of the underlying pathology that affects neuropsychological function in the TBI victim" (p. 108). This observation is supported by the study of Zubkov, Pilkington, Bernanke, Parent, and Zhang (1999) as well as that of La Fuente and Cervos-Navarro (1999), and Gennarelli and Graham (2005) go so far as to suggest that "it is the late recognition and treatment of intracranial haematoma that constitutes one of the most, if not the most, important avoidable factors in the management of TBI" (p. 31).

The former study noted that 45% of severe TBI victims showed vasospasm and deficits in the morphology of the vessels as postmortem (Zubkov et al., 1999). Of course, these results need to be leavened by the fact that the study was conducted postmortem and individuals who went on to survive the injury may not have been so affected. The study of La Fuente and Cervos-Navarro (1999) observed that microthrombi developed in the hemisphere contralateral to the hemisphere in which the contusions were noted on examination. This again underlines Bigler's point (2001) above that the extent of the injury in TBI is always greater that the identified lesion.

The effect of these secondary injuries, either intracranial processes, such as bleeding, or systemic processes, such as oedema result in the distortion, shift and herniation of the brain tissue and the production of secondary hypoxic or ischaemic events.

There are four types of brain herniation: (1) cingulate herniation wherein the cingulum is pushed across the midline with associated disturbance of the callosum and anterior commissure leading to disconnection syndromes; (2) temporal herniation where the uncus and hippocampus are pushed against the *tentorium cerebelli* causing compression; (3) tonsillar herniation in which the cerebellum is pushed through the foramen magnum causing the formation of "cerebellar tonsils," which, due to the effects of the raised intracranial pressure as a result of oedema, are "strangled" by the enlarged cranial volume; and (4) external herniation where tissue pushes through the bone flap created by open head injury or craniotomy. These problems come about as a result of the increase in cranial volume arising from haemorrhage or oedema in the wake of the initial injury.

Later changes associated with the injury include: raised intracranial pressure, secondary insult from extracerebral events, the systemic effects of multiple system injury such as hypoxia and fat embolism, degeneration of white matter (leukodystrophy), disturbed flow of CSF/hydrocephalus, and posttraumatic epilepsy from scar tissue formed during the injury. For example, in a study undertaken in Minnesota

(Annegers et al., 1998) it was noted that the 30-year cumulative incidence of post-traumatic seizure in patients without prior history of seizures or other brain trauma who sustained a nonfatal TBI was 2.1% for mild TBI, 4.2% for moderate TBI, and up to 16.7% for severe TBI. The principal risk factor for postinjury seizure was brain contusion and subdural haematoma, with a lesser effect of prolonged loss of consciousness and depressed skull fracture. Infarction has also been noted in the anterior lobe of the pituitary in 45% of cases (Harper, Doyle, Adams, & Graham, 1986).

Mortality following severe TBI has steadily fallen over the last century. Even over the last 25 years mortality following severe TBI has fallen from 36% in 1987 (Marshall, Gautille, Klauber et al., 1991) to 20–24% in a survey of head injury studies reported in 1997 (Bullock, 1997). Most of this improvement can be attributed to better primary healthcare and better control of secondary injury (Reilly, 2001). As a result, there are now an increasing number of individuals who survive these injuries with a range of TBI severity. In severe TBI, for example, between 23 and 50% of individuals will die with a proportion of about 40% being the most commonly reported mortality rate (Sherer & Struchen, 2004). The most common causes of death include brain swelling, traumatic axonal injury, and intracranial haemorrhage. In moderate TBI the mortality rate is less than 10% and usually due to the associated trauma of medical complications of the injury (Sherer & Struchen, 2004). Interestingly, male TBI victims are also more likely to die than are female victims (Gujral, Stallones, Gabella, Keefe, & Chen, 2006).

Recovery following moderate to severe TBI follows a negatively accelerating curve (Schretlen & Shapiro, 2003) that is most rapid in the first three to six months following the injury, but may continue for several years after injury. As a rule, most clinicians agree that the injury will be largely stabilized by about 24 months postinjury and any further improvement from this time on is more likely to be due to behavioural and emotional adaptation rather than to neural recovery.

Nonetheless, the recovery of neuropsychological, not to mention emotional or other functioning, is by no means uniform. Millis et al. (2001) note that for a subset of individuals with moderate to severe TBI, recovery may continue for several years after injury, with most improvement noted on tests of mental speed, visuoconstruction, and tests of verbal memory.

This is not to gainsay the possibility of regeneration of neurons in the hippocampus of the adult brain (e.g., Gurgo, Bedi, & Nurcombe, 2002; Kornack & Rakic, 1999; Kuhn, Dickinson-Anson, & Gage, 1996; van Praag et al., 2002), which holds out the promise of the prospect of manipulation of neuronal growth and the possible use of stem cells with a view to neural repair in these injuries within the foreseeable future.

With regard to the psychiatric and emotional residua of the injury, a number of stages of manifestation of the psychiatric injury have been described (Levin et al., 1982). Stern (1978) for example has suggested that psychiatric disturbance can occur at each phase of the recovery process following the injury. The first phase is noted in association with the recovery of consciousness and may persist for days or weeks following this time (Levin et al., 1982). The second phase is the subacute phase where the acute symptoms of the injury remit. This commonly is associated with the emergence from PTA, but the symptoms of the altered psychiatric state may persist after the PTA period. The third stage represents the more permanent changes in personality and affect associated with the long-term residual effects of the injury.

There is, however, a great deal of individual difference in recovery, and it is extremely difficult to predict the pattern, timeline, or ultimate extent of recovery for any given individual (Ponsford et al., 1995).

The neurological, neuropsychological, behavioural, and emotional consequences of TBI

The most common neurological symptoms following TBI include: headache, pain, nausea, dizziness or vertigo, unsteadiness or poor coordination, tinnitus, hearing loss, blurred vision, diplopia, convergence insufficiency, increased light and noise sensitivity, and altered sense of taste and smell. TBI has been noted to cause injury to each of the cranial nerves (Russell, 1960) with the concomitant disruption of the various sensory and motor functions of the head. Waddell and Gronwall (1984), for example, have noted significant increases in the sensitivity to light and sound stimuli following mild TBI.

The most common neuropsychological deficits include memory difficulties, decreased attention and concentration, decreased speed of information processing, compromise in working memory functioning, communication difficulties, difficulties with executive functions (including initiation and planning, concrete thinking, lack of initiative, inflexibility, the dissociation between thought and action, impulsivity, irritability and temper outbursts, interpersonal communication problems, socially inappropriate behaviours, self-centredness, changes in affect, lack of insight and of self-awareness and alterations in judgment and perception), fatigue and increased sensitivity to lack of sleep, stress, and increased use of drugs and alcohol (Groher, 1977; Levin et al., 1982; Morse & Montgomery, 1992; Pollens, McBrantie, & Burton, 1988; Ponsford et al., 1995).

The published research indicates that cognitive functioning recovers most rapidly during the first few weeks following a mild traumatic brain injury (MTBI) and effectively returns to baseline by one to three months postinjury in non-sports-related injuries (e.g., Iverson, 2005; Schretlen & Shapiro, 2003). The restitution of functioning in sports-related injuries tends to be more rapid, with decrements in neuropsychological test performance resolving in 5 to 10 days (Iverson, 2005). Cognition also improves over the first two years after moderate to severe TBI, but these individuals continue to show compromise greater than two years after the injury.

Depending on the focal point and severity of the injury, more specific deficits in visual, perceptual or language processing may also be added to this list. The language deficits following TBI include naming difficulties and diminution in fluency of speech.

Behavioural and characterological changes are often described in terms of loss of initiative, apathy, increased dependency, irritability, impulsivity, disinhibition, insensitivity to the need of others, childishness, poor judgment in social and financial matters, and either hypersexuality or hyposexuality, with an overall lack of insight into one's personality changes (e.g., Brooks, 1984; Wood, 1990).

Neuropsychiatric illness is a common concomitant of TBI (Jorge, 2005). Fann and colleagues (2004) compared the frequency of psychiatric diagnoses in 939 TBI patients and 2817 controls. The presence of any psychiatric diagnosis in the first year following the TBI was 49% in the moderate to severe group, 34% following an MTBI, and 18% in the controls. In patients without a prior diagnosis of psychiatric disorder, the adjusted relative risk for psychiatric illness in the first 6 months following a moderate to severe TBI was 4.0 (95% CI, 2.4–6.8). Following an MTBI it was 2.8 (95% CI, 2.1–3.7) in comparison to the noninjured controls. For those patients with a psychiatric diagnosis prior to the injury, the adjusted relative risk in the first six months postinjury was 2.1 (95% CI 1.3–3.3) for moderate to severe TBI and 1.6 (95% CI, 1.2–2.0) for MTBI. Prior psychiatric illness proved to be a significant predictor of psychiatric morbidity post TBI, and these problems tended to persist for these patients. This was particularly the case for patients with a previous history of mood or anxiety disorders or for those with a history of alcohol abuse (Dikmen, Bombadier, Machamer, Fann, & Temkin, 2004; Jorge, 2005; Wilde et al., 2004).

Behavioural disturbances such as impulsivity, poor self-control, inability to organise oneself to complete daily activities, and lack of flexibility (Proctor, Wilson, Sanchez, & Wesley, 2000), can have a devastating impact upon the individual in terms of reintegrating into their preinjury lives and functioning adequately and independently in society. In addition, these individuals may have diminished awareness and understanding of their impairments, which can affect their ability to engage in rehabilitation and learn compensatory strategies to enhance their ability to live independently.

The most common emotional and behavioural difficulties following TBI include emotional lability, irritability and aggression, change in personality, fatigue, decreased energy, anxiety, depression, apathy, disordered sleep, loss of libido, and poor appetite (Anderson, 1995). Fatigue, emotional distress and pain are each very common following TBI irrespective of severity.

As a result of the cognitive impairments such as slowed speed of information processing and attentional difficulties, many tasks that were once automatic for the individual, such as concentrating, monitoring ongoing performance, and warding off distractions, can now be completed only with deliberate effort (Lezak, 1995). This extra effort leads to the individual becoming more easily fatigued, further increasing the amount of energy that the individual has to expend to undertake the task in hand. This increasing effort and the resulting fatigue often leads to the individual becoming irritable, frustrated, and angry.

TBI can also result in a variety of neuropsychiatric disturbances ranging from subtle deficits to severe intellectual and emotional disturbances. In rare cases, it can result in chronic vegetative states. The neuropsychiatric disturbances associated with TBI include cognitive impairments, mood disorders, anxiety disorders, psychosis, and behavioural problems (Rao & Lyketsos, 2000).

The study of the nature of psychiatric illness occurring in the wake of TBI continues to expand our understanding of the brain, emotion, behaviour, cognition, physical illness, disability, and quality of life, and how these factors interact with each other. Because the brain is the common pathway by which are all humans experience well-being and suffering, the study of TBI thus provides the unique opportunity to enhance our understanding of all facets of the human experience (Fann, 1997).

Researchers have observed increased rates of depression, mania, generalised anxiety disorder, psychosis, behavioural dyscontrol, and cognitive deficits following TBI when compared to the rates in the general population. Others have also observed increased rates of obsessive-compulsive symptoms, posttraumatic stress disorder, depersonalisation, and personality disorder. Many of these syndromes are common both with the severely brain injured, as well as in the mildly injured subjects. While these disorders occur in the acute phase of TBI, delayed onset of symptoms also occurs. How these neuroanatomical, psychological, cognitive, medical, and social factors interact to determine the resulting psychopathology still needs to be clarified (Fann, 1997).

The residual emotional and behavioural difficulties that occur for individuals who have sustained a TBI have been well documented in the contemporary literature. Lishman (1997), for example, estimates that "the psychiatric consequences and their social repercussions may be judged to be significant in upwards of a quarter of patients who survive" (p. 161). These issues encompass a complex and interdependent set of variables that can lead on to a number of pathological states including substance abuse, depression, anxiety, chronic suicidal or homicidal ideation and action, poor impulse control, significant increase of frustration, and poor insight into behavioural and emotional processes as well as the numerous psychosocial complications associated with the injury (Delmonico, Hanley-Petersen, & Englander, 1998).

The majority of patients with mild TBI recover fairly quickly and are usually completely restored to their preinjury level of functioning in a relatively brief period of time following the initial injury (Mooney & Speed, 2001). However, a significant minority have prolonged, complicated or incomplete recoveries and display outcomes disproportionately worse than would have been predicted on the basis of the objective factors associated with the biomechanics of the injury. It is those individuals, who as a consequence of the injury, or the interaction of the injury with their preinjury state, have these disproportionately worse outcomes that constitute the principal focus of this discussion.

While it would be appropriate in a discussion such as this to include discussion of neurorehabilitation and the current pharmacological treatment approaches to the various conditions described herein, these are not discussed in detail in this volume for two reasons. The first is the sheer scope of an enterprise, which is beyond the cursory summary in this broader discussion of the complications themselves. As a result, the discussion of treatment is left largely untouched as it would require its own similar monograph to appropriately deal with the subtleties of this process. The reader is directed to a number of fine resources on this topic that have been produced over the last few years including the work of Ponsford (2004), Barbara Wilson (2004), and the comprehensive special issue of the journal *Neuropsychological Rehabilitation* edited by Huw Williams and Jonathan Evans (2003) as well as to some of our own foundation work on these topics (Curran, Ponsford & Crowe, 2000; Keppel & Crowe, 2000; Perlesz, Kinsella, & Crowe, 2000).

Jorge (2005) succinctly addressed the second issue with particular regard to pharmacological interventions with TBI in a recent review

> Although progress in basic research allows us to envision a promising future for therapeutic intervention following TBI, there is a lack of adequately controlled clinical studies to provide a solid scientific basis for neuropsychiatric treatment. Currently, treatment decisions are frequently made on the sole basis of clinical experience or with the limited support of open studies and anecdotal cases. (p. 295)

In their comprehensive review on this topic, Warden and colleagues (2006) noted

> Despite reviewing a significant number of studies on drug treatment of neurobehavioral sequelae after TBI, the quality of evidence did not support any treatment standards and few guidelines due to a number of recurrent methodological problems. Guidelines were established for the use of methylphenidate in the treatment of deficits in attention and speed of information processing, as well as for the use of beta-blockers for the treatment of aggression following TBI. (p. 1469)

Warden et al. presented recommendations for interventions with depression, anxiety and other conditions only as options.

Clearly we have much to learn and a long way to go in just characterizing the nature of the changes contingent upon the injury itself, much less in how to sensibly devise treatment strategies for these. Unfortunately, therefore, these discussions must be left to a possible further volume in the future.

Conclusion

The long-term outcome arising as a consequence of a brain injury and its behavioural and emotional consequences will be directly dependent upon the severity of the initial injury sustained. However, individual cases will each result in a different structural and behavioural pathology dependent upon the nature of the injury and the physical forces of the impact, as well as the age, sex, genetic endowment, and experience of the individual at the time of injury. Thus, while TBI can be treated as if it were a common diagnostic entity, the nature of the individual components in terms of the blow, the neural substrate, and the individual who sustains the injury, contribute unique variance to the explanation of the postinjury outcome. The variety of individual differences, environment, history, and injury-related factors following a TBI all interact to create a unique constellation of effects for each individual arising as a result of his or her injury. These factors and influences interact with the change in circumstances and life situation due to injury-related variables and combine to produce the variety of emotional and behavioural disturbances that occur subsequent to TBI. This complex interaction of forces is at its most exquisite and informative in the clinical state that follows the more mild forms of brain injury and the organic-psycho-syndrome referred to as the postconcussion syndrome.

2 The postconcussional syndrome (PCS)

The general public, fuelled by misrepresentations of these phenomenas by television and the cinema, operates under a sizeable number of misconceptions with regard to mild traumatic brain injury. These include the paradoxical notion that when an individual is struck on the head he or she will assume a fugue-like state until such time as all is set to rights again by a second blow. A second set of misconceptions constitutes

> what Evans has described as the Hollywood Head Injury Myth.... the depiction of head injuries on television and in motion pictures in two contexts. In fighting sequences of action, detective, cowboy and martial arts films, the portrayal of head trauma which would result in significant injury or death instead results in only a grunt, a grimace and a few bruises. The infliction of head trauma is also used for some of the funniest scenes in slapstick comedies and cartoons. (Evans et al., 1994, p. 272)

Perhaps the most common problem to emerge in research regarding brain injury is the lack of clear definitions surrounding the terminology used to describe these injuries (Hsiang, Yeung, Ashley, & Poon, 1997). Terms such as postconcussive syndrome, postconcussional disorder, mild head trauma, mild traumatic brain injury, traumatic brain injury, and closed head injury are often used interchangeably and it is difficult to ascertain what each of these terms mean, if indeed they represent differing phenomena. This lack of clarity contributes to at least some of the conflicting data published regarding brain injury and the cognitive deficits that may ensue as a consequence of them (Essleman & Uomoto, 1995). It thus seems worthwhile to clarify what these terms mean and how they have been applied.

Nosology

At the outset it is useful to draw a distinction between injury-related issues and those effects that occur as a consequence of the injury. So in the case of our list of entities detailed above, mild head trauma, mild traumatic brain injury, traumatic brain injury, and closed head injury would be considered injury-related descriptors. These should specify the nature of the injury that the individual has sustained (e.g., a blow to the head that resulted in a posttraumatic amnesia of one hour and a Glasgow Coma Scale (GCS) of 14 on initial presentation at the accident and emergency department).

The injury-related description is quite different from the behavioural or neurocognitive effects that have occurred as a consequence of the injury. Thus the individual may have a posttraumatic amnesia of one hour and a GCS of 14 on initial presentation at the accident and emergency department, but may also be showing a variety of cognitive and other symptoms such as headache, photophobia, heightened sensitivity to noise, dizziness, and lethargy that might lead to a diagnosis of the clinical syndrome of postconcussional syndrome or postconcussional disorder. The syndrome thus goes beyond the description of the injury itself to include aspects of the clinical presentation of the individual in the wake of the injury. As Silver and McAllister (1997) have noted:

> Mild TBI is not synonymous with terms such as post-concussive syndrome. The former simply refers to the less severe end of the spectrum of brain injury; the latter describes the cluster of signs and symptoms (usually including one or more difficulties from somatic, cognitive, and behavioral domains) that can be seen after TBI of any severity. (p. 103)

We must therefore be careful to ensure that in our discussions of these issues that the cause of the syndrome does not become conflated with its effect.

One useful place to begin our discussion is to define these states in terms of existing published resources. The term concussion is often used in the context of the discussion of traumatic brain injury (TBI). Wrightson (2000) observed that concussion describes a physical injury to the head that results in a short-lived impairment of neurological functioning (loss of consciousness or loss of conscious awareness (i.e., feeling dazed), with transient memory loss, and with the expectation of recovery within a week or two.

The *DSM-IV-TR* (APA, 2000), which is predicated upon a biopsychosocial model of psychopathology, adopts a multi-axial approach to the diagnosis of mental disorders and each of these axes refers to a different domain of information that may help in the planning of treatment and the prediction of outcome.

The clinical disorders and other disorders that may be the focus of clinical attention are represented on Axis I (for example, posttraumatic stress disorder; 309.81 and so on). Axis II focuses on the dispositional factors including issues such as personality disorder and mental retardation. On Axis III general medical conditions that may have lead directly or indirectly to Axis I or Axis II disorders are specified (for example, Disease of the nervous system 850.9, Concussion). Axis IV contains examples of psychosocial and environmental problems that may affect the diagnosis, treatment and prognosis of the mental disorder (such as negative life events, losses and lack of social support. Axis V includes a rating of the person's level of overall psychosocial functioning in the range from 0–100 in the form of the Global Assessment of Functioning (GAF) Scale.

The criteria presented in the *DSM-IV-TR* (APA, 2000) identify two entities that describe the diagnostic categories applying to head trauma. These are the Axis I Category 294.1: Dementia due to Head Trauma and a second category included in the Criteria Sets and Axes Provided for Further Study: Postconcussional Disorder.

The more severe entity described in the Manual (APA, 2000) is Dementia due to Head Trauma and indicates

> The essential feature of Dementia due to Head Trauma is the presence of a dementia that is judged to be the direct pathophysiological consequence of head trauma....Post-traumatic amnesia is frequently present, along with persisting

> memory impairment. A variety of other behavioural symptoms may be evident, with or without the presence of motor or sensory deficits. These symptoms include aphasia, attentional problems, irritability, anxiety, depression or affective lability, apathy, increased aggression or other changes in personality. (p. 164)

The Manual makes no stipulation as to the duration of the period of PTA, and focuses on the notion of the "dementia" occurring as a consequence of the head injury.

Over the last three decades, clinicians have become increasingly more interested in the less severe end of the TBI spectrum, and a number of terms to describe these more mild presentations have been proposed including: postconcussional disorder, postconcussional syndrome, and mild traumatic brain injury (MTBI).

The diagnostic category Mild Traumatic Brain Injury (Bernstein, 1999; Miller, 1996; Sweeney, 1992) has been a condition that has raised considerable debate over the last thirty years. Rimel et al. (1981) have defined mild traumatic brain injury as those injuries that feature a GCS between 13 and 15.

The definition of mild traumatic brain injury from the Mild Traumatic Brain Injury Committee of the Head Injury Interdisciplinary Special Interest Group of the American Congress of Rehabilitation Medicine (ACRM) (Kay, Harrington et al., 1993) proposes:

> A patient with MTBI is a person who has had traumatically induced physiological disruption of brain function, as manifested by at least one of the following: (1) any period of loss of consciousness; (2) any loss of memory for events immediately before or after the accident; (3) any alteration in mental state at the time of the accident (e.g., feeling dazed, disoriented or confused); and (4) focal neurological deficit(s) that may or may not be transient; but where the severity of the injury does not exceed the following: (1) loss of consciousness of approximate 30 minutes or less; (2) after 30 minutes, an initial GCS of 13–15; and (3) post-traumatic amnesia (PTA) not greater than 24 hours. (p. 86)

Many studies in the literature use the criterion of a GCS score of between 13 and 15 on first examination (Alexander, 1995) to classify an individual as having sustained an MTBI (e.g., Barth et al., 1983; Bohnen, Jolles, & Twijnstra, 1992; Levin, Mattis et al., 1987) regardless of the other features noted in the committee's definition.

A recent set of guidelines was developed by the Centers for Disease Control (CDC) and Prevention's Mild Traumatic Brain Injury Working group (2003). The criteria for MTBI are defined by:

> the occurrence of injury to the head arising from blunt trauma or acceleration or deceleration forces with one or more of the following conditions attributable to the head injury:

- Any period of observed or self-reported
    - Transient confusion, disorientation or impaired consciousness;
    - Dysfunction of memory around the time of injury; or
    - Loss of consciousness lasting less than 30 minutes.

- Observed signs or other neurological or neuropsychological dysfunction, such as:
  - Seizures acutely following the injury to the head;
  - Irritability, lethargy or vomiting following head injury, especially among infants or very young children; or
  - headache, dizziness, irritability, fatigue or poor concentration, especially among older children and adults. (p. 4)

The two definitions (CDC and ACRM) are consistent with each other, as both require that loss of consciousness (LOC) must last for less than 30 minutes, and that a disorientated or confused state as well as memory compromise are sufficient to satisfy the diagnosis without requiring a formal LOC. The differences include that fact that the ACRM criteria include GCS as an additional determinant of severity, while the CDC criteria concentrate more upon signs and symptoms. Unfortunately, this does include features that may overlap with the features of postconcussional syndrome (PCS) such as irritability, dizziness, headache, and compromise in concentration, conflating cause with effect and flying in the face of Sil'ver and McAllister's (1997) caution noted above.

In view of the imprecision surrounding the terms used to describe MTBI, Hsiang and colleagues (1997) undertook a study employing 1,360 participants who had been admitted to the neurosurgery service of the Prince of Wales Hospital in Hong Kong during the years 1994 and 1995 for the purposes of "redefining" MTBI.

After examining injury-related data such as GCS score, skull x-ray, and computed tomography (CT) scan findings, requirement for and level of neurosurgical intervention and 6-month postinjury outcome, Hsiang and colleagues (1997) found that 967 patients with GCS scores of 15 and no abnormalities demonstrated on radiographic investigations exhibited a good postinjury outcome. However, 108 of the patients with GCS scores of 13 or 14 with no acute radiographic abnormalities demonstrated a poor outcome. The researchers concluded that "patients with lower GCS scores tended to have suffered more serious injury" (p. 234).

While patients with GCS of 15 have a very low incidence of abnormal CT findings or need for surgical intervention (Gómez, Lobato, Ortega, & de la Cruz, 1996), neither history, physical examination, nor GCS can predict which patients will go on to have an abnormal CT scan following MTBI (Livingston, Loder, Koziol, & Hunt, 1991). Approaches based upon magnetic resonance imaging (MRI) with its improved quality of structural imaging are more likely to identify the pathological changes in these patients that may not necessarily be noted on CT (Bigler, 2001).

The incidence of intracerebral injury as revealed by CT scan in patients with GCS of 14 or 15 (i.e., the "complicated mild" TBI described in chapter 1) is relatively low (14% of 111 patients: Livingston et al., 1991 (GCS 14 or 15); 9.4% of 712 patients: Jeret et al., 1993 (GCS 15 only); 3.8% of 2481 patients; Gomez et al., 1996 (GCS 13, 14, or 15). Worse outcome was more likely to be noted with advanced age, lower GCS, and the presence of skull fracture (Jeret et al., 1993; Livingston et al., 1991).

A further problem often noted with current research and one that contributes to the variability of results seen in this literature is the classification of subjects primarily based on a GCS score. In most circumstances the GCS is administered through emergency departments, emergency medical centres, and trauma centres. This procedure in effect "misses" individuals who present to their general practitioners following the trauma to the head or who simply do not present for treatment at all. In these situations (if indeed they come to medical attention at all at the time of the injury) more subjective measures such as self-reported duration of loss of consciousness or posttraumatic amnesic (McAllister, 1994) are used to classify the severity of the injury. It is thus possible that there are intrinsic differences between the MTBIs diagnosed by these respective methods raising a possibility that we are not comparing the same things. An appropriate study that compares samples identified using each approach is long overdue.

Mechanism of injury has also been implicated in the likelihood of subsequent deterioration in MTBI. CT abnormality was more likely in cases of assault and for pedestrians struck by motorcars (Jeret et al., 1993). Baseball bat-induced injuries constitute a growing cause of head injuries. Adair (1990), for example, has noted that when swung by a major league player the end of a bat can reach speeds in excess of 60 miles per hour (mph), generating forces as high as 8,000 lbs at the time of impact with the ball. Groleau, Tso, Olshaker, Barish and Lyston (1993) have noted that in their series of 70 patients struck on the head with a bat, 45 (64%) experienced LOC. Nineteen of the 70 had no LOC and in six patients the presence of LOC was uncertain. In the study, 50% of the patients with intracranial haemorrhage initially had GCS scores of 15, while one in six of their patients with intracranial haemorrhage and one in four of their patients with acute subdural haematoma had either a negative or uncertain history of LOC and a normal GCS on arrival at the emergency room.

Ruff and colleagues (Ruff, Crouch et al., 1994) have noted that while one single uncomplicated mild brain trauma does not as a rule result in poor outcome with permanent functional disability, a minority of individuals continue to complain of persistent deficits months or years after the accident.

Postconcussional disorder is included in the *DSM-IV-TR* (APA, 2000) as a criteria set provided for further study and, as such, has no formal significance within the Manual. The Manual notes:

> Although there is insufficient evidence to establish a definite threshold for the severity of the closed head injury, specific criteria have been suggested for example, two of the following: (1) a period of unconsciousness lasting more than five minutes, (2) a period of post-traumatic amnesia that lasts more than 12 hours after the closed head injury, or (3) a new onset of seizures (or marked worsening of a preexisting seizure disorder) that occurs within the first six months after the closed head injury. There must also be documented cognitive deficit in either attention (concentration, shifting focus of attention, performing simultaneous cognitive tasks) or memory (learning or recalling information). Accompanying the cognitive disturbance, there must be three (or more) symptoms that are present for at least three months following the closed head injury. These include becoming fatigued easily; disordered sleep; headache; vertigo or dizziness; irritability or aggression on little or no provocation; anxiety, depression, or affective lability; apathy or lack of spontaneity; and other changes in personality (e.g. social or sexual inappropriateness).....This proposed disorder should not

> be considered if the individual's symptoms meet the criteria for Dementia Due to Head Trauma or if the symptoms are better account for by another mental disorder. (p. 760)

A number of concerns have been raised regarding the use of the term postconcussional disorder (PCD) by the *DSM-IV* (e.g., Anderson, 1996) as many investigators have noted that it is not an essential requirement for LOC or a lengthy period of PTA to occur for the PCD still to be diagnosed (e.g., Arciniegas & Silver, 2001; Lenninger, Gramling, Farrell, Kreutzer, & Peck, 1990; Ruff, Crouch et al., 1994; Ruff & Grant, 1999; Ruff & Jurica, 1999).

Ruff and Jurica (1999), in response to a number of the problems noted above with regard to the usefulness and applicability of the GCS in MTBI, attempted to create a synthesis of the criteria presented by the *DSM-IV* and the guidelines proposed by the ACRM (1993). These authors propose that patients affected by mild TBI represent a heterogenous population and that the use of a variety of discrepant criteria for diagnosis can only generate further inconsistency in the literature regarding these conditions.

Ruff and Jurica (1999) proposed three grades of severity of MTBI as drawn from the existing sources. Each of the categories features the presence of one or more neurological symptoms, and none of the participants had a GCS below 13. Their Type 1 group was based upon the ACRM criteria and featured an altered state of consciousness or a transient LOC, and an episode of PTA of 1 to 60 seconds duration. Their Type 3 category was based upon the *DSM-IV* category and featured an LOC of between 5 and 30 minutes and a PTA of greater than 12 hours. Their intermediate category (Type 2) featured definite LOC with time unknown or less than 5 minutes and a PTA between 60 seconds and 12 hours. All of the participants had sustained an MTBI according to the ACRM criteria, yet only 34% were classified as having a concussion under the *DSM-IV* criteria. Comparison between their 76 patients (i.e., 26 Type 1; 25 Type 2; and 25 Type 3) indicated no significant differences between the three groups with regard to the number of subjective complaints, neurocognitive performance on an extensive neuropsychological battery, or for preexisting risk factors. The authors contend that there is little benefit in slavishly adopting the *DSM-IV* criteria as a cutoff for the diagnosis of MTBI, as 66% of the patients studied presented with equal levels of emotional, physical, and cognitive complaint. The authors commended the less stringent ACRM guidelines for the diagnosis of MTBI due to the fact that they were the most inclusive.

In the European context, the International Classification of Diseases and Related Health Problems 10th edition Classification of Mental and Behavioural Disorders (ICD-10) (World Health Organization [WHO], 1992) describes a postconcussional syndrome. The criteria for this diagnosis include:

> **F 07.2 Postconcussional syndrome**: The syndrome occurs following head trauma (usually sufficiently severe to result in loss of consciousness) and includes a number of disparate symptoms such as headache, dizziness (usually lacking the features of true vertigo), fatigue, irritability, difficulty in concentrating and performing mental tasks, impairment of memory, insomnia, and reduced tolerance to stress, emotional excitement, or alcohol. These symptoms may be

accompanied by feelings of depression or anxiety, resulting from some loss of self-esteem and fear of permanent brain damage. Such feelings enhance the original symptoms and a vicious circle results. Some patients become hypochondriacal, embark on a search for diagnosis and cure, and may adopt a permanent sick role. The etiology of these symptoms is not always clear, and both organic and psychological factors have been proposed to account for them. The nosological status of this condition is thus somewhat uncertain. There is little doubt, however, that this syndrome is common and distressing to the patient.

Diagnostic guidelines: At least three of the features described above should be present for definite diagnosis. Careful evaluation with laboratory techniques (electroencephalography, brain stem evoked potentials, brain imaging, oculonystagmography) may yield objective evidence to substantiate the symptoms but results are often negative. The complaints are not necessarily associated with compensation motives.

Includes: postcontusional syndrome (encephalopathy), post-traumatic brain syndrome, nonpsychotic. (pp. 67–68)

The symptoms of the PCS can thus be grouped into three principal categories: cognitive complaints (decreased memory, attention and concentration), somatic complaints (headache, fatigue, insomnia, dizziness, tinnitus, heightened sensitivity to noise or light) and affective complaints (depression, irritability, and anxiety) (Levin, Gary et al., 1987; McAllister, 1994).

The criteria for the PCS have a considerable different tone in their description of the phenomenology associated with the condition than that used by either the *DSM-IV-TR* (APA, 2000) or the ACRM. The criteria focus much more upon the psychosocial effects of the condition than on the injury-related issues and mechanism and emphasise a more detailed account of the long-term disability that may be associated with the condition.

It is clear that from a nosological perspective considerable variability still pertains to the description of the milder end of the TBI spectrum and its diagnosis. Nonetheless, the available guidelines do outline a relatively consistent description that allows considerable agreement. The condition has three essential features: (1) a traumatic event of sufficient intensity to cause concussion; (2) a transient change to the mental state of the patient (i.e., LOC, PTA, confusion, somnolence); and (3) no evidence of focal brain damage, haemorrhage, or skull fracture on examination or on diagnostic evaluation (Bernstein, 1999). This entity should be distinguished from the "complicated" MTBI, which features an MTBI but with the additional feature of intracranial abnormality on neuroimaging including skull fracture. Iverson (2005) notes that "patients with complicated MTBIs perform more poorly on neuropsychological tests in the initial days and weeks after injury.., and they appear to have worse 6–12 month…and 3–5 year…outcomes than patients with uncomplicated MTBIs" (p. 302).

While Levin, Gary, and colleagues (1987) have noted that, as a rule, a single uncomplicated minor head injury rarely produces chronic disability or permanent cognitive impairment, this is not always the case. Alexander (1995) estimates that following a mild TBI 50–70% will be symptom free by three months postinjury, while 85–90% will no longer be limited by the effects of the injury by one year following the blow. Nonetheless, some individuals continue to report symptoms of PCS well into recovery (Suhr & Gunstad, 2002). Silver and McAllister (1997) have suggested that patients who experience postconcussive symptoms exceeding 12 months following the injury should be classified as having "chronic" or "persistent" postconcussive syndrome. Misclassification of patients presenting with postconcussive syndrome as having an MTBI, or vice versa, not only contributes to confusion in the brain injury literature, but also contributes to confusion regarding diagnoses should the presenting patient pursue a claim for compensation (Silver & McAllister, 1997). Once again the distinction between the nature of the trauma-related effects of the injury and the longer term clinical syndrome arising in the wake of the injury cannot be over emphasised.

PCS: Organic or functional?

In the history of psychiatry the lack of any obvious neuropathological signature of these disorders has resulted in years of delay and imprecise interpretations of these disorders that have their clearest manifestation in the use of the term "functional" disorder. A "functional" disorder is one for which there is overtly no "organic" cause. So, for example, epilepsy, Parkinson's disease, or an astrocytoma might be considered suitable organic causes for brain impairment. On the other hand, schizophrenia, depression, or obsessive compulsive disorder might be considered to be nonorganic or functional causes of a disorder. While many psychiatrists defend this distinction, it seems that delineating the contribution of "organic" causes of mental dysfunction from "functional" or psychiatric ones, has not proven to be a particular fruitful way to describe them.

Some of the difficulty is attributable to the mis-definition of the terms "functional" and "organic" according to McAllister and Arciniegas (2002). They contend that these terms were originally employed by Coombe, the originator of this distinction, as making a distinction between localised versus diffuse pathology rather than the more recent "mis-representation" of this concept as a distinction between biological versus psychological entities.

Time and again the literature has indicated that the effects of brain lesions are capable of influencing neurological functioning, neuropsychological functioning, and psychiatric symptomatology. Much of the disorder observed in psychiatric patients then is attributable to disruptions in the integrity of the cerebral systems and their consequent effects on cognition, affect, emotion, and reality orientation. In the context of our discussion of the behavioural and emotional consequences of TBI, the issue of whether PCS is a functional as opposed to an organic disorder has been vigorously debated.

The term *concussion* is often used in the context of the discussion of traumatic brain injury and is commonly considered to be a brief impairment of neurological and neuropsychological functioning, which resolves within 7 to 14 days (see definition from Wrightson [2000] above).

A number of symptoms, however, do persist beyond this period in a significant number of cases. These symptoms may be somatic (headaches, phonophobia, photophobia, insomnia, fatigue, blurred vision, and dizziness); cognitive (difficulty in concentrating, memory loss, decrease in speed of information processing, inability to multitask, and difficulty in initiating and planning) or neuropsychiatric (depression, irritability, anger, mood swings, and loss of libido). Usually there is a mixture of all three, constituting what has most commonly been called the postconcussional syndrome (WHO, 1992).

These issues become even more complex in the context of the dispute as to whether the PCS, although a commonly used and diagnosed clinical entity, actually represents a syndrome per se. As McAllister and Arciniegas (2002) note:

> Some experts regard the common signs and symptoms after brain injury as a "post concussive syndrome" that reflect a neurobiology and pathogenic process specific to TBI. Others regard the elements of this "syndrome" as merely co-occurring symptoms seen commonly after brain injury, each initiated by the same event (TBI) but produced by different underlying mechanism. (p. 265)

Mild head injuries have an estimated annual instance in the United States of somewhere between 100 and 392 per 100,000 individuals (Guerrero, Thurman, & Sniezek, 2000; National Institutes for Health [NIH] Consensus Report, 1998, 1999). These individuals commonly report headache, cognitive problems, dizziness, and affective disturbances in the wake of the injury (Suhr & Gunstad, 2002). The natural history of the disorder indicates that from 80 to 100% of patients suffering mild head injury will experience some or all of these symptoms in the first 6 to 12 weeks following injury (McClelland, 1996; Margulies, 2000; Rimel et al., 1981; Rutherford, Merritt, & McDonald, 1977; Wrightson & Gronwall, 1981).

Estimates of prevalence of these symptoms at three months posttrauma vary from 40–60% (Alves, Macciocchi, & Barth, 1993) to between 75 and 80% (e.g., Alves, Colohan, O'Leary, Rimel, & Jane, 1986; Rimel et al., 1981).

For the majority of individuals affected by an MTBI, a good recovery should be expected (Mooney & Speed, 2001), with the symptoms of the PCS in those individuals resolving over the weeks to up to three months following the injury (Iverson, 2005; Mooney & Speed, 1997; Schretlen & Shapiro, 2003). Nonetheless, there can be considerable diversity in the duration of the syndrome with reports indicating it can last as little as only a week to a few weeks (Cartlidge, 1977; Middleboe, Anderson, & Birket-Smith, 1992; Rutherford, Merritt & McDonald, 1979) to as much as five years after the injury (Edna & Cappelen, 1987; Masson, Maurette, & Salmi, 1996; Mazaux, Masson, & Levin, 1997). However, the majority of patients become asymptomatic over the ensuing months with only 30% symptomatic at 6 months (McClelland, Fenton, & Rutherford, 1994) to as low as only 15% remaining symptomatic at 12 months. Nonetheless, in some samples 35–50% of patients who have sustained an MTBI report symptoms for 1 to 3 years afterwards (Bohnen, Jolles, Twinjstra, Mellink, & Wijnen, 1995) and some continue to experience the syndrome up to 15 years following the injury (Rutherford, 1989).

The question thus arises: Is the residual effect of TBI in the form of the PCS an organic or biologically based entity, or a functional one and attributable to psychologically based causes, or is it something in between these two poles? Two camps in this debate have emerged: those who attribute the symptoms to neurological damage (e.g., Gronwall & Wrightson, 1974; Gronwall & Wrightson, 1975; Gronwall & Wrightson, 1980; Levin, High, Goethe et al., 1987; Wrightson, 1989) and those who contend that the symptoms are initiated by a physiological disturbance that tends to be transitory and that the symptoms are maintained by a psychological process (Lishman, 1988; Rutherford, 1989). Rimel et al. (1981) have contended that there are three possible causes for the PCS: (1) the effects of chronic and residual damage to the central nervous system (CNS); (2) secondary gain, and (3) an emotional response to the trauma or a posttraumatic stress disorder (PTSD).

Advocates of a biological cause of the PCS raise a number of issues in support of their explanation. The first is the manifest consistency in the reported symptoms suffered by individuals with the PCS. As Lishman (1988) has noted:

> Central to most descriptions are headache and dizziness, but these may be added abnormal fatigability, insomnia, sensitivity to noise, irritability, and emotional instability. Anxiety and depression are often prominent. Difficulties with concentration and memory may feature strongly among the complaints, and some degree of overt intellectual impairment may on occasion be detected. (p. 460)

It is this ubiquity of these reported changes that characterises the syndrome and as one of the great proponents of the PCS, Wrightson (1989) has observed, PCS "constitutes a syndrome as constant as any in clinical medicine" (p. 247).

These types of arguments lead to a consideration of the issue of sensitivity versus specificity of a clinical entity such as PCS. "Sensitivity refers to an instrument's ability to detect signs of behavioral dysfunction where it is present…In contrast, specificity refers to the "uniqueness" of particular scores, meaning that the test does not report an effect when it is absent" (Berent & Schwartz, 1999, pp. 11–12). So the real question for our discussion of the PCS is to what degree is the PCS a unique syndrome that occurs only in the context of mild TBI? One way we might respond to such a question is to consider a worst-case scenario.

The whiplash shake syndrome that occurs in abused children is considered to be a prototypical demonstration of the phenomena associated with head trauma and an illustration of the fact that central nervous system injury can occur even in the absence of direct head injury (Carter & McCormick, 1983). In most cases of this syndrome, there is a history of a minor accident or shaking of the child. The syndrome is characterised by respiratory depression secondary to the trauma. Physical findings include gastrointestinal symptoms including reduction in appetite, vomiting, and constipation as well as bulging of the fontanelle, a head circumference that exceeds the 90% percentile, and retinal haemorrhage. Subdural or lumbar puncture often reveals blood in the cerebral spinal fluid (CSF), and CT can show subarachnoid haemorrhage and cerebral contusion. The median age of children suffering from the syndrome is 5.8 months, mortality is 15%, and morbidity 50% (Mandel, 1989).

The longer term complications of the condition include blindness, visual motor impairment, seizure, and developmental delay. Follow-up CT studies have revealed cerebral infarction in the half of the children who survive, and cerebral injury is observed in all of them (Mandel, 1989).

The work of Dorothy Gronwall and her co-investigators (e.g., Ewing, McCarthy, Gronwall, & Wrightson, 1980; Gronwall & Wrightson, 1974; Gronwall & Wrightson, 1975; Waddell & Gronwall, 1984) has been particularly important in indicating subtle information-processing deficits in the PCS. These authors have contended that "concussion produces a persisting objective deficit, a decrease in the rate of information processing" (Gronwall & Wrightson, 1975; p. 995). They have demonstrated this deficit using a number of unique approaches, but most commonly using data obtained with the Paced Auditory Serial Addition Task (PASAT), a test that they developed. Waddell and Gronwall (1984) demonstrated that individuals with minor TBI featured lower thresholds for tolerance to light and also possibly to sound using measures administered one to three weeks following injury.

Data have also been gathered using positron emission tomography (PET) techniques that indicate that subsets of patients with persisting PCS have abnormalities on PET and single-photon emission computed tomography (SPECT) scanning (Umile, Sandel, Alavi, Terry, & Plotkin, 2002), although there were no differences between patients with persisting PCS and controls for resting glucose metabolism (Chen, Kareken, Fastenau, Trexler, & Hutchins, 2003). Gaetz and Weinberg (2000) noted that the greatest differences between patients with persisting PCS and controls was seen with visual event-related potentials (ERPs), leading the authors to conclude that their results provide some evidence of a difference between persistent PCS and controls supporting a neuropathological basis.

There is some evidence to suggest that repeated mild TBIs can cause permanent brain damage (Ewing et al., 1980; Gronwall & Wrightson, 1975). Gronwall and Wrightson assessed twenty young adults who were subjected to two successive concussive injuries and compared these to individuals who had had only a single concussion and to a nonconcussed control group. The patients who were subjected to the dual concussions featured a lower rate of information processing than that noted in controls or in subjects who were concussed once only. These patients also took longer to recover to the level of processing speed noted in those experiencing a single concussion. These investigators contend that concussion seems to be cumulative in its effect on performance of the PASAT. Soccer players who suffer repeated concussions perform worse on neuropsychological testing (Matser, Kessels, Lezak, Jordan, & Troost, 1999), and soccer players known for "heading" the ball have been reported to show a higher incidence of neuropsychological impairment than "non headers" (Tysvaer & Storli, 1989; Matser et al., 1999). Similarly, jockeys who report multiple previous injuries show decrements in response inhibition and less consistently compromise in divided attention in comparison to jockeys who report only a single prior injury (Wall, Williams, Cartwright-Hatton, Kelly, Murray, Murray, Owen, & Turner, 2006).

However, evidence against this notion has also been noted. National Football League (NFL) players (n = 685) who underwent baseline neuropsychological examinations before injury and then were reassessed (n = 95) in the few days postinjury did not show any observable decrement in performance at follow-up (Pellman, Lovell, Viano, Casson, & Tucker, 2004; Pellman, Lovell, Viano, & Casson, 2006). In fact, individuals who had had three or more concussions did not perform any worse than those with less than three "dings," undermining the notion of a dosage effect of injury.

Ewing et al. (1980) exposed patients to hypoxia a year or more after a minor TBI and found that after such a period these individuals still performed worse than control participants on memory and vigilance tasks.

There are, however, some problems with these studies that indicate that the conclusions should at least be carefully examined. These problems include: diagnostic uncertainty, reliance on self-reports of the injury, and the lack of medical validation of the diagnosis (McCrory, 2002). Some of the injuries examined in these series occurred as much as eight years after the initial injury. It is generally the case that sports-related injuries tend to be somewhat less severe and individuals usually recover more quickly, thus not requiring hospital admission (Iverson, 2005; McCrory, 2002).

Professional boxers are at risk of developing brain damage (Ryan, 1998) although the neuropathological changes associated with this process usually involve the proliferation of neurofibrillary tangles as seen in Alzheimer's disease (Hof et al., 1992; Roberts, Allsop, & Bruton, 1990; Tokuda, Ikeda, Yanagisawa, Ihara, & Glenner, 1991) rather than the traumatic axonal injury commonly associated with TBI. Some data are beginning to emerge on the incidence of the Apolipoprotein ε4 allele and its linkage with poorer outcome following TBI (Jorge, 2005), however, the support for this association continues to be equivocal. There have also been a number of observations in the literature that the serum protein S-100B may also be associated with PCS. However the data so far indicates that the protein may be specific but not a sensitive predictor of PCS (Savola & Hillbom, 2003). These results, however, are by no means clear-cut, with a number of studies reporting no long-term effects (Butler, 1994; Haglund & Bergstrand, 1990; Haglund & Eriksson, 1993; Haglund & Persson, 1990; Heilbronner, Henry, & Carson-Brewer, 1991; Murelius & Haglund, 1991).

Adherents of the "functional" explanation raise a number of points in response to the biological argument. Studies performed during the 1950s in which human volunteers were subjected to 40 g of sagittal deceleration using a linear decelerator, failed to produce any lasting neurological complications or evidence of permanent brain damage. Jet test pilots subjected to upwards of 450 g of deceleration showed no signs of concussion, and helmeted race car drivers often walk away from accidents involving deceleration over 200 g without brain injury. Falling into a fireman's net (20 g) or being subjected to the opening of a parachute (7 to 30 g) are not ordinarily associated with brain injury (Margulies, 2000). These observations have clear implications for the outcomes likely to occur as a result of the lower levels of deceleration noted with whiplash, for example.

While mild injury is a common disorder, it mostly affects younger male adults, but it is particularly amongst older adults and females that the middle phase of the postconcussion syndrome with its associated features of a physical symptoms, dizziness, irritability, fatigue, difficulty in hearing and vision, poor memory, poor concentration, anxiety, and depression tends to persist (McClelland, 1996). If this was a biologically determined entity, there would not be specificity in the manifestation of the condition in a particular demographic sample.

For example, studies tend to yield inconsistent results with regard to the risk factors for PCD and PCS such as psychological adjustment and premorbid psychiatric status (e.g., Cicerone & Kalmar, 1997; Fenton, McClelland, Montgomery, MacFlynn, & Rutherford, 1993; Karzmark, Hall, & Englander, 1995; McCauley, Boake, Levin, Constant, & Song, 2001; Pelco, Sawyer, Duffield, Prior, & Kinsella, 1992; Radanov, di Stefano, Schnidrig, & Ballinari, 1991; Robertson, Rath, & Fournet, 1994).

The interesting studies of Mickeviüiene and colleagues (Mickeviüiene et al., 2002; Mickeviüiene et al., 2004) are of particular note here. In their study, 300 participants with concussion were followed up for one year postinjury and examined with regard to the usual observed symptoms of PCS (Mickeviüiene et al., 2004). The study had the advantage of eliminating a number of the confounding factors associated with studies of PCS in the United States, United Kingdom, and Australia regarding compensation-related issues, as there was little possibility of economic gain associated with the injury in Lithuania (Mickeviüiene et al., 2002). After one year, the vast majority of symptoms demonstrated no difference between the injured and the control groups, with most of the concerns (e.g., headache, irritability, nausea, etc.) resolving by three months, but with some difference in memory, concentration, dizziness, and tiredness still noted at the one-year follow-up. The authors considered that the finding cast doubt upon the clinical utility of PCS for patients subjected to a LOC of less than 15 minutes.

The factors that tend to more consistently predict the condition include: female gender (Bazarian et al., 1999; Fenton et al., 1993; McClelland et al., 1994); advancing age (Dikmen, Temkin, & Armsden, 1989; Fenton et al., 1993; Radanov et al., 1991), stress and issues associated with postinjury socialization (Fenton et al., 1993; Moss, Crawford, & Wade, 1994; Radanov et al., 1991).

A wealth of literature also exists in describing the base rates at which the reporting of the clinical features associated with the PCS are noted in non-head-injured subjects. Gouvier, Uddo-Crane and Brown (1988), for example, have noted that no significant differences were found between the level of symptoms reported by a head injury group and uninjured controls. Both Iverson and McCracken (1997) and Gasquoine (2000) have noted that a similar level of symptom endorsement as that noted with PCS was also observed in a sample of patients suffering from chronic pain. Gasquoine suggested that the symptoms of PCS are not specific to concussion, but rather due to the effects of emotional distress more generally. Iverson and McCracken caution that levels of pain should be carefully considered in interpreting patients' physical, cognitive, and psychological complaints following head injury. Fox, Lees-Haley, Ernest, and Dolezal-Wood (1995) noted a similar coincidence of symptom reporting in psychiatric patients.

Mittenberg, DiGuilio, Perrin, and Bass (1992) have observed that, in a noninjured group of individuals asked to merely imagine the effects of a concussion, these individuals produced a profile of symptoms virtually identical to those observed in patients who had actually suffered head trauma. A similar finding was also observed by Iverson and Lange (2003) who noted that the PCS-type symptoms are not unique to MTBI, and that they are highly correlated with depressive symptoms.

It is clear on the basis of this evidence that the self-report of symptoms associated with PCS may well be sensitive to the injury. However, given that a variety of conditions including pain, psychiatric disorder, imagined injury or indeed no injury at all, produce similar levels of symptom endorsement, their specificity would appear to be quite poor. Elicitation of self-reports of behaviour, particularly in individuals who have been traumatised or are in the process of medico-legal disputes regarding these matters, must be treated with appropriate caution and symptom endorsement should be weighed appropriately in determination of diagnosis and causation.

Another interesting example of this phenomenon is the presentation of response bias in the elicitation of the examinee's history (Lees-Haley, 1992; Lees-Haley et al., 1997). Lees-Haley et al. (1997) gathered data on a total of 446 subjects (comprising 131 litigating and 315 nonlitigating adults from five locations across the United States) and noted that the litigating clients consistently reported themselves to be hypernormal before their injury. These differences applied to areas as diverse as life in general, concentration, memory, level of depression, level of anxiety, level of alcohol abuse, work or school performance, level of irritability, level of headache, level of confusion, level of self-esteem, fatigue, level of sexual functioning, quality of their marriages, and their relationships with their children. Only the level of drug abuse did not differ between the forensic group and the controls.

Overall, the individuals in the process of litigation perceived their functioning before the injury to be more satisfactory and trouble free than the level observed in equivalent noninjured individuals. This effect may occur as these individuals evaluate their present performance as a benchmark for the previous performance and this results in an overestimate of the level of premorbid function, the so-called "good old days" syndrome. This sort of evidence must sensitize the examiner to the possible inflation of the presently reported symptoms and concerns of the examinee to ensure that examinee bias in the presentation of the history and symptomatology is not reinforced in the reporting of the clinical state.

The study conducted by Mittenberg and colleagues (Mittenberg, Tremont, Zielinski, Fichera, & Rayls, 1996) presents a very interesting twist on the issue of cognitive behavioural intervention with the PCS. From studies as early as those performed by Schacter and Singer in 1962, it has been noted that individuals who did not have an explanation for their state of emotional excitation, as induced by the injection of a dose of adrenaline, tended to explain this emotional state by taking the cognitive explanation for the state provided by their environment. For example, if the individual with an unexplained arousal response was housed with an angry stooge he or she tended to report his or her emotional state as anger, while if he or she was teamed with a euphoric stooge, he or she tended to report his or her emotional state as euphoria.

Mittenberg and colleagues (Mittenberg, Tremont et al., 1996) exploited this phenomenon in the context of a previous observation by Kelly (1975) who observed that PCS symptom rates were higher when patients weren't given any explanation for their symptoms. Mittenberg et al. used a treatment group composed of 29 participants who had a GCS score between 13 and 15 on admission without any measurable period of posttraumatic amnesia. The investigators gave the treatment group a printed manual and they met with a therapist prior to hospital discharge to review the nature and incidence of expected symptoms, the cognitive-behavioural model of symptom maintenance and treatment, techniques for reducing symptoms, and instructions for the gradual resumption of premorbid activities. The control group received routine hospital treatment and discharge instructions.

The treatment group featured significantly shorter average symptom duration (33 versus 51 days) and significantly fewer of the 12 self-reported symptoms of the PCS (i.e., headache, light sensitivity, irritability, fatigue, memory problems, poor concentration, trouble thinking, blurred vision, noise sensitivity, anxiety, depression, and dizziness) at follow-up (1.6 versus 3.1). The treatment group also experienced significantly fewer symptomatic days (0.5 versus 1.3) and lower mean severity levels. The authors concluded that brief early psychological interventions can reduce the incidence and intensity of PCS.

Mittenberg et al. (1996) illustrates that the psychological management of the PCS can result in diminution of symptoms thus supporting the notion of significant psychological contribution to the manifestation of the syndrome. A subsequent report prepared by Mittenberg and colleagues (Mittenberg et al., 1996) reviewed the literature on controlled treatment outcome studies that indicated that a manualised, early, single-session treatment can prevent the PCS as effectively as traditional outpatient therapies, reducing symptoms by 0.32 of a standard deviation (i.e., 16% of untreated PCS patients would be symptom free if they had undergone the brief psychological treatment) (Mittenberg, Canyock, Condit, & Patton, 2001). A similar effect was noted in the study undertaken by Jennie Ponsford and colleagues (Ponsford et al., 2002) using a manualised intervention technique.

Unfortunately, to date there is no reliable evidence base to guide the management of the persisting postconcussion syndrome and there continues to be a lack of systematic follow up of MTBI and PCS cases in the period after one year postinjury (King, 2003). This area of intervention will continue to be one fraught with difficulty due to the diagnostic uncertainty, as well as to the issues associated with somatization, pain, and intercurrent depression in these individuals. This area continues to require more focussed study but the difficulties I am sure overwhelm almost anyone who has attempted to intervene with these very difficult cases. Hopefully, some brave soul will make some progress on this one in the future.

Gordon, Haddad, Brown, Hibbard, and Sliwinski (2000) examined a large sample of individuals with TBI (both mild and moderately severe), nonaffected controls, patients who were HIV-positive, patients with spinal cord injury, and patients who had had liver transplants. Individuals with mild TBI reported significantly more symptoms than did the other groups including those individuals with moderate/severe TBI and the MTBIs reported eight times the level reported by the individuals with no disabilities. The mild TBI subjects reported more cognitive, physical, and behavioural/affective symptoms than did any of the other groups, including those with moderate to severe TBI. It should be noted that the cluster of cognitive complaints was only observed with the TBI samples. The authors interpreted their results to mean that individuals with mild TBI have greater awareness of the functional limitations imposed by their brain injuries than did those whose injuries were more severe.

With regard to the issue of functional versus organic explanations of the PCS, it seems unlikely that a less severe injury would have a higher level of self-reported disability that a more severe one. This raises serious concerns about the dose/response relationship of brain injury. I will address this issue in more detail in the final chapter of this volume.

PCS and its evolution as a function of time

Lishman (1988), in his authoritative review on the physiogenesis and psychogenesis of PCS, noted that there seems to be a different pattern of the condition in the early stages following injury as opposed to those observed later in its development:

> Thus those who have pointed to organic influences have in general been undertaken within a few weeks or months of injury—those showing altered cerebral circulation, delayed evoked responses, impaired information processing, or early neurological impairment. By contrast, those who have highlighted non-organic factors have mostly dealt with patients in the chronic later stages—those drawing comparisons with non-head injured neurotic patients, uninjured twins or those showing no trace of relationship with severity of injury or indices of brain damage. (p. 468)

Lishman (1988) goes on to formulate a model of the PCS that proposes that early in the evolution of the disorder the cerebral dysfunction associated with the injury yields a group of nuclear symptoms including headache, dizziness, and fatigue. He contends these are firmly organic in origin.

As the process of recovery ensues, the organic symptoms recede as a consequence of the natural healing process. If the individual is left untroubled by them, recovery will proceed and the individual will not suffer any long-term consequences of the condition. If however, there are impediments to the natural process of resolution (and these impediments are considered by Lishman (1988) to be largely psychological in nature), then a more chronic course may develop. He contends that these psychological issues may lie in the patient's mental constitution, in a tendency to worry unduly, to acquire conditioning too rapidly, or to build anxiety around the symptoms.

They may also transpire in the wake of the handling that the individual receives following the injury. These might include other sources of distress such as domestic difficulties, financial hardship, resentment about the origins of the accident itself, ill effects of the attempt to struggle to cope too early or to face an uncongenial employment situation. The more substantial the obstacles, the more likely the individual will develop secondary depression or another form of neurosis.

Lishman (1988) contends that the symptoms of the PCS provide:

> the ideal nexus for neurotic elaboration—in contrast to physical disability, they are subjective, unverifiable, and irrefutable, and there is no way that the sufferer can reassure himself that they have disappeared. (p. 468)

Thus, according to Lishman (1988), the longer after the blow the PCS persists, the higher the likelihood that nonorganic factors feature in its maintenance. Early in the development of the condition (i.e., up to about 12 weeks postinjury) organic factors play a major role in the condition, but as the months ensue, the greater the likelihood that the condition is attributable to neurotic elaboration.

Nonetheless, the cautions raised by McClelland (1996) do need to be well heeded in any clinical situation:

> The postconcussional syndrome defies reductionist neuroscience. The efforts of physicians and lawyers to force the phases or indeed the whole syndrome exclusively into psychological or physical domains has more to say about pervasive dualism in medical thinking than about the syndrome itself....First, vulnerability to the development of PCS arises at both physical and psychological levels. Second, a head injury is a threatening life event as well as a physical trauma to the brain. The meaning of the life event matters—including the context of the event, responsibility for the event, and the perceived consequences. Third, the evidence for chronicity is far from one-sided. Persistence of the syndrome is more likely among those who become "cases." (p. 566)

Conclusion

What can we conclude regarding this fascinating clinical entity? It seems clear that the effects of an MTBI in most individuals will go on to complete resolution in the ensuing one to three months following the injury. For example, in the study by Ponsford et al. (2000), the symptoms of 84 consecutively admitted patients with MTBI noted that the symptoms noted at one week (i.e., headache, dizziness, fatigue, visual disturbance, and memory problems) had largely resolved (with the exception of headache and dizziness) by three months postinjury, and the symptom of concentration difficulty predicted only 3% of the variance of the correctly classified cases. In a minority of individuals, however, (i.e., approximately 10–15%), the condition may go on to become chronic and may last for a year or considerably longer. As the acute presentation becomes more protracted, psychological factors seem to overtake neurological ones and a condition characterized by somatization of the original symptoms may become entrenched. The self-reported symptoms of the PCS including somatic, cognitive, and psychiatric features are sensitive to the condition, but are relatively nonspecific, and similarly high levels of endorsement of these symptoms can be noted in a variety of other clinical groups including patients with pain, psychiatric disorders, or merely in intact individuals asked to imagine having sustained an injury.

The still unsolved question arising from this issue continues, however: Why does a similar intensity of injury affect one individual profoundly and yet leave another apparently similar individual untouched following a brief period of recovery? Clearly something more is at play here than is represented by a mechanico-physical description of the forces of rotation, acceleration, and deceleration associated with the blow. Lishman (1988) as indicated above is clearly of the view that it is psychological elaboration in the latter stages that leads to the prolonged symptoms of the chronic PCS.

One aspect of the relationship between traumatic brain injury and the emergence of the behavioural and the emotional disorder that has not been addressed so far is the relationship between these organic disorders and classic psychiatric syndromes.

The administration of clinical questionnaires, structured clinical interviews, and neurological or neuropsychological testing are not always sufficient to distinguish idiopathic from acquired forms of the various psychiatric disorders seen following TBI. As such, clinicians are thrown to their mettle to determine the respective origins of the disorders they seek to diagnose. Clearly, age of onset, a clinical history of sudden onset in the wake of the TBI and the absence of family history or other predisposing signals may orient the diagnosis in one way rather than the other (Etcharry-Bouyx & Dubas, 2000).

It seems clear that considerable caution must be exercised in the interpretation of the causes of the PCS. The aetiology is diverse and contribution of numerous aspects of the injury, the individual, their circumstances, the past history, and the handling of the condition subsequent to impact are all capable of influencing the development, elaboration, and persistence of this complicated condition. Postconcussion syndrome should be viewed as a psychological, neurological, and psychiatric state that can occur in the wake of a brain injury, but is separate from it. However, this process is set in train at the same time as the brain injury itself. PCS is the individual's psychological/neurological and physical response to the injury and should not be confused with the injury itself, which may be mild, moderate, or severe (Silver & McAllister, 1997).

This distinction is a worthwhile one and may usefully contribute to more appropriate classification of the conditions that occur following both mild and more severe TBI. Discussion and dispute still continue over the issue of MTBI, but for the purposes of this discussion it will be assumed that such a phenomenon does exist (just as severe TBI exists). Both conditions can, however, act as the precipitant of the response of the individual to the injury that constitutes the postconcussion syndrome.

3 Organic personality change

In their definitive textbook *Management of Head Injuries*, Jennett and Teasdale (1981) noted that personality change is "the most consistent feature of mental change after blunt head injury" (p. 294). In this chapter I survey the changes that can take place with respect to personality structure and function as a consequence of traumatic brain injury. Inevitably the notion of personality change following injury is intimately interlinked with the functions of the frontal lobe and the cognitive psychologist's notion of the executive system of the brain. Thus I begin with a survey of the frontal/executive systems and then attempt to connect these concepts with the structure of personality and how this might change as a consequence of injury.

Background

The first step in differentiating the subtle differences in approach to the functions of the frontal/executive system in more detail is to examine how these functions have been viewed in the theoretical literature. The model of brain functioning proposed by the Russian neuropsychologist Alexander Luria is a good place to begin.

Luria (1973) proposes that there are three slave systems within the working brain, each of which is hierarchically organised. These systems are the system for maintaining cortical tone and arousal (located in the brain stem), the system for gathering and retrieving information (located behind the central sulcus), and the system for motor planning and motor output (located before the central sulcus, i.e., the frontal lobe).

Each neuropsychological function is effected by a complex functional system incorporating a number of cortical zones and subcortical structures, each of which makes its own contribution to the performance of the function and supplies its own factor in the structure (Luria, 1973). The disruption of the function would thus occur irrespective of the site of the damage to the distributed system. However, the specific site of the lesion adds a characteristic flavour to the disruption of function based upon the area affected.

This notion of a coordinated set of independent brain regions that are connected to produce a given behavioural outcome has been termed modularity. The original notion of modularity comes from the work of the philosopher Jerry Fodor (1983, 1985, 2000). The basic premise of the theory is that there exist functionally isolated, specific cognitive processing systems in the brain. These components are independent of the other components of the operating brain and they can be selectively impaired by brain injury.

Fodor (1983, 1985, 2000) contends that there are two types of informational systems in the brain. These are informationally specific bottom up modules (such as some of the perceptual or motor systems) and diffuse nonspecific central systems. These latter systems are not associated with either top down or bottom up processing as within these systems the information flows "every which way" (Fodor, 1985, p. 4). Fodor contends that modular processing is genetically hardwired and the action of these modular systems is characterised by their rapid, automatic, and domain-specific processing.

The central systems on the other hand are slower, nonspecific, cognitively penetrable, and not fixed in their cognitive architecture. Fodor contends that the modules are special purpose devices suitable for obtaining specific information within their cognate domains, processing it rapidly and automatically, and then delivering the results of that processing for interpretation by the central processing systems.

The modules are characterised by the fact that top down processes such as the executive cannot interfere with their circumscribed functions with opinions, beliefs, or motivational factors. "It is the function of the central system to take the output of these processing systems and interpret this information and to relate it to the store of general knowledge" (i.e., sematic memory) (Fodor, 1983, p. 209).

Whilst Fodor's theory has been very influential, not everyone is a firm adherent. Elkhonon Goldberg (1995; also a major critic of the notion of double dissociation as evidence of cognitive specificity) contends that modularity theory has become popular because of its seductiveness and the illusory appeal of its instant explainability. Goldberg contends that each time the modularist encounters a new observation he or she can create a new module to explain it. As a result, modularity theory is not economical in that it increases rather than reduces the number of units of explanation. "Like the belief systems of antiquity, it merely relabels its domain by inventing a separate deity for every thing" (Goldberg, 1995, p. 194). He maintains that the key to the organization of the brain is not due to an assembly of modules but that the process emerges from the continuous, interactive, and emergent properties of complex neural organization.

A second problem for modular theory arises because of its apparent ability to conveniently explain double dissociation evidence, one of the methodological and theoretical cornerstones of contemporary neuropsychology. Double dissociation exists when two cognitive functions can be established to be independent of each other such that one individual may have a deficit in function X but not in function Y while another individual has the reverse pattern of deficit. Modular theory is often considered to imply the existence of separable cognitive components. Shallice (1988) points out the problem with this logic: If modules exist, then double dissociation is an excellent way of uncovering these. As the extensive neuropsychological literature can attest, double dissociations do exist, therefore modules exist.

The latter inference is only valid, however, if modular systems are the only systems that could produce double dissociations. A number of theorists however (e.g., Kimberg & Farah, 1993) clearly demonstrate that parallel distributed processing networks as modelled using artificial intelligence are equally capable of producing and explaining double dissociations. Despite its imperfections, and no one can deny that they exist, Fodor's modular theory can be of use, particularly in understanding the association between the frontal lobes and the executive systems of the brain.

A more recent approach to the localisation and explanation of the function of the various regions of the brain has been proposed by Marcel Mesulam (1985, 2000a). The "topologic approach" to brain function expands on the theories proposed by Luria

(1973) among others and presents them in what I believe to be the most satisfying model of the brain's function presented to date. The topological model (Mesulam, 1985, 2000a) proposes five functional areas of the brain that can be classified from those with closest connection to the internal environment to those areas that are responsible for the apprehension of stimuli in the extrapersonal space. The five areas are:

(1) Limbic areas including the septum, the substantia innominata, the amygdala complex, the hippocampal formation and the piriform complex. These areas are in closest association with the centres in the brain stem and hypothalamus that control homeostasis or maintenance of the internal state of the body.
(2) Paralimbic areas including the temporal pole, the orbito (i.e., ventromedial) frontal cortex, the insula, the parahippocampal gyrus, and the cingulum. These areas are responsible for the modulation of drive and control of the homeostatic urges as they impinge on the environmental demands, including emotion and memory.
(3) Unimodal (modality specific) association areas. These areas surround the primary reception and transduction areas and are responsible for attachment of meaning to the patterns of sensory activation: perception as opposed to sensation.
(4) Heteromodal (higher order) association areas. These areas are equivalent to Luria's zones of overlapping and are responsible for the integration of material from each of the sensory systems, and developing motor programs for responding to the implications of the sensory input.
(5) Idiotypic or primary sensory and motor areas, which are the primary sensory areas for vision, touch, hearing, and the other sensory and motor systems. These areas are in closest contact with the outside (extrapersonal) world.

Each of these systems has connections to the others either horizontally or vertically, although their connection is strongest with the immediately adjacent zone. The limbic areas are unique insofar as they are the only regions of the brain to have a direct connection to the hypothalamus, the head ganglion of the internal milieu.

Methodological issues

While there is no question that the frontal lobes play a crucial role in the formulation and execution of behaviour, there can be a tendency on the part of investigators in this area to imbue these brain regions with an almost mystical quality. Anthony David has sounded an excellent commentary and cautionary note on this issue in his paper *Frontal Lobology: Psychiatry's New Pseudo-Science* (1992):

> The frontal lobes are the most evolutionarily advanced organ of the body. Herein lie the highest functions: thought, intellect, creativity, self-control and social interaction (Kolb & Whishaw, 1990; Lishman, 1987; Milner & Petrides, 1984; Russell & Roxanas, 1990). As one recent reviewer notes (Reading, 1991), it is hard to avoid "sounding metaphysical" when going through such a list...All

> psychiatry, not to mention human life, is there. Psychiatric disorders are, by definition, problems at the highest levels of thought, so how does it help us to state that they are, by analogy and implication the surface manifestations of frontal lobe neuropathology? (p. 244)

One cannot help but agree with David's opinion as well as the caution echoed by Goldberg (1995) above concerning the tendency of the modularists to generate a new entity to describe each newly discovered function. How does it help us if we are merely renaming psychiatric deficits "frontal" deficits and providing no greater explanation or prediction than the tenuous notion of some sort of unspecified phrenology. Clearly the depth of our explanations must go further than this.

Two further issues also need clarification with regard to the roles of the frontal lobe in executive and personality function. The first of these is the sheer size of the frontal lobe. As Mesulam (2000a) has noted: "This surely is a fine piece of real estate." Nonetheless, "localizing a disturbance to this region is rather like a person directing a visitor to an address marked 'Europe'" (David, 1992, p. 244). Thus, appropriate description of the regions of the frontal lobe must be based on their specification with regard to appropriate neuroanatomical and functional landmarks.

The second problem for this area has been identified by Martha Farah and her associates in noting that "attempts to provide unified accounts of frontal functions usually depend on central executives that are dissociated from the mechanism used to perform the tasks themselves" (Kimberg & Farah, 1993, p. 411). This presents a problem to arguments about localization of function and the correlation between neuroanatomical lesion and the behavioural alteration, as further regions are implicated in yet further functions such as describing the executive and the problem associated with homuncular views and the internal regress (i.e., a little executive in each of our heads controlling and directing behaviour and a yet smaller executive inside their heads who are doing the same and so on). Clearly, the most economical view is to begin with assuming a direct association between the neuroanatomical locus and the behavioural change and only when this direct association between the two has proven untenable should the hypothesis invoke other constructs and other regions.

One final issue associated with this area is that while the notions of executive function and frontal lobe function are often used interchangeably, it is clear there are differences between these two constructs, which will be explored in more detail below. It is also the case that the notion of personality change and the impairment of frontal/executive functioning have been used as if they actually refer to the same thing in frontally injured individuals. Certainly much of the literature on traumatic brain injury (TBI) has assumed that personality change subsequent to the TBI and the executive deficits associated with the injury share a common cause and are treated as if they are identical. Clearly this is not the case and caution in the attribution of functional change to neuroanatomical cause is one that needs to be clearly specified. Data provided in the study of Golden and Golden (2003), for example, clearly indicate that in their survey of 320 chronic TBI patients, the observed cognitive deficits and the personality dysfunction were independent of each other.

It is clear that concise formulation of the various roles of the frontal lobes is necessary and the recourse to concepts like the executive creates even more difficulty in defining the concepts necessary to detail the various roles these regions would perform and how these might be dissociated from each other. That being the case, it is necessary to determine if there is more than one frontal lobe syndrome. If so then how many frontal lobe syndromes are there? What techniques can we use to characterize these conditions, and is there any validity to these techniques? Hopefully in this chapter the respective contributions of each of these sources of variance will be more clearly apportioned. Before we do this, though, it is a good time to focus upon issues of definition and how these various constructs may relate to each other.

Phenomenology and nosology of postinjury personality change

Perhaps a good place to begin with a discussion of personality change as a consequence of TBI is to decide what exactly personality is. Prigatano and colleagues (Prigatano, Fordyce et al., 1986) have proposed the following definition:

> Personality is defined as patterns of emotional and motivational responses that develop over the life of the organism; are highly influenced by early life experiences, are modifiable, but not easily changed by behavioral and teaching methods; and greatly influence (and are influenced by) cognitive processes. In humans, these patterns of emotional and motivational responses are in part self-recognized, but they may remain outside the individual's realm of conscious awareness. Others who are familiar with the individual's daily behavioral characteristics may recognize emotional and motivational responses that the person may not be fully aware of or be able to report subjectively. Finally, the form of a given emotional or motivational response is highly dependent on the environmental consequences as well as the biological state of the organism. (p. 30)

The *DSM-IV-TR* (APA, 2000) indicates

> The essential feature of Personality Change Due to a General Medical Condition is a persistent personality disturbance that is judged to be due to the direct physiological effects of a general medical condition. The personality disturbance represents a change from the individual's previous characteristic personality pattern....Common manifestations of the personality change include affective instability, poor impulse control, outbursts of aggression or rage grossly out of proportion to any precipitating psychosocial stressor, marked apathy, suspiciousness, or paranoid ideation....Although it shares the term "personality" with the Axis II Personality Disorders, this diagnosis is coded on Axis I and is distinct by virtue of its specific etiology, different phenomenology, and more variable onset and course. (p. 187)

The Manual contends that there are eight subtypes of organic personality change: labile, disinhibited, aggressive, apathetic, paranoid, other (i.e., not any of the previously mentioned subtypes), combined, and unspecified. The presentation will be contingent on the nature and localization of the pathology; for example, frontal lobe injuries may yield symptoms including lack of judgment or foresight, facetiousness, disinhibition, and euphoria. Head trauma is included as one of the types of neurological and other general medical conditions that can culminate in the organic personality change.

While many forms of personality change could occur as a result of TBI in line with the suggestions of the *DSM-IV-TR*, only a few types, most notably the disinhibited, aggressive, and apathetic patterns most commonly occur following TBI.

How many frontal lobe syndromes are there?

Teuber (1964), after extensive study of lesions of the frontal lobe, has said: "I started out by trying to find a unitary concept, but as I moved along, it became clear that no single hypothesis could carry far enough to cover all the manifestations of frontal lobe lesions" (p. 410). Numerous theorists have addressed this issue in the ensuing decades, but definitive evidence to support dissociation between the various syndromes and symptoms associated with pathology of the frontal lobes remains elusive.

Prigatano (1992), in his comprehensive review of the personality changes associated with TBI, classified these changes into two groups of symptoms: active versus passive disturbances, a categorization originally proposed in the work of Eames (1988). Within the active group of symptoms Prigatano (1992) includes: irritability, agitation, belligerence, anger, abrupt and unexpected acts of violence or episodic dyscontrol syndrome, impulsiveness, impatience, restlessness, inappropriate social responses, emotional lability or rapid mood changes, sensitivity to noise or distress, anxiety, suspiciousness or mistrust of others, delusional phenomena, paranoia and mania or manic-like states. In the passive group he includes: aspontaneity, sluggishness, loss of interest in the environment, loss of drive or initiative, tiring easily, depression, childishness including self-centredness, insensitivity to others, giddiness, over talkativeness and exuberance/euphoric behaviour, helplessness, and lack of insight or awareness of behavioural limitations. He noted that of all of the symptoms, irritability was the single most common complaint identified by both the patient and the family (Prigatano, 1992).

The notion of grouping the features of the personality change following TBI into two spheres of change along a spectrum of positive versus negative symptoms as originally proposed by John Hughlings Jackson (1875) has been numerously reported in the literature. For example Luria (1969; 1973) has described two variants of the change in personality mediated by the frontal lobe: one characterized by euphoria, disinhibition, impulsiveness and inadequacy of action and the other featuring a narrowing of interest and emotional indifference. These descriptions are similar to those described by Blumer and Benson (1975) in their description of the pseudodepressed versus the pseudopsychopathic patterns of personality change following frontal injuries. The division of the changes into two groups of symptoms has also been made by Wood (1987) (i.e., positive versus negative); the description by Eames noted above (1988: i.e., passive versus active) and the disorders of control and drive proposed by Robyn Tate (1987).

Tate (1987) characterized the symptoms noted in individuals with frontal injuries into disorders of drive and disorders of control, respectively. If we consider a

Table 3.1 The Two Functional Syndromes Associated with Frontal Compromise

Disorders of Drive	*Disorders of Control*
Apathy	Restlessness
Inertia	Hyper-reactivity
Lack of initiative	Disinhibition
Inflexibility	Impulsivity
Rigidity	Irresponsibility
Cognitive slowing	Cognitive acceleration

number of the commonly encountered changes that can occur following frontal injuries including TBI, they constitute a continuum of behaviour ranging from too little of a particular feature through to too much. The normal or unimpaired state can thus be considered as the middle ground between these two extremes. Table 3.1 illustrates some possible examples of the extremes on this continuum.

Using this scheme it is possible for us to make some tentative connections between the neuroanatomical features of the injuries to the frontal lobe and the observed behavioral changes.

Cummings (1985; Lichter & Cummings, 2001) has described three major frontal lobe syndromes: (1) a dorsolateral prefrontal cortical cortex (DLPFC) syndrome featuring compromise in executive functions including decreased verbal and design fluency, abnormal motor programming, impaired set shifting, reduced learning and memory retrieval and poor problem solving; (2) an orbital prefrontal cortex syndrome (OPFC) featuring disinhibition, irritability, impulsivity, emotional lability, poor insight, poor judgment, and distractability; and (3) a medial prefrontal cortical (MPFC)/anterior cingulate syndrome featuring apathy and diminished initiative (abulia). He has called these syndromes, respectively, the disinhibited, apathetic, and akinetic frontal lobe syndromes.

More recently, Damasio (1994, 1996) and his colleagues have moved away from describing the disinhibited group as "orbitally" lesioned and instead prefer the description of this area as the ventromedial prefrontal cortex. This has some appeal due to its better anatomical consistency thus allowing a comparison between ventromedial prefrontal lesions with those that are dorsolateral. For the purposes of this discussion, the term ventromedial will be used in preference to orbital.

This description of the ventromedial-lesioned individuals is reminiscent of the observation by Burgess and Shallice (1996). Their anterior-lesioned group showed a higher tendency to guess than did their nonlesioned controls and were more likely to abandon a correct rule once it had been attained. Burgess and Shallice concluded that this was attributable to the fact that these patients had an exaggerated willingness to adopt bizarre hypotheses. One might perhaps more prosaically refer to this behaviour as disinhibition. Burgess and Shallice did note, however, that there were no differences between the two groups in their level of perseverative responses.

If we consider the operations necessary for the execution of an action from the original idea through to its completion, the steps in this process might look something like the following (Luria, 1973):

IDEA → intention → programming → regulation → verification → OUTCOME.

In comparison to the types of frontal lobe syndromes presented by Cummings (1985; Lichter & Cummings, 2001), the intention and programming dysfunctions are most clearly associated with the pseudodepressed/apathetic/akinetic-type syndrome or a disorder of drive, and include features such as high levels of apathy and indifference and concreteness in program development. On the other hand, the regulation and verification components of the process seem to be associated with the pseudopsychopathic/disinhibited-type syndrome or a disorder of control. Hence, if we described the deficits featured by these individuals in terms of Luria's typology outlined above, compromise in the area of intention and programming would produce the clinical presentation of disinhibition, impulsivity, and distractability, whereas deficits in the area of regulation and verification might lead to poor error utilization (Crowe, 1992).

This scheme is also reminiscent of the suggestions made by Gray (1987) in the context of his behavioural inhibition system model of approach versus avoidance. In the model, a nonspecific arousal system receives convergent input from a behavioural activation system and a behavioural inhibition system. The arousal system is associated with the activation of the behaviour to be rewarded whereas the inhibition system is associated with suppression or termination of the behaviour in anticipation of punishment. Overactivation of the arousal system produces impulsive behaviours (undue focus upon an advantage at the cost of potential disadvantages) as could an underactive inhibitory system (a failure to focus upon a disadvantage).

It is difficult to determine how the often noted frontal lobe sign of perseveration might fit into these various schemes. It may be that perseveration represents a deficit in programming such that only one possible behavioural option (i.e., the perseverated theme) is considered an appropriate solution to the task, and is, therefore, concretely perseverated. On the other hand, it may represent a dysfunction in the regulation and verification components of the task as a previously tried theme is retried again and again, rather than being discarded either as unsuccessful or of having already previously been employed. As yet, the evidence for each explanation seems equal.

A similar suggestion has also been applied to the description of impulsivity. Brunas-Wagstaff, Bergquist and Wagstaff (1994) have contended that impulsivity may be viewed as an inability to inhibit an inappropriate response and also as an increase in the speed at which information processing occurs. Subsequent studies (e.g., Rieger & Gauggel, 2002) have raised doubts about the degree to which TBI patients have difficulty in their ability to inhibit ongoing responses, which the authors propose are not very common after TBI, and the pervasive observation that speed of information processing following TBI is slowed rather than accelerated. Clarification of the various possible mechanisms of the construct of impulsivity is reviewed in Enticott and Ogloff (2006).

In my series of studies that attempted to dissociate these two patterns of responding on the commonly used "frontal" lobe task of phonemic verbal fluency (Crowe, 1992, 1996; Crowe & Bittner, 2006), I compared these two frontal lobe syndromes in subjects putatively lesioned in the ventromedial areas of the frontal lobe with those lesioned in the dorsolateral areas. While the study did find support for the dissociation of the two syndromes (putative involvement of the DLPFC leading to impairment in the level of response generation and putative involvement of the ventromedial prefrontal cortex [VMPFC] leading to impairment of selectivity and rule governance of response), there were a number of inconsistencies in the data.

The deficit in the area of response generation noted with the TBI participants who were deemed to feature lesions to the base of the forebrain in line with the suggestions of Courville (1942), did not do so consistently. Whilst a proportion of the group did feature higher levels of error (as revealed by scatter plot), the overall group result did not prove to be significantly different from the controls.

In a subsequent study (Crowe, 1996) I investigated the possible reason for not finding a specific deficit in the head injured/VMPFC group, which it was hypothesized arose from the fact that not all closed head injuries necessarily result in damage to the VMPFC. It thus seemed possible that the problem with the earlier study (Crowe, 1992) may have been that the injuries for all subjects were diffuse, thus contaminating the picture of which components of the behavioural outcome were due to generalised damage throughout the brain and which were due to specific effects on the VMPFC.

Malloy and colleagues (Malloy, Bihrle, Duffy, & Cimino, 1993) have described an orbital medial frontal syndrome and they note that these individuals feature a syndrome characterised by anosmia, amnesia with confabulation, difficulties with response inhibition as measured by Go-No-Go task deficits, personality changes, and hypersensitivity to pain. They contend that this condition is associated with poor social and vocational adjustment and that the condition is distinct from the pattern emerging following dorsolateral frontal damage.

Damage to the orbital frontal area is a common sequelae of TBI. Because the olfactory nerves are located directly below the VMPFC, posttraumatic anosmia is a common effect of these injuries (Martzke, Swan, & Varney, 1991), particularly if the blow is sustained as a result of the patient falling backwards and striking the occiput against a firm surface (O'Shanick & O'Shanick, 2005). Estimates of the frequency of posttraumatic impairment of smell have been estimated to be as high as 20–30% of survivors of trauma (Costanzo & Becker, 1986; Levin, High, et al., 1985). As expected, the impairment of the sense of smell is closely correlated with the severity of the injury. In mild head injuries anosmia varies from 0–16%, in moderate injuries from 15–19% and in the more severe cases may be as high as 24–30% (Costanzo & Zasler, 1992).

Damage to the olfactory apparatus following TBI may stem from three principal causes: injury or tearing of the olfactory nerves; damage to the nose or the nasal passages; or contusion or brain haemorrhage to the olfactory parenchyma (Costanzo & Zasler, 1992). Jennett and Teasdale (1981) have noted that shearing and abrasion of the olfactory nerve is often associated with contusion and laceration of the surrounding orbital cortical areas, a finding also supported by other researchers (Costanzo & Zasler, 1991; Malloy et al., 1993). These researchers have even gone so far as to suggest that "olfactory function in and of itself seems to be a relatively good marker for associated neuropathological abnormalities in the medial frontal and anterior temporal lobes" (p. 21).

The establishment of the convergent validity of traumatic anosmia as a sign of damage to the orbital frontal area of the brain has been attempted by a number of investigators. Varney (1988; Varney & Menefee, 1993) has found that patients with severe or total posttraumatic anosmia have a high rate of chronic unemployability (92%) and that even those subjects with mild forms of dysnosmia were chronically unemployed (64%). These latter findings were made despite the fact that these subjects had no clear neurological, intellectual, or memory deficits that explained their unemployment. Varney (1988) also noted that these subjects had other cognitive and emotional problems including absentmindedness (100%), poor planning and anticipation (95%), indecisiveness and poor decision making (93%), perplexity responses (83%), unevenness in the quality of work output (80%), unreliability (74%), inability to learn from mistakes (74%), and an inability to get along with fellow employees and supervisors (60%).

There has, however, been dispute in the literature (Greiffenstein, Baker, & Gola, 2002, 2003; Varney, 2002) suggesting that the relationship between posttraumatic anosmia and late psychosocial and neuropsychological outcome may be artefactual (see Greiffenstein et al., 2002), due to the fact that the patients described as anosmic by Varney were identified on the basis of self-report.

Given that traumatic anosmia has been proposed to be a relatively reliable indicator of ventromedial frontal involvement (Costanzo & Zasler, 1992), the aim of the subsequent study my group undertook using the phonemic fluency task (PFT) was to compare two groups of TBI participants who differed with respect to their olfactory status. To ensure that the problem was not identified as a result of abnormal symptom endorsement, all the patients in the study had been identified as anosmic by either a neurosurgeon, a neurologist, or an ear, nose, and throat (ENT) physician. It did indeed prove to be the case that those participants with loss of sense of smell were significantly more prone to disinhibited responding on the PFT than were the nonanosmic TBIs (Crowe, 1996).

The groups did not, however, differ in terms of their level of production on the task, supporting the notion that a generalised effect of damage as a consequence of TBI can lead to both diminution of level of response as well as disinhibition and impulsivity in selection of the response and that these effects can to some extent be dissociated depending upon the localisation of the damage within the frontal lobe.

Malloy and colleagues (1993) and Tate (1999) found compromise in control of responding noted in their studies with TBI participants using rule breaking errors on fluency measures as an indicator of impaired control of responding. In the latter study, Tate administered the Current Behaviour Scale (CBS) (a series of 25 bipolar adjectives which are rated on a 7-point scale) (Elsass & Kinsella, 1989) to the relatives of the patients with TBI on admission (in the attempt to rate preinjury character) and again at six months posttrauma. The TBI group featured increases in the loss of emotional control and loss of motivation items on the CBS following the injury.

The TBI participants who were identified as having a high level of rule breaking on the basis of neuropsychological measures (i.e., breaking the designated rules on the word fluency and design fluency tests, rule breaking errors on the first five trials of the Milner maze, and perseverative errors on the Wisconsin Card Sorting Test [WCST]) showed significant posttraumatic increases in the loss of emotional control variable of the CBS. Tate argued that "rule breaking errors on fluency tests have clinical utility in documenting the types of changes in everyday (dyscontrolled) behaviours as observed by relatives" (1999, p. 49).

While there is some support for the notion of specific indicators of impaired responding in TBI patients, the evidence is by no means universal. Anderson, Bigler, and Blatter (1995) have noted that tests that are traditionally classified as measures of "frontal lobe" damage such as the Halstead Category Test (HCT) and the WCST do not distinguish frontal from nonfrontal performance and "do not add anything unique about frontal integrity and neuropsychological functioning in TBI patients" (p. 900).

Anderson et al. (1995) further note:

> While HCT and the WCST performance is altered by brain injury, it does not appear to be related to volume of focal frontal damage, presence or absence of frontal damage or to the degree of non-specific structural (atrophic) changes. These findings indicate that the important variable in HCT and/or WCST performance in TBI patients is the injury itself regardless of the location or amount of structural damage. (p. 906)

This data adds yet more weight to the observation made in chapter 1 that the relationship between neuroanatomical locus, neuropsychological deficit and postinjury changes to personality is by no means straightforward.

Perhaps recognition of the caution noted by Cummings (Lichter & Cummings, 2001) that the frontal lobe extends beyond its cortical representation into an extensive subcortical network underpinning the frontal regions that can be identified at each of the levels of the striatum, the pallidum, and the thalamus, is a worthwhile observation to make here. Damage to the subcortical circuitry that connects the various regions of the frontal lobe (i.e, OPFC, VMPFC, DLPFC, and the MPFC) at the level of the striatum, the pallidum, and the mediodorsal thalamus each produces an identical presentation to that noted with the damage to the cortical areas, perhaps accounting in part for the observations noted by Anderson et al. (1995) above.

Regarding the specifics of change to personality following TBI, Tate (2003) has noted that change to personality can and does occur as a consequence of the injury on various dimensions of personality, including features such as increases in neuroticism, addiction, and criminality as well as a trend towards decrease in extraversion that occurs as a result of TBI. Nonetheless, these changes tend to be largely independent of the premorbid personality structure of the individual, supporting Lishman's (1997) observations of the existence of consistent pattern of frontal lobe personality changes that occur independent of the personality of the individual before the injury.

Based on this review, it seems reasonable to conclude that there are at least two patterns of personality change that can occur either independently or in concert following injury to the frontal lobe either as a consequence of lesions or vascular events in these regions or due to the second effects of trauma. In considering the frequency with which these types of personality changes occur it seems worthwhile to examine them within the context of the two frontal/personality alterations that have been discussed within the literature variously described as disorders of drive and disorders of control (Tate, 1987).

Prevalence and incidence of secondary organic personality change following TBI

In their review of the incidence of organic personality disorder (OPD) in their final sample of 28 TBI patients interviewed within two weeks of the injury and subsequently at six months postinjury using a structured clinical interview based upon the International Classification of Diseases (ICD)-10 criteria, Franulic, Horta, Maturana, Scherpenisse and Carbonell (2000) diagnosed 32% of their sample with OPD. Unfortunately however, they did not indicate a breakdown of the types of OPD observed. However, the authors did note that using the neurobehavioural rating scale developed by Levin, High, Goethe et al. (1987) that the OPD patients differed from the non-OPD patients on measures of cognition and energy, preoccupation with somatic and anxiety-related concerns, and language. The participants with OPD predominantly had frontal injuries. Once again in common with a number of observations in the literature, they noted that the difference in behavioural outcome was independent of the cognitive impairments.

Streeter, van Reekum, Shorr and Bachman (1995) noted that in a comparison of 54 males with borderline personality disorder to 49 psychiatric control patients there was a much higher incidence (42%) of TBI in the borderline group as compared to the controls (4%). As the TBI had occurred before the full expression of the personality disorder, the authors felt that the TBI had been a cause rather than a result of the TBI. Hibbard, Bogdany et al. (2000) noted that using the Structured Clinical Interview for the *DSM-IV* on 100 participants recruited from a larger pool of 438 TBI patients, 24% of the sample could be diagnosed with a personality disorder prior to the TBI, whereas 66% met the diagnostic criteria for at least one personality disorder after the injury. The most common forms of post-TBI personality disorder were borderline (34%), avoidant (26%), paranoid (26%), obsessive-compulsive (27%), and narcissistic (14%). Those patients who had had personality disorder before the TBI were more likely to show personality disorder afterwards.

Many investigators agree that the most commonly reported personality change following TBI is increased irritability (Prigatano, 1992) accompanied by the associated features of frustration, aggression, egocentricity, impulsiveness, impairment of judgment and insight, and inappropriate expression of affection (Franulic et al., 2000). These changes seem to generate greater distress for patients in the period more than six months following the injury rather than in the acute stage.

Haboubi, Long, Koshy, and Ward (2001) report that irritability is the third most commonly reported complaint in their large cohort of patients assessed 6 months postinjury. At one year, a number of investigators (e.g., 30–35%: Deb, Lyons, & Koutzoukis, 1998, 1999; 33.3%: Kim, Manes, Kosier, Baruah, & Robinson, 1999; 32%: van der Naalt, van Zomeren, Sluiter, & Minderhoud, 1999) note approximately one-third of patients complain of irritability in the year following the injury with the highest level of endorsement being in the mild to moderately injured group and the lowest being in the severe patients. In summarizing this data, Alderman (2003) has noted that "studies are in general agreement that about a third of patients with mild head injuries report irritability. However, this symptom also remains a persistent complaint in the longer term" (p. 212).

Some investigators have expressed the opinion that the individuals who make the best recovery post-TBI are those who show a high level of agitation postinjury (O'Shanick & O'Shanick, 2005). For example, there is a high correlation between the level of the catecholamines and their measured metabolites and quality of outcome post-TBI (Clifton, Ziegler, & Grossman, 1981; Woolf, Hamill, Lee, Cox, & McDonald, 1987).

Injury to the frontal lobe as a result of TBI can exist with relative preservation of performance on standardized tests of frontal functioning. Satish, Streufert and Eslinger (1999) have noted their study of a 48-year-old woman who was involved in a motor vehicle accident (MVA) that culminated in a 2-week period of posttraumatic amnesia (PTA) and damage to the ventral frontal region involving the lateral orbital gyrus including Brodmann's Areas (BA) 12 and 13 and extending into the deep white matter to the tip of the frontal horn. While most of her scores on intelligence, memory, language, spatial and perceptual functioning were in the normal range, she did demonstrate mild attenuation in her performance on the WCST, Trail Making Test Part B and the Paced Auditory Serial Addition Task (PASAT).

Her living circumstance, however, underwent a much more profound change. She was demoted to routine office work whereas before her injury she had been an independent telephone company service operator with high skill in computer processing for the five years preceding her injury. Following the injury, she demonstrated marked difficulty in tracking information changes, completing tasks with efficiency, and organizing herself.

Assessment of this woman using a tool employed in industrial and organizational psychology in the form of the Strategic Management Simulation technique revealed impaired scores on a variety of decision-making measures. These included impairment in initiative, information utilization, breadth of strategy development, and the ability to opportunistically and flexibly deal with rapidly changing situations. She did, however, demonstrate better performance on tasks within context and when she was required to focus on only one aspect of the situation (Satish et al., 1999).

The pattern of impulsivity following TBI can also be extended to the issue of increase in aggression subsequent to the injury (Kim, 2002). Impulsive aggression (IA), either physical or verbal, is a common sequela of TBI (Eslinger, Grattan, & Geder, 1995). In their study of this phenomenon in 45 severe TBI participants, Greve et al. (2001) have noted that 26 of their sample (i.e., 58%) had persisting problems with aggression. This group had a higher incidence of premorbid aggressive behaviours and tended to be younger and were more irritable, impulsive, and antisocial than the nonaggressive controls. Interestingly, the researchers noted once again that the level of IA was not related to self-regulatory behaviour as assessed by measures of neuropsychological functioning as there were no differences between the IA and non-IA-head-injured controls. The authors contend that their finding supported the notion that "the brain injury did not cause a personality change, but simply further disinhibited an already impulsive and aggressive individual such that they continued to have aggressive outbursts, even in a highly structured and controlled environment" (p. 260).

This notion of the preexistence of antisocial tendencies in the impulsive aggressive individual following TBI supports a number of other findings in the literature regarding aggression. Rosenbaum and Hoggs (1989) note that of 31 consecutive patients referred for evaluation of marital violence, 19 (61.3%) had prior histories of severe TBI. Of this group, a large percentage (48.4%) had coincidental high levels of alcohol abuse. The suggestion that TBI and impulsive aggression may be implicated in forensic presentation was also observed by Allgulander and Nilsson (2000) in their epidemiological study of 1739 homicides between 1978 and 1994 in Sweden. They found that TBI, physical abuse, alcohol dependence, and criminal recidivism increased the risk of being murdered.

Blair (1995, 2001, 2004; Blair & Cipolotti, 2000; Blair, Jones, Clark, & Smith, 1997) has raised an interesting explanation for why this result might occur. His contention is that the notion of "acquired sociopathy" as originally proposed by Damasio, Tranel and Damasio (1990) may develop as a consequence of brain injury.

Blair (1995) proposes a violence inhibition mechanism wherein submissive social cues from a victim inhibit the expression or proliferation of the violent behaviour on the part of the perpetrator. Blair contends that moral socialization of the individual reduces aggressive behaviour on the part of the individual as a result of the convergent behavioural modification techniques of aversive conditioning and instrumental learning.

Blair (2004; Blair, Mitchell, & Blair, 2005) contends that the role of the VMPFC in impulsive aggressive behaviours is twofold: (1) the VMPFC is responsible for calculating the expectation of reward attached to the behaviour (an observation consistent with the work of Edmund Rolls (2000) who contends that rather than being an inhibitory mechanism per se, the VMPFC involves the learning of stimulus-reward associations and the alteration of responses on the basis of alteration of behavioural contingencies); and (2) the VMPFC is responsible for the recognition of social cues related to aggression, a process Blair refers to as "social response reversal." Social cues (e.g., disapproval by others, shame, embarrassment, etc.) often serve to modulate the expression of reactive aggression. However, if this system is impaired the impulsive aggression becomes more likely.

One of Blair's (Blair & Cipolotti, 2000; Blair, 2004; Blair, Mitchell, & Blair, 2005) patients, JS, a 56-year-old electrical engineer who was found unconscious with evidence of trauma to the right frontal lobe, shows this pattern of change. On presentation JS had a Glasgow Coma Scale (GCS) of 9, and an enhanced computed tomography (CT) scan showed low-density abnormalities involving the orbital prefrontal cortex (i.e., the VMPFC) as well as the left temporal lobe almost certainly involving the left amygdala. This case presents a graphic illustration of the types of changes associated with the construct.

> JS "failed to conform to social norms" and was notably "irritable and aggressive." His episodes of property damage and violence were frequent and were elicited after little provocation; e.g., an alteration in routine. He was "reckless regarding others personal safety;" on one occasion he continued to push around a wheel-chair bound patient despite her screams of terror. His "lack of remorse"

> was striking; he never expressed any regrets about the nurses he hit. He failed to accept responsibility for his actions, justifying his violent episodes in terms of the failure of others (e.g., they were too slow). (Blair & Cipolotti, 2000, p. 1124)

JS also demonstrated failure to plan ahead and an inability to sustain consistent work behaviour. He fulfilled all of the criteria for acquired sociopathy with the exception of premorbid aberrant behaviour (Blair & Cipolotti, 2000).

Blair and Cipolotti (2000) subjected JS to a number of tasks designed to specifically identify the nature of the deficits in social cognition associated with the behavioural change. These included tasks aimed at assessing reversal learning (i.e., tasks including the Iowa Gambling Test (IGT); tasks that assess the ability to recognize emotional expression and emotional responding including tasks of processing of facial expression, autonomic responses to environmentally salient visual stimuli and face processing tasks; social cognition tasks including tasks of verbal comprehension, emotional attribution, theory of mind, moral/conventional distinction tasks, and social situations tasks.

Blair and Cipolotti (2000) observed that the consistent pattern of deficit noted in JS' case was his impairment in recognizing and responding to angry and disgusted expressions and his poor performance in tasks that assessed the ability to deal with social situations; most notably, an inability to appropriately attribute the emotions of fear, anger, and embarrassment to protagonists in a story and the ability to identify violations of social behaviour.

Blair and Cipolotti (2000) further proposed that as a consequence of his injury, JS had sustained damage to a brain system responsible for apprehending the angry expressions and concerns of another that would ordinarily result in cessation of the aberrant behaviour and an inability to be able to modify his behaviour in response to these signals.

This observation fits in quite well with observations made by Grattan and Eslinger (1989) who noted that brain-injured subjects displayed significantly lower scores on Hogan's Empathy measure than did the comparison group. The impaired empathy performance relates to impairment in neuropsychological tasks of cognitive flexibility, however, not to tasks of abstraction abilities. This seemed to be particularly the case for injuries associated with the right hemisphere.

Blair et al. (1997) also support the notion of brain injury culminating in impairment of empathy. Their study investigated the psychophysiological responsiveness of psychopathic individual to the distress cues and to threatening or neutral stimuli. Relative to the control sample, the psychopathic individuals showed reduced electrodermal response to distress cues. Blair (2001) considers that acquired sociopathy is most likely the consequence of impairment in the brain systems that respond to threat. He contends that these behaviours are

> a consequence of inability to socialize due to an impairment in the capacity to form associations between emotional unconditioned stimuli (particularly distress cues) and conditioned stimuli (specifically representations of transgressions). If the person is raised in a social environment (for example, poverty) where there are advantages for engaging in antisocial behaviour, they will

> engage in this behaviour but will not experience aversion to the distress of their victims. (p. 730)

A number of studies have attempted to identify which brain regions are activated during social reasoning tasks. Social reasoning causes activations of the left superior frontal gyrus, the orbitofrontal gyrus, and the precuneus in tasks that required the subjects to engage in empathic and forgiveness-related responding. Activation associated with empathy was also noted in the left anterior middle temporal and left inferior frontal gyri, whereas forgiveness caused activation of the posterior cingulate (Farrow et al., 2001).

The association between executive deficits and antisocial behaviour (including criminality, antisocial personality disorder, and psychopathy) has received further endorsement from the meta-analysis undertaken by Morgan and Lilienfield (2000), which supported a correlational link between these phenomena. They noted a moderate to large effect size (0.62) between the two, and the relationship was not moderated by age, gender, level of intelligence, or ethnicity. They noted their largest effect size was observed with the Porteus mazes test and the smallest with the Stroop test.

It is not always the case that the personality changes associated with TBI are a bad thing. Lishman (1987) has noted that "occasionally patients indeed could be said to have shown improvement in personality, in that they were now less prone to worry and were more outgoing and sociable" (p. 161).

In their report of three cases showing marked changes following brain injuries, Labbate, Warden and Murray (1997) describe a case in which a 20-year-old soldier who reported shyness, blushing, and anxious feelings as a child and a teenager, and who used alcohol to help his social anxiety, needed to drink fluids to the point of pain to successfully complete the mandatory urine drug testing in the army. He was subsequently hit in the forehead with a brick causing a brief loss of consciousness (LOC) and six hours of PTA. Subsequent to the blow, he met *DSM-IV* criteria for personality change due to traumatic brain injury, disinhibited type. After his injury he felt more comfortable in group settings, rarely blushed, and became unconcerned about public urination. The changes related to his social anxiety continued at follow-up, seven months postinjury.

The second type of pattern of organic personality change to emerge following TBI is the apathetic/pseudodepressed/abulic/negative symptom/disorder of drive syndrome and is characterized by apathy or lack of motivation not attributable to intellectual impairment (i.e., not dementia), emotional distress (i.e., not depression) or a diminished level of consciousness (i.e., not delirium) (Marin, 1991).

The second and third cases described by Labbate et al. (1997) again prove interesting. The second case involved an initial presentation of a man with antisocial personality disorder, including an extensive forensic history involving incarceration for a hit-and-run offence, theft during his youth, heavy drinking, and a dishonorable discharge from the navy, featured complete remission of his sociopathic tendencies following a motorcycle accident in which he sustained a severely contused frontal lobe and the removal of a volume of his right frontal and temporal areas.

The third case in this series featured a woman who had had a long history of anger dyscontrol, including argumentativeness and rapid resort to physical violence. She was struck by a truck while jogging and suffered six days of PTA, and the magnetic resonance imaging (MRI) revealed bilateral frontal contusion. Subsequent to her recovery, she reported marked personality change, and after the injury she no longer felt angry, did not engage in arguments, and was able to calmly register her complaint about ward nurse behaviour.

Clearly in these last two cases the previously high levels of aggressive and antisocial behaviour were overcome as a result of the effects of the TBI on premorbid personality consistent with the notion of an increase in apathetic responding, in line with the extensive literature on the prefrontal leucotomy and lobotomy procedures (Stuss & Benson, 1986; Valenstein, 1986).

Kant, Duffy, and Pivovarnik (1998) using standardized evaluation tools (Clinical Neuropsychiatric Examination, the self- and family-member-rated version of the Apathy Evaluation Scale [AES]) (Marin, 1991; Marin, Biedrzycki, & Firinciogullari, 1991) and the Beck Depression Inventory, noted that of 83 consecutive TBI patients seen at a neuropsychiatric clinic, 10.84% had apathy without depression, an equivalent percentage had depression without apathy, and another 60% of the patients exhibited both. Younger patients were more prone to apathy and depression than the older patients, and the patients with the more severe injuries were more likely to reflect apathy alone. Interestingly family members observed the apathy syndrome more than the patients themselves, possibly indicating a decrease in the level of self-awareness following the injury.

While these data do indicate that there is overlap between apathy and depressive mentation, these are separable constructs, and the implications of each are quite different in the treatment and management of patients following the TBI (Levy et al., 1998). Recent literature places the conditions associated with diminished motivation on a spectrum spanning from apathy at the least severe end through abulia to akinetic mutism at the most severe end of the disruption of behavioural responding (American Congress of Rehabilitation Medicine [ACRM], 1995; Fisher, 1983; Marin, 1997; Marin & Chakravorty, 2005; Mega & Cohenour, 1997).

Akinetic mutism is characterized by impaired initiation of behaviour and cognition with preservation of visual tracking (ACRM, 1995). Essentially the patient is mute and motionless despite being awake. The symptoms of abulia are similar but somewhat less severe than those of akinetic mutism with poverty of behaviour and speech, lack of initiative, blunting of emotional responding motor slowing, and delay of speech production (Fisher, 1983; Mega & Cohenour, 1997). Apathy is a diminution of motivation in the presence of normal consciousness and other forms of cognition, but with diminution in the quantity rather than the quality of behavioural responding (Marin & Chakravorty, 2005).

In a subsequent replication and extension of the Kant et al. (1998) study discussed above, Andersson, Gundersen and Finset (1999) investigated the levels of apathy and psychophysiological reactivity in a sample of thirty severe TBI participants. Using a cutoff score of 34 on the AES, they noted that 66.7% of the sample featured self-reported levels of apathy above the cutoff. This compares quite favorably with the level noted in the Kant et al. (1998) study that noted an overall level of 71.1%. A subsequent study by Andersson and Bergedalen (2002) noted a level of 62.3%, although an earlier study (Andersson, Krogstad, & Finset, 1999) noted a somewhat lower level of 46.6%. Nonetheless, it is clear that in the range of 47–71% of severe TBI participants feature supra-cutoff levels of apathy in the period following TBI.

A large percentage of these participants will also feature reduced self-awareness as this phenomenon appears to be closely related to levels of motivation and emotional responsivity (Andersson, Krogstad et al., 1999) in this patient group. From a neuropsychological perspective the apathetic pattern of personality change in TBI is commonly associated with compromise in memory functioning, including impairments of acquisition and recall of information, as well as with compromise in executive functions and diminution of psychomotor speed (Andersson & Bergedalen, 2002). It has been reported that stimulant medications such as amantadine, amphetamine, bromocriptine, buproprion, methylphenidate, and selegeline may be useful in treating this syndrome (Kraus & Maki, 1997a, 1997b; Marin, Fogel, Hawkins, Duffy, & Krupp, 1995; Warden et al., 2006).

Evolution of secondary organic personality following TBI

The emergence of the personality change following TBI is a difficult matter to precisely describe. Personality changes are reported to be the most significant problems noted both by caregivers and, to a lesser extent, the individual him or herself at 1, 5, and 15 years postinjury (Livingston, Brooks, & Bond, 1985a; 1985b; Thomsen, 1984; Weddell, Oddy, & Jenkins, 1980), and these are often described as consistent with the notion of an exacerbation of premorbid traits (O'Shanick & O'Shanick, 1994).

Paradoxically, while individuals are sometimes reported as showing more intense versions of their premorbid selves, Varney and Menefee (1993) have noted in their extensive review of 98 TBI affected individuals that "it was not uncommon for family members to use the expression 'invasion of the body snatchers' in reference to their head-injured relative. That is, they looked the same, but had become totally different persons" (p. 41). Clearly, the changes to the personality associated with TBI are, at the very least, complicated.

Another variant of this theme is represented by the suggestion that these individuals actually regress as a consequence of the injury. Childish behaviour following TBI may represent the regress to earlier forms of behavioural responding including awkward responding in social exchanges such as not taking turns in conversation, not sharing, interrupting and not inviting expansion on a conversational topic, which is relatively common in teenage communication patterns (Ehrlich & Sipesk, 1985; Szekeres, Ylvisaker, & Cohen, 1987). Similarly, inappropriate infatuation with caregivers in the healthcare setting often represents a misinterpretation on the part of the patient of the helping role of the healthcare professional, and irritability and aggressive behavioural may arise from an inability to filter environmental noise in association with inability to be able to inhibit behavioural response sets (O'Shanick & O'Shanick, 2005).

Lesion location and mechanism of the secondary organic personality following TBI

As noted in chapter 1, the location of the frontal and anterior temporal regions proximal to the bony protrusions and cavities of the skull overlying the orbits and the anterior temporal fossae contribute to their vulnerability to bleeding, bruising, or swelling, particularly when rotational acceleration is applied to the freely moving head. This problem is exacerbated by the complex series of forces that occur within the brain following head injury that leads to the development of distortion, twisting, and stretching of the neurons culminating in the generalized effects of traumatic axonal injury occurring throughout the brain (Bigler, 2001).

In one of the earliest reported studies of this phenomenon, Courville (1937) autopsied 40 consecutive cases of TBI and discovered a high frequency of injury, haemorrhage, or contusion in the orbital frontal, frontal polar, and anterior temporal regions. In a similar series, Nevin (1967) also emphasized the preponderance of lacerations and contusions in these regions. Other investigators using a variety of techniques (e.g., Stuss & Gow, 1992) have replicated these findings.

Adams and his coworkers in Glasgow (Adams, Graham, Scott, Parker, & Doyle, 1980) obtained strong support for the notion of the vulnerability of the frontal lobes to injury in TBI. Adams et al. developed a contusion index following fatal head injuries that was based upon the size and depth of contusion to the brain substance and found that the contusion index was largest in the frontal lobes, followed closely by the anterior temporal region.

In a magnetic resonance imaging study of mild to moderately head-injured subjects Levin, Williams, Eisenberg, High, and Guinto (1992) reported a series of 50 consecutively referred TBI patients at a trauma treatment centre. They noted that the frontal lobes were the most common site of focal lesions. Interestingly, the study also observed that both the abnormality of signal on MRI and the level of neurobehavioural impairment resolved in parallel over the one to three months following injury in the mild to moderate TBI group, supporting the notion of relatively rapid recovery of gross neural function in the 4 to 12 weeks following injury.

Despite the obvious vulnerability of the anterior regions of the brain to injury in TBI, it has only been since the mid-1980s that the notion of frontal lobe compromise as a result of TBI has become widely accepted (Fisher, 1985). Up until then, the emphasis of most investigations had focused on the pervasive compromise in memory, attention, and intelligence associated with the injury (Levin et al., 1982).

During the mid-1980s, a series of studies associating the deficits arising from TBI with those attributable to frontal lobe compromise emerged (e.g., Bond, 1984; Dikmen, Reitan, & Temkin, 1983), changing the focus of the field to the anterior regions of the brain and their effects upon cognition, emotion, behaviour, and personality structure.

Lezak (1995; Lezak, Howieson, & Loring, 2004) argued that in individuals with severe TBI, compromise in three major spheres of behavioural functioning will be noted. These are: cognition, executive functioning, and emotion. Executive functions are those abilities "that enable a person to engage successfully in independent, purposive, self-serving behaviour" (Lezak et al., 2004, p. 35). Impairment in executive functions reduces the individual's ability to generate new solutions to problems and to adaptively and appropriately use previously acquired knowledge and skills to achieve a desired aim. These deficits particularly pertain to the ability to carry out the functions of daily living or to prevent the individual from engaging in harmful or maladaptive behaviour. This includes the notion of cognitive flexibility, which is "the capacity to generate a diversity of ideas, consider behavioural alternatives and respond to changing complex configural patterns, be they sensory-perceptual, linguistic, emotional or social" (Grattan & Eslinger, 1989, p. 176). For example, the individual with damage to the frontal lobes may have difficulty planning, recognising, and choosing between alternatives of action or tasks (Lezak, 1995) or may behave in a pragmatically inappropriate manner (Proctor et al., 2000).

A particularly compelling description of some of these behavioural and personality changes is provided by Damasio and colleagues in their description of EVR (Damasio, 1994; Eslinger & Damasio, 1985):

> Elliot was able to recount the tragedy of his life with a detachment that was out of step with the magnitude of the events. He was always controlled, always describing scenes as a dispassionate, uninvolved spectator. Nowhere was there a sense of his own suffering...Elliot was exerting no restraint whatsoever on his affect. He was calm. He was relaxed... He was not inhibiting the expression of internal emotional resonance or hushing inner turmoil. He simply did not have any turmoil to hush....He needed about 2 hours to get ready for work in the morning, and some days were consumed entirely with shaving and hair washing. Deciding where to dine might take hours, as he discussed each restaurant's seating plan, particulars of menu, atmosphere, and management. He would drive to each restaurant to see how busy it was, but even then he could not finally decide which to choose. Purchasing small items required in-depth consideration of brands, prices, and the best method of purchase. He clung to outdated and useless possessions, refusing to part with dead houseplants, old telephone books, six broken fans, five broken television sets, three bags of empty orange juice concentrate cans, 15 cigarette lighters, and countless stacks of old newspapers. (Damasio, 1994, pp. 44–45)

Certainly, it could be argued that this behaviour is mere eccentricity or just poor housekeeping. However, the drastic contrast between Elliot's behaviour before his injury and his current state clearly indicates that something more is at work (Damasio, 1994). Premorbidly he was a well adjusted and successful accountant, but following the bilateral ablation of his orbital and lower medial frontal lobes due to a meningioma, he changed completely. He made impulsive investments culminating in bankruptcy, could not sustain a job due to his tardiness and absenteeism, and divorced twice (the second marriage, which was to a prostitute, only lasted six months) due to his personality change. Interestingly he also indicated normal performance on an extensive battery of neuropsychological tests including the WCST, the word fluency test, and the Category Test (Damasio et al., 1990).

The frontal lobes constitute about one third of the brain's substance and it is broken into several distinct regions: the motor areas (the motor strip [Brodmann's area (BA)] 4), the lateral premotor cortex and supplementary motor area (SMA) (BA 6), the frontal eye field area (BA 8), Broca's area (BAs 44 and perhaps 45), the posterior region of the cingulate cortex, and the premotor cortex (which is commonly referred to as the frontal agranular cortex due to its distinctive microscopic appearance). There are three regions of the prefrontal cortex: the dorsolateral prefrontal cortex (DLPFC) including the lateral aspects of BAs 9 to 12, all of BA 45 and 46 and the superior portions of area 47. The medial prefrontal cortex (MPFC) including the anterior cingulate (including BAs 24, 25 and 32) and the ventromedial prefrontal cortex, which is more commonly labeled the orbital prefrontal cortex (OPFC) and includes the inferior portions of BA 47, and the medial parts of BAs 9 to 12 (Gazzaniga, Ivry & Mangun, 2002).

As noted above, Lichter and Cummings (2001) have described at least five major frontal subcortical circuits: a motor circuit originating in the SMA, an oculomotor circuit originating in the frontal eye fields, the circuits of the prefrontal cortex including: a DLPFC circuit that mediates "executive" functions; an anterior cingulate circuit that is involved in motivational mechanisms, and an orbital frontal circuit including: (1) a medial orbital frontal circuit that allows integration of visceral-amygdalar states ("somatic markers"—see below), and (2) a lateral orbital frontal circuit involved in integration of limbic and emotional information into contextually appropriate behavioural responses.

The somatic marker hypothesis: Cognition meets emotion

Speculation about the functioning of the frontal lobe has undergone a massive resurgence over the past decade as a result of an intriguing and sophisticated hypothesis developed by Antonio Damasio and his colleagues (Bar-On, Tranel, Denburg, & Bechara, 2003; Bechara, Damasio, & Damasio, 2000; Bechara, Tranel, & Damasio, 2000; Damasio, 1994; Damasio, 1996; Damasio et al., 1990; Tranel, Bechara, & Damasio, 2000). This renewed interest has lead to a concentrated focus on the regions of the frontal lobe and the contribution that each of these regions makes to planning and error utilization.

The contribution that emotion makes to reasoning and decision making has been an enduring fascination for psychology. While each of us can attest to the fact that emotions can and do influence our judgments, there has been a lack of agreement in the literature as to how and where in the processing of this information this influence actually occurs.

In the psychological literature, the concepts of reasoning and decision making are intimately entwined. However, the exclusive reliance on reasoning and the complete disregard of the role of emotions is not always conducive to successful decision making. In the social domain for example, complex outcomes are often required and these decisions can have life-defining ramifications. These situations are characterised by uncertainty and a myriad of response choices, and the possible outcomes associated with each choice must be considered and evaluated to make the best of the situation. To best achieve this outcome, some mechanism for making these choices in real time must be invoked to prevent the "dead air" of each of the parties sitting pensively like Rodin's thinker as they cruise the supermarket shelves on market day, incapable of deciding whether to buy tinned spaghetti rather than tinned baked beans.

The somatic marker hypothesis (SMH) proposed by Damasio and his colleagues (Bar-On et al., 2003; Bechara, Damasio et al., 2000; Bechara, Tranel et al., 2000; Damasio, 1994; Damasio, 1996; Damasio et al., 1990; Tranel et al., 2000), proposes that effective decision making is crucially dependent upon emotional processing. Damasio proposes that the emotions are physiological signals from the body (the soma) that arise in response to stimuli encountered in the environment. These signals, or somatic markers, act as biasing devices in the consideration of options and outcomes by attaching either positive or negative emotional weighting to a particular course of action (Damasio, 1994). This biasing device acts to constrain the field of search from the multiple options and future outcomes possible, to a much more narrow choice thus allowing logic-based, cost-benefit analysis (Damasio, 1994) to apply to the small final set of possible options. This allows the individual to decide on the course of action within a short time interval (Damasio, 1996), allowing continuity of behaviour and action in a changing environment.

The SMH (Damasio, 1994) makes four basic assumptions: (1) reasoning and decision making operate at a number of levels of neurobiological functioning, some of which are conscious and others of which are not; (2) cognitive operations rely on different cognitive modules of the working brain including at least attention, working memory, episodic and semantic memory, and language functioning irrespective of the content of images; (3) reasoning and decision making depend upon the knowledge an individual has about his or her previous experience of situations, actions, options for actions, and outcomes that are factored into each newly encountered situation; and (4) this knowledge is mediated by the higher-order cortex and various subcortical nuclei which bring a variety of possible sources of information (i.e., prior knowledge about the world, bioregulatory processes, and bodily states in the form of emotions, all of which are brought together into a multifaceted decision-making space) (Bechara, Tranel, & Damasio, 2002).

Two sets of events are implicated in the establishment of the somatosensory patterns that relate to previous experiences (Bechara et al., 2002). The first, the "body loop," occurs when a true somatic state is activated in the body, the second constitutes the "as if body loop." Once an emotion has been experienced, representations or memories of this experience can be formed. By the latter means it is possible to circumvent the body loop and directly activate the insular and somatosensory cortices once an emotion has been learned, effectively producing the emotional effect of an experience without having actually undergone this experience (at least on this occasion). This activation of the "as if body loop" produces an image of an emotional body state that is fainter than would be the case if it were in fact expressed in the body (Bechara et al., 2002), but one that can be effectively recruited for information processing and decision making.

Thus somatic markers are feelings that are experienced prior to the occurrence of conscious reasoning and function as bioregulatory responses to the environment, either external or internal, which aim to maintain homeostasis (Bar-On et al., 2003). These signals involve at least musculoskeletal, visceral, and internal milieu components, all of which are included in the definition of a somatic state (Damasio, 1994; 1998). Once established, these signals can be activated by either primary or secondary inducers, each of which is sustained by an independent functional network (Bar-On et al., 2003; Bechara, 2003).

Primary inducers are unconditioned stimuli that are innately pleasurable or aversive. For example, encountering a snake poised to strike can automatically elicit the somatic response of fear (LeDoux, 1996). The amygdala is crucially involved in this response, and once these signals are relayed to higher centres they can remain covert, only penetrating to the level of the brain stem, or become overt, when relayed to the parietal cortex (i.e., the insula and SI, SII), where they are perceived as a feeling (Bechara, 2003; Damasio et al., 2000).

Secondary inducers are generated by the recall or the thought of a particular action or stimulus that induces a somatic response when it is retrieved into working memory. For example, the thought of encountering the snake can trigger a somatic response. The VMPFC is the structure crucially activated by the secondary inducers (Bar-On et al., 2003; Bechara, 2003; Damasio, 1995).

Damasio (1994) contends that the machinery of "primary emotion," which is responsible for the generation of somatic markers, is innate. This system is programmed to process information relating to the personal and social domains, and has the ability to attach adaptive somatic responses to varying social settings. For example, when a situation arises that has some salient previously encountered aspects, this leads to an activation of higher-order association cortices resulting in recall of pertinent associated facts, which are experienced in the form of images. Simultaneously, the VMPFC and the emotional disposition apparatus are activated. This combined activation results in a reconstruction of previous relevant experience. Depending upon the nature of the previous experience, signals relating to these images act upon the VMPFC, which has previously created the link between the current situation and the somatic state. This state then becomes active, reactivating the somatic pattern that orients or biases behaviour towards the appropriate action (Bechara et al., 2002), the so-called gut feeling that occurs in a previously unencountered but similar situation.

Somatic markers thus do not act in an all or none manner and exercise a biasing role in decision making. The establishment of somatosensory patterns regarding a particular situation act to "mark" it in a particular way (Damasio, 1998). The process of decision making, however, is a complex and interactive one and dysjunctions can occur between primary and secondary, or secondary inducers only. Despite the redundancy, once triggered, somatic states are implemented in the body, irrespective of the origin of the induction. All somatic inputs, both positive or negative, are averaged into one overall somatic state (Bar-On et al., 2003; Bechara, 2003; Damasio, 1994) that acts as the weight applied in the decision-making process (Bechara et al., 2002; Damasio, 1994; 1998). Thus the markers can lead to the elimination of particular response options or highlight the positive aspects of others, leaving the decision maker with fewer response choices to consider. The individual can then make a cost-benefit-type analysis on the much reduced pool of options that remain. On the other hand, the absence of somatic markers retards both the speed and accuracy of the decision-making process (Damasio, 1994; 1998).

Overt biasing in favour of a particular plan of action is seen at the level of the VMPFC and the anterior cingulate. When enlisted as part of overt process, the somatic state acts as an inducement or an alarm signal, engaging the individual to commence either approach or withdrawal behaviours, respectively (Bar-On et al., 2003; Bechara, 2003; Damasio, 1994). The biasing signal can, on the other hand, occur covertly, at the level of the striatum. Covert somatic markers also produce approach or withdrawal behaviours, however, the decision maker remains unaware of these signals and does not act with a conscious decision to do so (Bar-On et al.,

2003; Bechara, 2003; Damasio, 1994; 1998). This is the so-called "gut feeling" that many of us encounter when things just do not seem quite right, but we can't quite put our finger upon why this is the case.

This suggestion is quite similar to the formulation of frontally mediated decision processes developed by Rolls and his colleagues (Rolls, 1999; 2000; Rolls, Hornak, Wade, & McGrath, 1994) who have argued that the role of the ventral frontal and orbitofrontal cortex is in the rapid learning or reversal of stimulus-reinforcer associations. These authors contend that impaired decision making of VMPFC patients is not due to defects in the emotional processes responsible for somatic marker activation, but more to a failure to alter behaviour following a change in environmental reinforcement contingencies. In either case, the final result seems to culminate in the same behavioural outcome.

Initial investigations by Damasio and colleagues employed skin conductance response measures (SCR: Damasio, 1994; Damasio et al., 1990) in reaction to emotionally laden stimuli as a measure of the somatic marker response. This data indicated that individuals with compromise of the VMPFC featured a blunted response to the stimulus material in comparison to unimpaired controls (Damasio & Anderson, 1993; Eslinger & Damasio, 1985). These impairments existed despite preserved intelligence, language, memory, perception, executive functions, and social knowledge (Eslinger & Damasio, 1985; Saver & Damasio, 1991). Damasio (1994; Saver & Damasio, 1991) has proposed that VMPFC-lesioned patients make choices that have high immediate reward but severe delayed punishment because they have a "myopia" for the future. They seem to be guided only by the immediate prospects of the gain associated with the stimulus, whatever that might be, and are insensitive to the ultimate consequences of the behaviour. The evidence suggests that these patients have access to the relevant knowledge needed to consider options for actions and scenarios for future outcomes, thus their defect seems to be at the level of applying such knowledge (Saver & Damasio, 1991).

Subsequent investigation with the SMH have largely relied on the development of a novel gambling task [the Iowa Gambling Task (IGT)], an empirical test of decision making developed to assess an individual's ability to balance immediate rewards against long-term losses (Damasio, 1994; Bechara et al., 2001; Grant, Contoreggi, & London, 2000).

The IGT was developed to simulate a complex, real-life decision-making situation that relied upon uncertainty of outcomes in the form of rewards or punishment, somewhat like the more open-ended form of the Wisconsin Card Sorting Test. The goal of the IGT is to maximize profit on a loan of play money, where response is guided by various schedules of immediate reward and delayed punishment (Bechara, Damasio, Damasio, & Anderson, 1994). The participant has to select a card from one of four seemingly identical decks of cards and the object of the task is to make as much money as possible. Each selection yields a certain amount of money, but two of the decks pay out more than the other two. Unbeknownst to the participant, selecting cards from the different decks yields different outcomes. Selections from decks A and B are disadvantageous, as these decks yield higher immediate rewards but also higher penalties. In contrast, selecting from decks C and D is advantageous. These decks yield lower immediate rewards but lower penalties (Bechara, Damasio, Tranel,

& Anderson, 1998; Bechara, Damasio, Tranel, & Damasio, 1997; Bechara, Damasio, Damasio, & Lee, 1999; Bechara, Tranel & Damasio, 2000; Damasio, 1994). During the task, participants cannot predict what will happen, nor can they keep an exact tally of their gains and losses due to the sheer enormity of the possible interacting effects of the rewards, the decks, and the need to generate the responses.

Unimpaired participants gradually learn to avoid the disadvantageous decks and select from the advantageous decks, while patients with focal VMPFC lesions fail to shift their behaviour towards more advantageous responding, and persist with the disadvantageous decks (Bechara et al., 1994; Bechara, Tranel, Damasio, & Damasio, 1996).

Studies of substance abusers who exhibit qualitatively similar decision-making deficits to VMPFC-lesioned individuals provide convergent validity of the role of the VMPFC. For instance, impairments on the IGT and related decision-making tasks have been reported in chronic alcohol, cocaine, amphetamine, and opiate abusers (Bechara, Dolan et al., 2001; Grant et al., 2000; Rogers et al., 1999). These decision-making deficits are particularly notable in abusers of those substances that affect the dopaminergic reward systems of the prefrontal cortex (i.e., the ventral tegmental area and the nucleus acumbens), such as alcohol, cocaine, and amphetamines (Rogers et al., 1999; Volkow & Fowler, 2000).

Neural systems, including the VMPFC, the amygdala, the insula and SI/SII parietal cortices have a strong influence in the establishment and efficacy of somatic markers throughout the decision-making process. The VMPFC, particularly BA 25, lower 24 and 32, and the medial aspects areas 11, 12, and 10, have been associated as the critical neural network for the acquisition of somatic markers (Bechara, 2002). These studies have highlighted the specificity and the severity of the deficits found in patients with VMPFC lesions (Bechara et al., 1997, 1998, 1999, 2000; Damasio, 1994, 1998). Damage to the VMPFC of an individual often results in marked difficulties for the subject in reexperiencing (recalling) happy and sad events, and subjects demonstrate difficulty in reexperiencing emotions via the recall of emotional events, consistent with the predictions of the somatic marker hypothesis.

The amygdala also plays a crucial role in the somatic marker hypothesis (e.g., LeDoux, 1996). Somatic responses can be activated by the amygdala, a central autonomic structure, in the viscera, the vascular bed, the endocrine system, as well as other nonspecific neurotransmitter systems (Bechara et al., 2002, Damasio, 1998). Moreover, the amygdala exhibits a central role in emotion. Research has demonstrated that deficient performances on the IGT can result from damage to the amygdala (Bechara et al., 1999). For example, the performances of four participants with bilateral amygdala damage and 13 matched controls on the IGT indicated that the amygdala-lesioned participants selected more cards from the disadvantageous decks and fewer cards from the advantageous decks, similar to bilateral VMPFC participants (Bechara et al., 1999). Despite the presence of hippocampal damage in most of these participants, their poor performances were demonstrated to be specific to lesions involving the amygdala, supporting the notion that the amygdala is a crucial structure in the decision-making process.

Despite the similar IGT performances of the bilateral VMPFC and bilateral amygdala-lesioned participants, these two regions perform different roles. Amygdala damage prevents the development of conditioned emotional responses to aversive stimuli (Le Doux, 1996) and therefore results in coupling information from the outside world with somatic states generated by primary punishment (Bechara et al., 2002). For example, individuals with amygdala damage no longer elicit appropriate somatic states in response to the concept of winning or losing money.

Conversely, VMPFC damage does not affect this form of conditioning. Individuals with VMPFC damage have the capacity to generate somatic states in response to the feedback, but do not appear to use them effectively (Bechara et al., 2002). The visceral and somatosensory projection systems are also crucially involved in the generation of somatic markers, especially the insula, and the SI and SII cortices, which receive signals from the body (e.g., Bechara et al., 1997).

The dopaminergic and serotonergic neurotransmitter systems of the prefrontal cortex (PFC) have also been implicated as mediators of decision making (Bechara, 2003; Bechara, Damasio et al., 2000), with the blockade of both dopamine and serotonin interfering with the selection of advantageous decks of cards. These results underline the relationship between covert biasing of decisions and the dopaminergic system, and conversely the relationship that biasing of overt decisions has with the serotonergic system (Bechara 2003; Bechara, Damasio et al., 2000).

Tranel and colleagues (2002) investigated the contribution of the side of lesion of the frontal lobe and its implication to the SMH. They found that the right orbitofrontal cortex is crucial for successful performances on the IGT, while the left orbitofrontal cortex seems to be of less importance. As the task progresses, participants with unilateral left VMPFC lesions gradually shift their preferences from the disadvantageous decks to the advantageous decks. This same shift has been displayed by nonlesioned participants (Bechara, Damasio et al., 2000; Bechara, Tranel et al., 2000). In contrast, participants with unilateral right VMPFC lesions failed to demonstrate this change from disadvantageous to advantageous decks, similar to participants with bilateral VMPFC damage (Bechara, Damasio et al., 2000; Bechara, Tranel et al., 2000).

Clearly, a whole new chapter in the development of localization of functioning of the frontal has been opened by Damasio and his colleagues, and this has illuminated the way in understanding frontal injuries per se as well as the effects of conditions such as TBI, which have a more diffuse mechanism of injury on these regions of the brain (Levin & Kraus, 1994).

With regard to the specific effects of brain injury following TBI, the direct association of these changes to behavioural outcome have been considerably more difficult to characterise. Stuss and Gow (1992) provide a compromise in this dilemma in their emphasis on the "frontal system" rather than the direct attribution of the changes to the frontal lobe. They contend that this approach allows a more accurate characterisation of the network of regions implicated in these behaviours, and they emphasize the reciprocal nature of the connections of the frontal lobe with other brain regions (not the least of which the limbic circuit as well as the frontal subcortical circuits).

At first blush, the compromise in brain functions is attributable to two sets of compromise (i.e., positive versus negative; pseudopsychopathic versus pseudodepressed; disorders of control versus disorders of drive) making it possible to offer some tentative localisations of these presentations in TBI. Fuster (1989, 2003) has characterised the two syndromes as due to impaired inhibitory control mechanisms in the case of lesions of the orbital prefrontal cortex (OPFC) and to an inability to initiate and carry out new and goal directed behaviours in the case of damage to the medial and dorsolateral prefrontal cortex (M&DLPFC).

Gualtieri (1991) associated irritability with damage to the anterior regions of the brain including the anterior temporal lobe and the OPFC. Eames (1990) also emphasized the later suggestion, particularly the connection between the OPFC and the limbic areas. Starkstein and Robinson (1991) also contend that the symptom may be attributable to damage to the feedback loops connecting the two regions.

The apathetic/abulic/negative/disorder of drive pattern of personality change has been noted in a number of neuropsychiatric conditions including TBI, stroke, Parkinson's disease, Huntington's disease, Alzheimer's disease, and disorders involving the frontal-subcortical circuitry including the thalamus, and the basal ganglia (Lichter & Cummings, 2001; Crowe & Hoogenraad, 2000), as well as compromise of the dorsolateral prefrontal cortex.

However, Stuss and Gow (1992) sound a note of caution with regard to specifying localization of particular forms of personality change following injury to the frontal lobe in TBI:

> We propose that "frontal dysfunction" in TBI as a psychological concept should be at least partially dissociated from frontal localization. Frontal dysfunction refers to alteration in abilities such as decision making, planning, focusing selectivity and monitoring of performance. Their frequent theoretical and experimental association with focal frontal lobe lesions has led to the common use of the term "frontal dysfunction." Frontal (executive, control, supervisory) dysfunction, however, may be secondary to multiple etiologies, of which frontal lobe disturbance may well be most prominent. To minimize the confusion between brain localization and psychological construct, we suggest using a generic term such as "executive control function" during this period of theoretical development. (p. 278)

Conclusion

Speculation about the functioning of the frontal lobe has undergone a massive resurgence over the past decade as a result of an intriguing and sophisticated hypothesis developed by Antonio Damasio and his colleagues. This has led to a concentrated focus on the regions of the frontal lobe and the contribution that each of these regions makes to planning and error utilization. This speculation is now further permeating the long-standing discussion of how best to characterise the changes in behaviour and cognition associated with TBI.

While no one would dispute that personality change is "the most consistent feature of mental change after blunt head injury" (Jennett & Teasdale, 1981, p. 294), exactly what personality is and how this emerges from the brain, and how this ephemeral construct might be affected by TBI and its associated injury to the frontal lobe remains something of a mystery. We stand on the threshold of an exciting and informative new chapter in this story that should prove to be more concise and informative than the historical descriptions of loose categories of behaviour changes as either too much or too little of some particular target behaviour. Perhaps we will finally come to a more clear understanding of the role that the frontal lobe subserves and how these behaviours and dispositions might change as a consequence of development or damage. The future is clearly a bright one.

4 Anxiety disorders

Given the enormous neurological, neuropsychological, psychological, emotional, economic, and social upheaval that occurs for the individual following a traumatic brain injury it is not surprising that traumatic brain injury (TBI) often leads to the development of clinical states of anxiety. The cognitive specificity hypothesis proposed by Beck and colleagues (Beck, Brown, Steer, Eidelson, & Risking, 1987) suggests that schemas developed across the lifespan may be activated by environmental stimuli, drugs, and endocrine factors and, as a result, lead to biased information processing that tends towards a particular direction (Beck, 2005). These specific biases in the case of depression tend to focus upon themes of loss and devaluation of the self and, in the case of anxiety, they centre on themes of threat and vulnerability (Beck et al., 1987). Thus, in depression the cognitions invariably focus upon regrets and recriminations about what has been, whereas the focus of the thinking associated with the anxiety disorders is based upon trepidation in anticipation of what is to come and the fear associated with confronting it. Individuals who have suffered from a serious traumatic brain injury would surely be entitled to both schemas. Some investigators estimate that the incidence of measurable anxiety may be as high as 30% of TBI-affected individuals (Epstein & Ursano, 1994).

Background

Fear is one of man's basic emotions and has been a crucial mechanism for our survival both as individuals and as a species. If danger did not rapidly induce an unpleasant mental state and avoidance behaviour, animals might quickly be overwhelmed by a hostile environment. Although human beings still face dangers, the modern environment is usually relatively safe. Yet the neurobiology that induces the fear response persists. Taken to excess, however, these undue concerns about particular objects or situations and the over anticipation of the future become pathological and are reflected in the various clinical states that occur in association with the TBI.

In nature, the response of an organism to a perceived stressor can be broken down into a number of steps that are recognised as the fight/flight (or the fight/flight/freeze) response. These steps include:

(1) The initial recognition of the threat of the present situation.
(2) The appraisal of this situation as threatening.
(3) The development of a state of arousal proportionate to the nature of the perceived threat.
(4) Preparation for reaction to the threat by way of activation of the muscles and increased alertness.

(5) Response to the threat either by avoiding it, confronting it, or by psychologically controlling either of these responses.
(6) And finally with the resolution of the conflict, the dissipation of the arousal and return to the baseline state.

Some investigators consider that the nature of the fight/flight/freeze response is predicated upon the proximity of the threat to the individual. For example, a lower level, distant threat causes an animal to freeze. A higher level, closer threat causes an animal to flea. Only at the highest levels, where the threat is very close and escape is impossible, will the animal display reactive aggression and attack the feared object (Blair et al., 2005; Blanchard, Blanchard, & Takahashi, 1977).

It is well established that fear, pain, sexual activity, and emotional stress induce high levels of stress and arousal resulting in abnormal activity in the neocortex and the limbic system and, as a direct result, disrupt learning and memory (Crowe, Ng, & Gibbs, 1989a; 1989b; 1990; Joseph, 1998). This disruption probably occurs as a direct effect of these processes on long-term potentiation (e.g., Diamond, Fleshner, & Rose, 1994; Shores, Seib, Levine, & Rose, 1989).

As a part of the fight/flight/freeze response the hypothalamic-pituitary-adrenal (HPA) axis prepares the brain and the body for the possible catastrophic consequences that may arise as a result of the exposure to the stressor by secreting large amounts of adrenaline and noradrenaline, corticotrophin-releasing factor (CRF) and corticosteroids from the adrenals. These stress hormones potentiate the behavioural and autonomic reactions that occur following an injury, thus providing a protective as well as an activating influence on the organism and enabling it to continue to function and thus escape or fight for its life (Joseph, 1998).

However, the high levels of the corticosteroids have also been established to injure hippocampal pyramidal neurons (Packan & Sapolsky, 1990), to kill cells in the dentate gyrus and Ammon's horn (Lupien & McEwen, 1997), and to induce hippocampal atrophy (Gilbertson, Shenton, Ciszewski et al., 2002; Sapolsky, 1990; 1994; 2000; Uno, Tarara, Else, Suleman, & Sapolsky, 1989). This effect is exacerbated by activation of the Type II adrenal steroid receptors that abound within the hippocampus (Lupien & McEwen, 1997; Sapolsky, 1990). The overproduction of corticosteroids is directly correlated with hippocampal atrophy, and memory loss has been noted in individuals with Cushings syndrome, for example, who feature excessive levels of corticosteroids as a consequence of the condition (Starkman, Gebarski, Berent, & Schteingart, 1992).

Clearly under excessive and prolonged levels of stress, excitation, and arousal, learning and memory—not to mention numerous other higher level intellectual functions (e.g., attentional mechanisms) (Crowe et al., 2000)—may become compromised, resulting in amnesia as well as in other neurocognitive difficulties. Excessive arousal and prolonged stress coupled with other predisposing factors may well explain some of the disturbances of memory noted in traumatic amnesia, and the trauma-induced repressed memory syndrome that affects individuals subjected to sexual abuse, rape, physical assault, frontline combat, and natural disasters (Joseph, 1998).

Following a single terrifying event these effects would be devastating, but when combined with a previous history of emotional trauma or hippocampal compromise, these individuals are at further risk of memory loss due to the additive effect of the contemporary high levels of corticosteroids combined with the previous inoculation.

Discussion of the effects of prolonged levels of arousal as reflected by posttraumatic stress disorder (PTSD) has resulted in a large literature on the effects of these conditions on cognition and the integrity of neural structure. In their extensive evaluative review on these matters, Horner and Hamner (2002) note:

> On the whole, there is evidence for at least mild impairment in attention and immediate memory associated with PTSD; 16 of the 19 studies reviewed in this paper reported evidence of attention and immediate memory deficit (or both). However of these 16 studies, at least 15 have included PTSD patients with a significant psychiatric comorbidity, reflecting the extreme difficulty of recruiting "pure" samples of PTSD patients. At present, the literature supports the conclusion that deficits in attention and immediate memory are seen in PTSD patients who also manifest other psychiatric disorders; the extent to which the observed deficits are specifically attributable to PTSD remains unclear. (p. 26)

Horner and Hamner (2002) further note that in the large population-based study by Barrett, Green, Morris, Giles and Croft (1996), PTSD alone was not associated with cognitive deficits, but it was when the PTSD was associated with other psychiatric disorders.

The nature of changes on structural and functional imaging associated with a diagnosis of PTSD has been discussed at some length in the literature. Reduced hippocampal volume has been reported in individuals suffering from chronic PTSD (Bremner et al., 1995). These investigators measured hippocampal volume using magnetic resonance imaging (MRI) in 26 combat veterans with PTSD and compared them with 22 gender matched healthy controls. Bremner et al. noted that there was an 8% reduction in hippocampal volume in the PTSD-affected subjects as compared with the healthy controls.

Bremner et al. (1997) also noted a similar level (12%) of reduction in volume in the left hippocampus in 17 adult survivors of childhood abuse. A similar result (5% decline in volume of the left hippocampus and a nonsignificant trend for the right hippocampus) was noted in 21 women with a history of sexual abuse (Stein, Koverola, Hanna, Torchia, & McClarty, 1997). More recent reviews including the meta-analysis of Smith (2005) indicate that on average PTSD sufferers had a 6.9% smaller left hippocampal volume and a 6.6% smaller right hippocampal volume in comparison to controls.

Gurvits and colleagues (1996) found a similar pattern of change in their seven combat veterans with PTSD when they were matched to combat and non-combat-involved controls. Gurvits noted a 26% reduction of hippocampal volume and the result remained significant after adjustment for age, brain volume, alcohol abuse, and combat exposure.

In their longitudinal study of trauma survivors, Bonne and colleagues (2001) noted that at one week and six months following a trauma, there was no reduction in hippocampal volume. They noted that a smaller hippocampal volume is not necessarily a risk factor for developing PTSD and that, in those cases in which brain abnormality may subsequently emerge, it more commonly occurs in individuals with a chronic or complicated PTSD.

To date, two studies (Bremner et al., 1995; Gurvits et al., 1996) have noted correlations between the diminution of hippocampal volume and neuropsychological tests performance (i.e., Wechsler Memory Scale, Benton Visual Retention Tests, Arithmetic subtest of the Wechsler Adult Intelligence Scale-Revised [WAIS-R]). However, the subsequent investigation by Bremner et al. (1997) did not indicate a correlation between cognitive measures and the hippocampal volume. Clearly the relationship between these variables is not a direct one.

A number of functional neuroimaging studies have also been conducted with PTSD-affected individuals (e.g., Bremner et al., 1997; 1999a; 1999b; Liberzon et al., 1996; 1997; Rauch et al., 1996; 2000; Semple et al., 1996; Shin et al., 1997; Zubieta et al., 1999). These studies are "consistent with altered regional brain activity in PTSD patients in areas implicated in emotional regulation, learning and memory" (Horner & Hamner, 2002, p. 25). These investigators particularly stressed the role of the anterior cingulate, which plays a crucial role in facilitating exaggerated emotional and behavioural responses particularly in the context of fear conditioning. This region has also been implicated in a number of other psychiatric conditions including schizophrenia (Yücel et al., 2001, 2002) and the affective disorders (see Mayberg, 2001).

Methodological issues

The acute stress response is the normal reaction to a stressor that can be either external (a bully kicking sand into your face) or internal (the thought of Christmas with your family). This reaction has two components: one physiological and the other psychological. The gamut of these responses both physiological and psychological is largely mediated by the adrenergic neurotransmitter system. The changes associated with activation of adrenaline and noradrenaline in the acute stress response include: increased heart rate, dry mouth, piloerection (hair standing on end), sweating/clammy palms, paraesthesia (sensory loss or numbness usually of the hands and feet), nausea and headache, increase in urinary frequency, and hypersensitivity to sensory stimuli.

These changes may be doubly manifest for the individual who develops an anxiety state within the context of the changes associated with TBI. People with TBI may become easily confused and/or overwhelmed by complex or highly stimulating settings. If reasoning is impaired, they also may become very anxious and agitated about their decision-making processes. These individuals are thus more likely to either "blowup" or "shutdown" when their ability to process their experiences has been stretched too far (Contole & PACS Team, 1996).

An individual with a TBI who may already feature a compromise in attention and speed of processing due to the inability to generate and execute strategies to deal with distraction, or to deal with more than a single sensory input at any one time, may find the effects of anxiety doubly debilitating.

Near-death experiences (NDEs)

One aspect of survival of TBI that has not been discussed to any great extent in the literature is the degree to which survival following a serious injury may constitute an NDE. People who have been faced with an unavoidable outcome of death, but through some means have avoided this outcome, have reported NDEs (Stevenson & Greyson, 1979).

Each NDE is comprised of a set of unique and a set of common elements. The commonly described elements include: feeling "out" of the body, feeling of passing through a tunnel, entrance into an unearthly realm, meeting with other people or beings, seeing a light, and replaying of one's significant life events (Greyson & Stevenson, 1980). The experience is commonly reported to be profound and to have immense and life-changing effects (Parnia, Waller, Yeates, & Fenwick, 2001).

Numerous methodological difficulties surround the description of these events, including the lack of a standardized definition of the NDE phenomenon and agreement as to its exact nature (Kellehear, 1993); difficulties and inconsistencies associated with measurement and classification of the experience (Greyson, 1998); sampling of participants (Greyson, 2001); and the comprehensiveness of the possible data collection associated with the experience (Kelly, 2001).

Clearly the personality and beliefs of the individual who experiences an NDE significantly colour the nature of the experience and the way in which it is interpreted (Gabbard, Twemlow, & Jones, 1981). Similar to the experience of recalling dreams, distortions can quickly creep in and these are confounded and multiplied by retelling the story of the experience, quickly altering the original content (Gabbard et al., 1981). Various social psychological phenomena also apply to the description and interpretation of these experiences, including social desirability in shaping the recall of the event (Greyson et al., 1983), fear of rejection and ridicule, concerns regarding sanity, and the desire not to burden those around them (Hoffman, 1995).

Verifiability is also an important concern here. Owens, Cook, and Stevenson (1990) found that of the 58 patients they studied who reported NDEs, 30 of them (52%) were not near death at the time of their NDE and of these, 21 erroneously believed that that their death was imminent or had already occurred. Stevenson, Williams-Cook, and McClean-Rice (1989) reported a similar figure of 55% of their 107 NDE patients not close to death with some only having minor illnesses. It may well be that the *expectation* of dying rather than the *actual risk* of dying per se initiates the NDE, indicating the vulnerability of this effect to personal belief.

A further aspect of the NDE occurs when the individual in question survives the accident or event but a significant other involved does not. This situation, referred to as survivor guilt (McMillan, 1996), adds to the emotional burden of the surviving individual, possibly acting as a further focus for posttraumatic stress. McMillan (1996) noted that 4 individuals featured this symptom in the sample of 10 cases in whom PTSD had emerged following mild to severe closed head injuries. Two of these emerged because of NDEs in the accident (one in which the individual's child was involved in the accident and might have been killed, and the second in which passengers were injured while the individual was driving).

McMillan (1996) also noted that the patients reported a number of consistent themes relating to their distress: confrontation with death, realization of their own physical vulnerability, loss of control, and adjustment to the "amnesic gap" in their lives. McMillan raised the possibility of irrational survivor guilt. In a single case report of PTSD following a severe head injury, McMillan noted that the young woman in question, who had been a passenger in the vehicle driven by a friend, developed the irrational belief that she had somehow caused the accident or failed to prevent it.

While few TBI sufferers report NDEs, the issue is one that must at least be considered in the evaluation of the individual in the wake of what is clearly a life-threatening event, and the implications of this to that individual may have significant, long-term and life-changing effects (Martin & Kleiber, 2005).

Phenomenology and nosology of the secondary anxiety disorders

Anxiety consists of apprehension, tension, and undue concerns about a perceived danger. It is usually accompanied by signs associated with the activation of the sympathetic nervous system and is described as free-floating anxiety when there is no conscious recognition of the specific threat. Anxiety is regarded as the chief characteristic of all of the neurotic disorders, and can be differentiated from normal or adaptive fear in that: (1) it is not related to a perceived realistic threat or at least is out of keeping in degree with the level of threat that such an object or event actually would pose; (2) it results from some form of intrapsychic conflict; and (3) it is not relieved by the amelioration of the objective situation.

Spielberger (Spielberger, Lushene, & McAdoo, 1977) divided anxiety into two distinct forms: trait anxiety and state anxiety. State anxiety is that level of anxiety that all individuals experience from time to time in response to a real or perceived threat. This is responsive to the presence of the perceived environmental cue and varies as a function of time. Trait anxiety, on the other hand, is a dispositional pattern of responding to a variety of evoking stimuli that is typically associated with the anxiety disorders.

The *DSM-IV-TR* (APA, 2000) divides the anxiety disorders into a series of subdisorders including panic attacks, agoraphobia, panic disorder with and without agoraphobia, the specific phobias, social phobia, obsessive-compulsive disorder (OCD), posttraumatic stress disorder, generalised anxiety disorder (GAD), anxiety disorder due to a general medical condition, substance-induced anxiety disorder, and anxiety disorders not otherwise specified. Readers are encouraged to consult *DSM-IV-TR* for the full details of the diagnostic criteria for each of the anxiety conditions.

Each of these disorders is characterised by a pattern of anxiety inappropriate to the environmental cues elicited by the stimuli in normal individuals. Within the context of this discussion, I will concentrate particularly upon PTSD because it has generated a huge volume of literature in the area of TBI, particularly in the attempt to dissociate the effects of minor traumatic brain injury from PTSD (if, indeed, such a split is actually possible). The overlap between these conditions is clearly not unexpected as inevitably the sort of injury that would result in a mild to an extremely severe TBI would, of necessity, be associated with an "exposure to an extreme traumatic stressor involving direct personal experience of an event that involves actual or threatened death or serious injury, or other threat to one's physical integrity" or that of another (APA, 2000, p. 463).

In this section, I also focus on the other anxiety disorders that occur in association with TBI including the generalised anxiety disorder, panic disorder, phobia, and obsessive compulsive disorder, although these tend to be less commonly encountered in TBI populations. In their compilation of 12 studies concerning the incidence of anxiety disorders in association with TBI, Epstein and Ursano (1994) noted that the study "of the 1199 patients from 1942 to 1990, revealed that approximately 29% of head injury patients were diagnosed with clinical anxiety following TBI" (p. 286). A similar incidence has been noted by Silver and colleagues (Silver, Kramer, Greenwald, & Weissman, 2001) who noted that in their community sample of over 5000 adults, 361 (7.2%) had suffered TBI and of this subsample, 11% suffered major depression, 11% phobic disorders, 5% OCD and 3% panic disorder. Koponen and colleagues (2002) noted similar rates and observed that of their 60 TBI patients, 8% featured panic disorder. Fann, Katon, Uomoto, and Esselman (1995) noted that 24% of their sample of 50 patients features GAD and in the study of Hibbard, Bogdany et al. (2000) 27% of their 100 patients featured obsessive compulsive personality disorder following injury. Mooney and Speed (2001) noted that 24% of their mild TBI patients were classified as having developed an acquired anxiety disorder following their injuries.

Consistent estimates of the rate of the emergence of anxiety disorders following TBI garnered from a variety of sources indicate that the incidence post-TBI are between 3 and 28% for GAD, between 4 and 17% for panic disorder, between 1 and 10% for phobic disorders, between 2 and 15% for OCD, and between 3 and 27% for PTSD (Hiott & Labbate, 2002; Koponen et al., 2002; Moore, Terryberry-Spohr, & Hope, 2006). Generally speaking, the most commonly noted anxiety symptoms noted following TBI include: free-floating anxiety, fearfulness, intense worry, generalised uneasiness, sensitivity in interpersonal situations, and anxious dreams (Rao & Lyketsos, 2002).

Acute stress disorder

Acute stress disorder (ASD) is the development of anxiety and dissociation as well as other symptoms of a stress reaction that occur within the first four weeks following an extreme traumatic stressor (APA, 2000). As for a diagnosis of PTSD, the condition consists of dissociative, reexperiencing, avoidant, and arousal symptoms. The main difference between ASD and PTSD is that for the diagnosis of ASD three dissociative symptoms must be present, and that the symptoms occur one month after the exposure to the traumatic stressor.

A particular problem pertains to the diagnosis of ASD in the context of MTBI because there is considerable overlap among the symptoms associated with each condition. The dissociative symptoms of reduced awareness, depersonalization, derealization, and amnesia are commonly noted during both posttraumatic amnesia (PTA) and postconcussional syndrome (PCS) (Bryant & Harvey, 1998). The major goal of the task force responsible for developing this diagnosis for the *DSM-IV-TR* was to identify individuals in the posttrauma phase who would be likely to subsequently develop PTSD (Bryant & Harvey, 2000).

To satisfy the criteria for the diagnosis of ASD, the individual must display acute dissociation (emotional numbing, derealization, depersonalization, reduced awareness of surroundings, dissociative amnesia), reexperiencing phenomena (intrusive memories, nightmares, flashbacks), avoidance (effortful avoidance of thoughts, conversations or places reminiscent of the trauma), and arousal symptoms (insomnia, heightened startle response, concentration deficits) (Bryant, 2001). Due to the difficulties associated with the issue of PTA and the reexperiencing of the event, some investigators (e.g., Warden et al., 1997) have proposed that the criteria for the diagnosis of PTSD be modified in the context of TBI to exclude the reexperiencing phenomena.

Posttraumatic stress disorder (PTSD)

Posttraumatic stress disorder is characterised by the development of characteristic anxiety symptoms following exposure to an extreme traumatic stressor. The revision of the criteria included in the *DSM-IV-TR* (APA, 2000) includes the fact that the individual should experience fear, helplessness or horror at the time of the event (Harvey, Brewin, Jones, & Kopelman, 2003).

PTSD is defined (APA, 2000) by the following criteria (APA, 2000):

(1) The individual must have been exposed to or witnessed a threatening event involving death or serious injury or a threat to the physical integrity of self or others.
(2) The individual's response must have involved intense fear, helplessness, or horror.
(3) The individual must display reexperiencing symptoms that may include intrusive memories, nightmares, feelings as if the event were reoccurring or distress when reminded of the trauma.
(4) The individual engages in attempts to avoid the thoughts, feelings, or reminders of the trauma.
(5) The individual suffers from high levels of arousal that may take the form of insomnia, irritability, difficulty concentrating, hypervigilence, or an exaggerated startle response.
(6) These disturbances must go on for more than one month.
(7) The symptoms must cause impairment in the individual's ability to function.

Harvey et al. (2003) contended that the features of PTSD exist along a continuum and that

> Many patients are seen in clinical practice who show several features of PTSD, but who fall just short of a strict formal diagnosis in some way....PTSD is essentially a syndrome or cluster of symptoms whose number and severity vary along

> a continuum, and that strict hard-and-fast categories (PTSD/no PTSD) may miss important pathology and may be the source of apparent conflicts in the literature. (p. 664)

Although approximately 69% of the population will be exposed to a traumatic event in their lifetimes (Norris, 1992), the lifetime prevalence for PTSD is only 7.8%. Using the *DSM-IV* definition, the American Psychiatric Association (1994) estimates the prevalence rates between 3 and 58% depending upon the nature of the traumatic event. PTSD has been reported in 39% of survivors of motor vehicle accidents (Blanchard et al., 1996), 16% of firefighters (McFarlane, 1988), and 38% of assault victims other than sexual assault (Riggs, Rothbaum, & Foa, 1995). A diagnosis of ASD has been reported to be 19% following assault (Brewin, Andrews, Rose, & Kirk, 1999) and 13% following a motor vehicle accident (MVA) (Harvey & Bryant, 1998).

The fact that not all individuals who are subjected to a life-threatening event go on to become traumatized has lead Sbordone and Guilmette (1999) to argue that exposure to the event may be a necessary, but not a sufficient, condition for the development of PTSD. The prevalence of PTSD across the lifespan is 5% for males and 10% for females (Foa, Keane, & Friedman, 2000). Kessler, Berglund, Demler, Jin and Walters (2005) noted a similar figure of 6.8% in community-based studies and, given a similar trauma, women are reported to be four times more likely to develop PTSD than are men (Resick, 2001a, 2001b). While estimates vary, approximately 39% of road traffic accident victims, 24% of young urban adults, and 15% of Vietnam veterans meet the criteria for PTSD (Bryant & Harvey, 1999).

The frequency with which ASD and PTSD occur following the survival of an motor vehicle accident (MVA) (i.e., without TBI) has also been a matter of some dispute. Motor vehicle accidents are a relatively commonly encountered life-threatening event and cause significant psychological distress (Breslau, Davis, Andreski, & Peterson, 1991). MVAs are recognised as *the* most common precipitant of PTSD (Blanchard & Hickling, 1997; Norris, 1992).

Estimates of the level of PTSD following MVA range from 10 to 46% (Blanchard, Hickling, Taylor, Loos, & Gerardi, 1994; Blanchard et al., 1996; Brom, Kleber, & Hofman, 1993; Mayou, Bryant, & Duthie, 1993), and between 18 and 42% of survivors display severe acute stress reactions (Bryant & Harvey, 1995, 1996; Harvey & Bryant, 1998c; Mayou et al., 1993).

Harvey and Bryant (1998a, 1998b) have noted that in their group of 92 MVA survivors measured at one month following injury, 13% developed ASD, and a further 21% had subclinical levels of ASD. At a 6-month follow-up, 78% of the ASD participants (i.e., 10% of the initial sample) and 60% of the subclinical group (i.e., 12.6% of the initial sample) met the criteria for PTSD. Bryant and Harvey (1999) also compared individuals with and without mild traumatic brain injury (MTBI) at 1 and 6 months postinjury and noted comparable rates of ASD and PTSD. It is thus clear that a sizeable percentage of individuals involved in a MVA (approximately 20%) will go on to develop PTSD. The interesting question to ask is to what degree will individuals who also suffer brain impairment in the injury either increase or decrease the level of this diagnosis?

One particular issue of concern here is the degree to which an individual, particularly one in the context of some form of medico-legal dispute, might be able to feign the symptoms of PTSD for the purposes of increasing the likelihood of a successful settlement. Lees-Haley and Dunn (1994) found that 99% of untutored (and uninjured) undergraduates could achieve a performance satisfying *DSM-IV* criteria on a symptom checklist. Burges and McMillan (2001) noted a similar level of endorsement when they observed that 94% of their sample of 136 further education night-class college students could satisfy the criteria of PTSD on the Posttraumatic Symptom Scale Report (PSS-SR) (Foa, Riggs, Dancu, & Rothbaum, 1993) after listening to a vignette describing a man assaulted by three youths when walking home from work. The participants (half of whom were administered the PSS-SR and the remainder a checklist containing bogus items not normally associated with PTSD) were capable of satisfying the criteria for PTSD using the standard checklist by guessing. Clearly it is possible for even relatively untrained participants with little or no knowledge of PTSD to fake responses on symptom checklists sufficient to achieve the diagnosis.

Posttraumatic stress disorder and its distinction from TBI

Considerable controversy has surrounded the issue of differential diagnosis of the organic sequelae associated with a TBI and PTSD, and whether indeed these two conditions can coexist. Both Price (1994) and Sbordone (1991) have argued that "PTSD and MTBI are mutually incompatible disorders since patients who sustain PTSD simply cannot 'forget' the traumatic event, whereas patients who sustain MTBI (e.g., cerebral concussion) have no recollection of the traumatic event.... Thus, patients who sustain PTSD, if given the opportunity, can provide exquisite and highly detailed chronological, as well as emotionally charged, recollections of the traumatic event in comparison to patients who sustain MTBI, who have no recollection of the traumatic event" (Sbordone & Liter, 1995, p. 406).

Warden et al. (1997) have noted no cases of PTSD that met full criteria in their sample of 47 TBI-affected active duty military personnel, although they did note that 6 met the avoidance and arousal criteria and of these 5 also had organic mood or anxiety disorders. These researchers noted that "even in the face of potentially life threatening injuries, amnesia for the event greatly decreases the likelihood of developing PTSD" (p. 20) and further that "the lack of intrusive memories and reexperiencing phenomena is due to the neurogenic amnesia" (p. 21). A similar view is expressed by Boake and Bontke in the Controversies Debate in the *Journal of Head Trauma Rehabilitation* (Bontke, 1996).

Multiple factors determine whether an individual will develop PTSD following a traumatic event. These predisposing factors include: female gender, social disadvantage, childhood adversity, genetic predisposition, and substance abuse (Sbordone & Guilmette, 1999). A previous exposure to trauma, early separation, or a family history of anxiety or PTSD could also be convincingly added to this list (Resick, 2001a, 2001b). McMillan and colleagues (MacMillan, Williams, & Bryant, 2003) noted that "if the event is unanticipated and not preventable, involves actual or threatened fear of death, and is outside the person's control, then development of PTSD symptoms is likely" (p. 151).

A number of investigators have reported the incidence of PTSD in head-injured victims to range from 20 to 40% (Bryant & Harvey, 1995; Hickling, Gillen, Blanchard, Buckley, & Taylor, 1998; Ohry, Rattock, & Solomon, 1996; Rattock & Ross, 1993). McMillan et al. (2003) provides a comprehensive discussion of the incidence of PTSD following mild to severe TBI and codes the studies for their controlled versus uncontrolled methodology. They conclude that the studies reviewed

> overall support the case that PTSD can develop after minor or severe TBI in children and adults, despite loss of consciousness and post-traumatic amnesia. Some caution is required when comparing studies, given that different assessments of PTSD have been used, the severity of brain injury is not always clear, several studies are retrospective, and because relatively few are well controlled and none incorporate assessment of PTSD that is blind to group membership. (p. 156)

Blanchard and colleagues (Blanchard, Hickling, Taylor et al., 1996) noted in their study of 158 MVA victims assessed one to four months postinjury, 62 (39%) met the *DSM-III-R* (APA, 1987) criteria for the diagnosis for PTSD. They found that 70% of the participants could be classified as PTSD sufferers (or not) based on four variables: prior major depression, fear of dying in the MVA, the extent of the physical injury, and whether or not litigation had been initiated. Eight variables including the presence of litigation, prior mood disorder, fear of dying in the MVA, ethnicity, road conditions responsible for the MVA, extent of injury, prior history of PTSD, and the presence of a whiplash injury accounted for 38.1% of the variance observed on the clinician-administered PTSD Scale (Blake et al., 1990).

Another factor that is a very interesting explanatory variable in accounting for postinjury distress is allocation of the blame for the event. Delahanty and colleagues (1997) noted that in those situations in which others were responsible for the MVA, they demonstrated increased distress 6 and 12 months postaccident. In those situations in which the individual himself or herself was responsible, the participants used more self-blame coping, although in the self-responsible group, self-blame was associated with more distress.

Contrary to the issues raised by Sbordone and colleagues (Sbordone, 1999) are the numerous reports in which evidence of PTSD has been reported following TBI (e.g., Bryant, Marosszeky, et al., 2000; Feinstein, Hershkop, Ouchterlony, Jardine, & McCullagh, 2002; Grigsby & Kaye, 1993; Hickling et al., 1998; King, 1997; McMillan, 1996; McNeill & Greenwood, 1996; Ohry et al., 1996; Williams, Evans, Wilson, & Needham, 2002). The series of studies conducted at the Westmead Hospital in Sydney, Australia presents a wealth of evidence supporting the coexistence of the two conditions. These studies were mostly limited to individuals with mild TBI and record the presence of ASD and PTSD in this subset of brain-injured patients. In the acute phase of recovery following the injury (Bryant & Harvey, 1995a), fear and intrusive recollections of the accident were noted in both head-injured and noninjured individuals. These symptoms were, however, much more common in the nonhead-injured individuals.

Mayou et al. (1993) noted that in their 188 consecutive cases of MVA victims who were admitted to emergency rooms with loss of consciousness (LOC) less than 15 minutes after their injuries, 11% of the total sample featured a diagnosis of PTSD in the year following the accident. The study conducted by Feinstein et al. (2002) indicated that in a sample of 282 outpatients assessed a mean of 53 days following their injuries and stratified based on the duration of their PTA, the symptoms of PTSD occurred in all groups. However, when the PTA extended beyond one hour, symptoms of reexperiencing the event and avoidant behaviour were endorsed significantly less often. Feinstein et al. concluded "...irrespective of the mechanisms involved, symptoms of PTSD may occur across the full range of head injury severity" (p. 29).

Williams et al. (2002) investigated the prevalence of PTSD in a community sample of 66 severe TBI patients. The authors found a prevalence rate of 18% for moderate to severe PTSD in the brain-injured sample. These authors also noted that a diagnosis of PTSD may be less common in severe as compared to mild brain trauma. A similar observation was made by Glaesser, Neuner, Lutgehetmann, Schmidt, and Elbert (2004) who proposed that the effect of a less coherent memory of the events surrounding the injury may make this material less available to fuel intrusive thoughts and avoidance.

In assessing the possibility of the emergence of PTSD in the context of a significant LOC one must ask: To what degree it is possible for a PTSD to emerge if the trauma cannot be recalled? A number of possible mechanisms have been proposed to determine how such a process might be physically possible. It has been suggested that an implicit, rather than an explicit, memory of the trauma could have formed in response to the traumatic event (Layton & Wardi-Zonna, 1995; Schachter, 1992). This process would rely on the development of a fear-conditioning process causing exaggerated emotional and behavioural responses to conditioned stimuli (Brewin, Dalgleish, & Joseph, 1996; Hamner et al., 1999). A similar sort of suggestion has also been made by Bryant (1996) in his observation that patients with MTBI and LOC or PTA may develop "pseudomemories" of the trauma. He describes two case reports in which the participants developed delayed onset PTSD following significant periods of PTA, but based upon their "memories" garnered from newspaper clippings, police reports, and self-generated imagery.

A second possibility relies on the notion of the formation of explicit memories that form during the windows of recall in PTA (see chapter 1) where elements of the experience excluding the blow and the associated LOC itself act as the trauma (i.e., due to the brief retrograde and anterograde amnesia the individual might recall the imminent collision, blood trickling down the face, and "coming to" in the vehicle). It is also possible that self-generated/imagined experiences of the trauma (Bryant, 1996; Hickling et al., 1998; McMillan, 1996, 2001; McMillan & Jacobson, 1999) could possibly emerge in the more severe TBI spectrum. Unfortunately to date no clear conclusion can be drawn regarding which, if any, of these mechanisms pertain in this context, and clearly further experimentation and observation regarding this fascinating prospect is worthwhile.

In their comprehensive consideration of the mechanisms by which the coexistence of PTSD and TBI might be possible Harvey et al. (2003) argued that there are two possible resolutions of the debate:

> One resolution involves accepting that TBI patients do not experience a particular set of symptoms that are common among non-TBI patients with PTSD, but that this is nevertheless no barrier to them receiving a PTSD diagnosis....The second resolution involves accepting that TBI patients do experience the same symptoms as other PTSD patients, but that there may be crucial differences in symptom content....At present the kind of detailed information about symptoms that would enable us to choose between these various possibilities has not been collected." (p. 672)

Nonetheless, it is the case that having amnesia for the event, although not necessarily protective against the development of PTSD, seems to decrease the severity of the diagnosis and is particularly protective against the intrusive symptoms of the condition (Turnbull, Campbell, & Swann, 2001).

Generalised anxiety disorder (GAD)

GAD is characterised by excessive anxiety and worry occurring on more days than not for a period of at least six months (APA, 2000). The person finds it difficult to control this worry and is distressed by it and, as a consequence, is compromised in their daily functioning. Lewis and Rosenberg (1990) report that TBI patients often experience anxiety of a generalised and free-floating type consisting of persistent tension, worry and fearfulness, which is experienced in an intense and overwhelming way but without much comprehension due to their inability to understand or adapt to these external and internal stimuli.

GAD in the TBI-affected patient is also frequently associated with depression (Jorge, Robinson, Starkstein et al., 1993) with comorbidity rates ranging from 33 to 65% (Stavrakaki & Vargo, 1986). For example, Jorge, Robinson, Starkstein et al. (1993) studied a mixed TBI sample, all of whom were diagnosed with GAD (n = 7) and also met the criteria for major depression. Merskey and Woodforde (1961) noted that of their 27 cases of minor TBI referred for assessment in the absence of medico-legal considerations, 7 cases (25.9%) had endogenous depression while 9 cases (33.3%) featured a diagnosis of mixed anxiety and depression. Van Reekum, Bolago, Finlayson, Garner, and Links (1996) assessed 18 subjects (10 with severe TBI and 8 with mild or moderate TBI) an average of 4.9 years following the TBI using the SADS-L (Endicott & Spitzer, 1978). Of the sample, 11 (58%) received a post-TBI diagnosis of major depression. Bipolar affective disorder was found in three subjects (16%) and cyclothymia in a further 2 subjects. Seven subjects (37%) received a diagnosis of anxiety disorder, with 5 of the 7 featuring generalised anxiety disorder. The remainder had panic disorder (1), with the others having mixed phobias and obsessive compulsive disorder. Four of the seven developed their anxiety states following the injury.

Fann, Uomoto, and Katon (2000) evaluated 50 consecutive patients referred to a university brain rehabilitation clinic and noted that 24% of these patients had a diagnosis of GAD at the time of interview. Thirty-four percent of the patients had had a previous history of GAD. Only 2% of the sample featured panic disorder, a level consistent with that observed in the uninjured population.

As a rule, the likelihood of GAD following a TBI is fairly low and in those cases in which it does occur, the diagnosis commonly occurs in association with depression or a prior history of the condition.

Panic disorder

Panic disorder is characterised by the presence of recurrent, unexpected panic attacks followed by at least one month of persistent concern about having an attack (APA, 2000). In a comparison of agitated versus nonagitated patients following traumatic brain injury, Levin and Grossman (1978) noted that patients who experienced screaming, combativeness, and other signs of sympathetic arousal in the acute confusional phase following the brain injury tended to display significantly higher levels of anxiety, depression, and thought disturbance after stabilization or improvement in orientation. The symptoms did not appear to be related to the side of the injury but correlated with acute aphasic symptoms and the appearance of auditory or visual hallucinations (Epstein & Ursano, 1994). Schuetznow and Wiercisiewski (1999) report a single case of panic disorder featuring anxiety symptoms regarding health, and fear of suffering a heart attack following TBI. Again, panic is a relatively uncommon presentation following TBI in most of the published literature, but can occur comorbidly with PTSD (McMillan et al., 2003).

Phobias

Phobias are characterised by a persistent fear of a clearly discernible circumscribed object or situation (APA, 2000). Not uncommonly, individuals develop phobic responses subsequent to TBI and these symptoms often emerge in the context of PTSD. In non-TBI samples, the most commonly occurring phobic objects include insects, heights, confined spaces, or receiving injections (APA, 2000). Generally phobic concerns are relatively rarely reported following TBI although there are certainly a number of cases of specific aversion to motor vehicles and of being a passenger in a car in those individuals who have been involved in MVAs (Blanchard & Hickling, 2004). Deb, Lyons, Koutzoukis, Ali, and McCarthy (1999) reported a single case of specific phobia in their sample of 196 TBI cases, while van Reekum et al. (1996) noted one case out of their sample of 18. Mayou et al. (1993), however, noted a much higher incidence of 7% in their sample of 188 cases, with all of these related to travel. However, the latter sample was identified from motor accident victims only while the other studies identified their samples from a range of situations (Moore et al., 2006). Overall, the condition is probably best considered within the context of PTSD and as a specific stress response to particular aspects of the injury or its sequelae (McMillan et al., 2003; Williams, Evans, & Fleminger, 2003).

Social phobia

Social phobia is characterised by "a marked and persistent fear of social or performance situations in which embarrassment may occur" (APA, 2000, p. 450). As Moore et al. (2006, p. 127) noted: "despite its status as the most common of all anxiety disorders, social phobia has received very little attention in TBI research." These researchers go on to calculate the incidence of this condition post-TBI as extrapolated from the observations of van Reekum et al. (1996), insofar as these investigators note that there is a 89% comorbidity between social phobia and avoidant personality disorder and in van Reekum et al.'s study the incidence of the latter diagnosis was 17% (i.e., an approximate incidence of social phobia was about 15%).

Obsessive-compulsive disorder (OCD)

OCD is characterised by the presence of recurrent obsession or compulsions (APA, 2000). Obsession are persistent ideas, thoughts, or experiences that are experienced as intrusive and inappropriate, while compulsions are repetitive thoughts (i.e., praying, counting, repeating words silently) or behaviours (such as hand washing, checking, ordering or adjusting things), the goal of which is to reduce anxiety or distress (APA, 2000).

The symptoms of OCD need to be distinguished from the phenomenon of "organic orderliness" associated with TBI. Brain-injured individuals often tend toward increased rigidity in their behaviour and to intolerance of the disruption of their routines (Williams et al., 2003) following injury. This requirement for order is perhaps not too difficult to understand as a means of coping with the neuropsychological and psychological deficits encountered following a TBI including memory disorders and problems with planning and categorization. The notion of the reestablishing some form of control in a world that has spun out of control as a result of the effects of the injury also probably underlies this type of response.

OCD following traumatic brain injury tends to be relatively rare in the literature, but at least 57 cases have so far been described: 5 cases (Lewis, 1942); 7 cases (Anderson, 1942); 1 case (Adler, 1945); 14 cases (Hilbom, 1960); 2 cases (Lishman, 1968); 4 cases (McKeon, McGuffin, & Robinson, 1984); 1 case (Khanna, Narayan, Sharma, & Mukundan, 1985); 1 case (Kettl & Marks, 1986); 1 case (Jenike & Brandon, 1988); 1 case (Drummond & Gravestock, 1988); 1 case (Laplane, Boulliat, Baron, Pillon, & Baulac, 1988); 1 case (Lewis & Rosenberg, 1990); 1 case (Donovan & Barry, 1994); 1 case (Max et al., 1995); 4 cases (Childers, Holland, Ryan, & Rupright, 1998); 1 case (Khouzam & Donnelly, 1998); 10 cases (Berthier, Kulisevsky, Gironell, & Lopez, 2001); and 1 case (Williams et al., 2003).

In the large sample assembled by Berthier et al. (2001), they noted that the patterns of OCD symptomatology (e.g., contamination, somatic symptoms, requirement for symmetry, cleaning, and checking) were well specified and associated with cognitive deficit and MRI evidence of disruption of the frontal-subcortical circuitry.

The time when obsessive compulsive behaviours are observed following the traumatic brain injury varies considerably in the published literature spanning from days to years following the impact, and often worsening over time (Etcharry-Bouyx &

Dubas, 2000). Following head injuries the duration with which these problems can emerge may be as little as 24 hours (McKeon et al., 1984) to three or more years after the injury (Khanna et al., 1985).

The mechanism by which OCD develops following TBI has been a matter of considerable speculation in the literature. Baxter and colleagues (1992) have found significant correlations between the activity of the orbital prefrontal cortex with that of both the caudate nucleus and the thalamus in those individuals who received treatment for their OCD, but not following treatment in those who responded. They also found that changes in metabolic rate as measured by cerebral blood flow in the head of the caudate on the right directly correlated with successful treatment. Rauch, Jenike, Alpert, and colleagues (1994) found an increase in relative cerebral blood flow during an OCD symptomatic state in the right caudate nucleus when compared with the resting state. These patients also featured activation of the left anterior cingulate cortex and the bilateral orbital frontal cortex.

These findings support the neuroanatomical theory of OCD (Insel, 1992a, 1992b) that suggests the involvement of a reverberating circuit consisting of increased glutaminergic neurotransmission from the orbitofrontal and cingulate cortices, the caudate nucleus and the ventral striatum followed by increased GABAergic inhibitory neurotransmission to the globus pallidus followed by decreased inhibitory neurotransmission to the thalamus.

Based on this theory it is expected that only lesions of the pallidum, striatum, and thalamus are necessary to produce OCD. However, there is clear evidence to support the notion of frontal lobe pathology variously in the development of this condition (Donovan & Barry, 1994; Eslinger & Damasio, 1985). In support of the organic basis of this diagnosis, it should be noted that individuals who develop OCD following brain injury tend to have a negative family history for the condition and a later age of onset of the condition than do noninjured control subjects with the diagnosis (Berthier, Kulisevsky, Gironell, & Heras, 1996).

My previous work with the condition (McLaren & Crowe, 2003), supports the notion of a number of predisposing psychological factors to the emergence of OCD in susceptible individuals. In both a clinical and nonclinical sample the development of OCD-like symptomatology occurs in the context of a significant uncontrolled stressful life event in association with the individual's previous disposition to demonstrate the overly sensorious constraint on internal cognitions labelled thought suppression. This is best illustrated by of the example of requesting an individual *not* to think of a white bear, which in most cases produces the opposite effect. Clearly the constellation of factors that occur following head injury constitute a marked uncontrollable stressful life event, and the suggestion arising from our previous investigation would indicate that a predisposing tendency towards thought suppression would result, indeed, in the individual demonstrating OCD-like symptomatology if they had this predisposition.

Prevalence and incidence of secondary anxiety disorders including demographic and psychiatric correlates

Anxiety disorders are common in patients with TBI and range in frequency from 11 to 70% (Klonoff, 1971; Lewis, 1942). In their review of 12 studies conducted between 1942 and 1990, Epstein and Ursano (1994) noted that in a total sample of 1,199 subjects, most of whom had featured only minor head injuries, 29% of postinjury subjects featured anxiety disorders.

Deb, Lyons, Koutzoukis, Ali et al. (1999) followed up 196 patients who were admitted to the hospital between July 1, 1994 and June 30, 1995 with a traumatic brain injury. Each of these patients had a period a loss of consciousness, radiological evidence of brain assault, or a GCS of less than 15. Of the 120 patients interviewed between the ages of 18 and 64, 26 (21.7%) had an International Classification of Diseases (ICD)-10 diagnosis of psychiatric illness. Of this group, 17 patients (14%) had diagnoses of anxiety disorder including 11 (9%) with panic disorder, 3 (2.5%) with generalised anxiety disorder, 1 (0.8%) with phobic disorder, and 2 (1.6%) with OCD.

Despite the likely association between TBI and the anxiety disorders there is still some inconsistency in this literature. One of the most notable inconsistencies is in the dose response relationships of the presence and severity of the anxiety disorders relative to the severity of injury. Sir Austin Bradford Hill first proposed the concept of the "biologic gradient" in 1965. He proposed that one of the criteria for a causative rather than a correlational relationship between a particular clinical entity (in this case post-TBI anxiety disorder) and the putative cause (i.e., the injury) was the degree to which the severity of the causative entity correlated with the severity of the presentation. This effect is often reported to be inconsistent across studies and in many cases paradoxically, the relationship operates in a manner featuring a negative gradient, with often less severe injuries (i.e., MTBI) resulting in more anxiety symptoms than either moderate or severe TBI (Rapoport, McCauley, Levin, Song, & Feinstein, 2002; van Reekum, Cohen, & Wong, 2000). Clearly any direct association between the two phenomena cannot easily explain this type of data and many factors that mediate the relationship between the two conditions, including the PCS discussed in the last chapter, must significantly colour the expression of the pathology.

Evolution of secondary anxiety disorders following TBI

While the presence of psychiatric disorder is major determinant of outcome following TBI (Mooney & Speed, 1997), predicting which individual will go on to have an uncomplicated recovery and which will never recover remains a significant diagnostic dilemma. Certainly the evolution from the ASD to PTSD follows a reasonably predictable course, but ultimately which individual will develop and sustain the diagnosis of posttraumatic anxiety and the PCS is less predictable.

Fenton et al. (1993) note that of the 39% (n = 45) of their sample of MTBI patients who demonstrated psychiatric caseness at six weeks postinjury, nearly half demonstrated four times the average level of social difficulties noted with controls at six months postinjury. Similarly, Merskey and Woodforde (1972) noted that even at four years postinjury, 50% of their MTBI sample who reported psychiatric sequelae demonstrated no improvement in PCS symptoms. Clearly these conditions do resolve in many patients following the injury, but as yet the literature is still not clear on how quickly they will, the trajectory of the recovery, whether it returns to the preinjury level, and why it is that some individuals will go on to have long-term psychiatric morbidity from the injury.

Lesion location and mechanism of secondary anxiety disorders

Grafman, Vance, Weingartner, Salazar, and Amin (1986) conducted a study of 52 veterans who suffered penetrating missile wounds that caused damage to the orbitofrontal cortex during the Vietnam War. Grafman et al. found that the patients with left-sided or bilateral wounds showed no differences in mood states when compared with the control participants. However, patients who had right-sided orbitofrontal lesions initially manifested anger that later gave way to panic, lassitude, general anxiety, and edginess. As a result Grafman et al. contended that the right orbitofrontal cortex plays a critical role in the regulation of anxiety states. Specification of the site and side of lesions and their contribution to the development of psychiatric state must be interpreted with the utmost caution. This matter is addressed in more detail in the discussion of the mood disorders in chapter 5.

The effects of brain injury and their implication to the emergence of anxiety disorders was reviewed by Wise and Rundell (1999). This review indicates that lesions affecting the temporo-limbic areas, most notably the amygdala, the basal ganglia, and the frontal lobe—particularly the cingulate cortex—are implicated in the post-traumatic development of anxiety disorders. It has also been suggested that right-sided lesions (e.g., Grafman et al., 1986) may increase the likelihood of development of these conditions. This observation is supported by the functional neuroimaging studies that indicate increased activity in the orbitofrontal and insular cortices as well as in the basal ganglia in anxiety-prone individuals subjected to provocation in the scanner.

Gray and McNaughton (1996) proposed a model of the neuroanatomical underpinning of anxiety that has proven helpful in understanding a number of aspects of this presentation. They propose that anxiety emerges when the "behavioral inhibition system" (i.e., the septo-hippocampal systems but also the anterior thalamus, the circuit of Papez, the cingulate cortex, and the noradrenergic system) becomes dysfunctional and the individual becomes sensitized to particular environmental stimuli. This is particularly the case for individuals who may have developed effective coping strategies following stressful life events predating the TBI but who once again become sensitized as a result of the advent of the TBI (Ruff, Camenzuli, & Mueller, 1996).

Conclusion

Perhaps there is little to add to this discussion beyond the observations of Epstein and Ursano (Epstein & Ursano, 1994) in their review of this literature:

> Approximately 30% of TBI patients have clinically measurable anxiety. Clinicians should be especially alert to anxiety, because it does not always present in an overt fashion. The interrelationships between anxiety and TBI are multifactorial, and the effect of specific tissue damage upon the nature of the symptomatology remains uncertain. (p. 306)

Clearly Epstein and Ursano's observations are just as true today.

5 Mood disorders following Traumatic Brain Injury (TBI)

The association between TBI and the mood disorders has a long history. Perhaps of all the psychiatric and emotional alterations associated with TBI it is depression that occurs most commonly (e.g., Grant & Alves, 1987). The issues that immediately come to mind in this discussion include:

(1) How frequently do changes in mood occur following TBI?
(2) Are these changes sufficient to meet a *DSM-IV* diagnosis of major depression or bipolar disorder?
(3) What clinical variables associated with the TBI (i.e., injury-related variables, neuroanatomical locus, neuropsychological status), if any, predict the development of the affective disorders?
(4) What course do the affective disorders follow subsequent to a TBI?
(5) What is the relationship of the physical and most notably the neuropsychological, emotional and behavioural effects of affective disorder in association with TBI on the evolution and presentation of the condition?

Each of these issues will be addressed in turn, but perhaps first it will be worthwhile to summarise what we know about the affective disorders in the absence of TBI as a framework upon which we can hang the added complication of the affective disorder occurring in the context of TBI.

Background

Mood disorders or affective disorders are those conditions in which a disturbance of mood is the predominant clinical feature. The understanding of the affective disorders must take place at three different levels of inquiry. These include: (1) the experience of the mood disorder, which refers to the conscious feeling of depressive affect or sadness at one end of the continuum or of elation and euphoria at the other; (2) the outward expression of the affective disorder including changes in the level of activity and neurovegetative functioning; and (3) the cognitive components of the disorders characterised by the either unduly negative or unduly positive appraisal of internal or external events.

Kraepelin (1910) originally proposed the unitary notion of the mood disorders and combined a number of previously unconnected mood disorders including mania, depression, depression with mania, and elderly depression under a single diagnostic umbrella. This monolithic conception was challenged through the 1950s by Sir Martin Roth and his group (Roth, 1955) at Newcastle, who proposed that depression should be divided into either severe psychotic or endogenous (melancholic) versus a more mild neurotic or reactive form of depression. Roth proposed that reactive depression was caused by ambient life stressors and was dominated by psychological-type factors, while endogenous (melancholic) depression was biological in origin and was characterised by loss of interest, loss of appetite and weight, deceased interest in sex, sleep disturbances, psychomotor retardation, and agitation.

Paykel (1974) considerably clarified the nature of the relationship between endogenous and reactive depression. He noted that only 15% of a clinically depressed sample evidenced a lack of precipitating (depressogenic) events in the two years or more before the onset of the problem (Brown, Harris, & Hepworth, 1995; Paykel et al., 1969). Clearly based on this evidence, the vast majority of individuals (85%) who would go on to have a major endogenous depression would have had a reactive depression first. Thus the issue is really one of why most individuals who sustain a significant life stressor go on to recover, while others go on to develop a major depressive state.

Gilbert (1989) notes that depressogenic events include: (1) direct attacks on a person's self-esteem that force him or her into a subordinate position; (2) events undermining a person's sense of rank, attractiveness, or value (particularly with regard to his or her core roles); and (3) blocked escape. It is clear, therefore, that a major stressful life event such as sustaining a TBI, affecting each of these aspects of functioning, would comfortably fit within the category of a depressogenic event.

Contemporary psychiatry (e.g., Sadock & Sadock, 2004) postulates that there are two major forms of affective disorder: unipolar affective disorder or depression without mania, which features a depressive state that is continuous and unremitting and may come in episodes; and bipolar affective disorder, which features an alternation of mania and depression. This mania generally lasts for a few days to several months, but usually for about a few weeks. These periods are interrupted by episodes of depression that last up to three times longer.

The major depressive episode is characterised by at least 2 weeks during which there is depression of mood or loss of interest or pleasure in most activities. Other features noted include changes in neurovegetative functioning including changes in appetite, sleep (duration and architecture) and activity pattern, decreased energy, feelings of worthlessness or guilt, difficulty thinking, concentrating and making decisions, recurrent thoughts of death and suicidal ideas, planning, or attempts (APA, 2000).

The presentation of depression can differ considerably with age with conditions such as anaclitic depression noted in infants, increased activity, aggression, and acting out behaviours noted in children, and distractibility and memory problems more commonly noted in older adults. Childhood depression also differs from the adult presentation in that there is a higher frequency of suicide attempts and guilt noted in younger depressive patients, while the rates of neurovegetative change (i.e., disruption of eating, sleeping, and activity levels) are higher in older depressive patients.

The common presentation of depression is a state characterized by depressed mood, loss of interest or enjoyment, reduced self-esteem, feelings of guilt or worthlessness, a pessimistic world view, ideas or acts of self-harm, disturbed sleep, disturbed appetite, decreased libido, reduced energy, and reduced concentration and attention. The atypical presentation features a reactive mood (i.e., the individual brightens during or in anticipation of positive events), increased appetite or weight gain, excessive sleepiness, leaden feelings of arms or legs, and a lifelong trait of sensitivity to personal rejection. The atypical presentation is more commonly noted in younger patients and in female patients (Hunt, Andrew, & Sumich, 1995).

The severity of depression ranges from mild depression to severe depression. Mild depression features symptoms such as requiring extra effort to do the things that need to be done and minor impairment of social or occupational functioning. Moderate depression involves impairment of social or occupational functioning and levels of effort midway between mild and severe and symptoms that prevent the individual from doing the things that need to be done. Severe depression features marked impairment of social and occupational functioning and levels of effort and may include psychotic symptoms (i.e., hallucinations and delusions either mood congruent or incongruent) including impairment of the usual activities of daily living and somatic features (i.e., disturbance of eating, sleeping, sexual functioning, and motivational state) are nearly always present.

Dysthymia, a dispositional condition of depression, has also been noted. Over periods of years this involves the individual experiencing depressed mood, loss of interest or energy, social withdrawal, poor concentration and memory, feelings of inadequacy, low self-esteem, and feelings of guilt, irritability, anger, hopelessness, and despair (APA, 2000).

The spectrum of the bipolar affective disorders has been a matter of considerable dispute and debate within the psychiatric literature. Krauthammer and Klerman (1978) made this point well and note: "Although diagnostic problems still exist regarding the boundaries of mania with schizophrenia (schizoaffective states), with depression (mixed manic-depressive states), with confusional states ("delirious mania") and with normality (cyclothymia and mild hypomania), the symptoms of mania are widely accepted" (p. 1333).

In the bipolar disorders, mania is defined by the presence of a persistently abnormal elevated, expansive, or irritable mood that must go on for at least one week unless it leads to an earlier hospitalisation and must be accompanied by at least three additional symptoms including inflated self-esteem or grandiosity, decreased need for sleep, pressure of speech, flight of ideas, distractibility, increased interest in goal-directed activities or psychomotor agitation, and excessive involvement in pleasurable activities with a high potential for painful consequences. The condition must also be sufficiently severe to cause marked impairment of social or occupational functioning (APA, 2000).

Patients who suffer from mania progress through stages of the condition. Stage I mania manifests as hypomania with mild euphoria or irritability, expansive speech, and increased energy and usually, a reduced need for sleep. Stage II features grandiosity, euphoria, increased energy, impulsivity, increased sexuality, increased rate of speech and interpersonal interaction, frank insomnia, paranoia, and irritability. Stage III features clear psychotic symptoms including hallucinations and delusion, confusion, incoherent speech, agitation, or catatonia, in association with insomnia. The majority of patients passes through these stages in sequence and recovers in the reverse sequence (Gerner, 1993).

Depression affects about 13–20% of the population of the United States at any given time, and 2–3% are hospitalised or seriously impaired because of depression. In addition, about 1% of the adult population (0.65% men and 0.88% women) have acute bipolar illness (APA, 2000; Calev, Pollina, Fennig, & Banerjee, 1999; Gold, Goodwin, & Chrousos, 1988). The lifetime risk is 3–4% in men and 5–9% in women. The risk of depression is two to three times higher among women than men (Young, Schefter, Fawcett, & Klerman, 1990). The incidence of affective illness in an individual also raises the risk of a similar diagnosis in a first degree relative by two to three times (Young et al., 1990), but such findings are by no means straightforward and considerable dispute exists (McGuffin & Katz, 1989a; 1989b). The incidence rises to one third of the population in those over age 65.

The average untreated episode of depression lasts 6 to 8 months or more, and if left untreated, 25–30% of adult depressives will attempt suicide (Richelson, 1993). About 65–70% of patients respond to antidepressant drug therapy and will go on to complete recovery. Electroconvulsive therapy (ECT) works in a further 10–15% of patients, leaving about 20% of individuals relatively intractable to treatment (Richelson, 1993).

As noted above, depression affects a variety of systems and behaviours. These include:

- Physical functions: including appetite, activity levels and sleep, which tend to respond best to antidepressant medication;
- Cognitive and behavioural functions: which tend to respond best to psychological strategies (i.e., increasing activity, structured problem solving, CBT, assertiveness and communication training).

Appetite and sleep tend to improve first during recovery followed by behaviour, while thoughts and feelings tend to improve last.

There are five effective treatments for depression: (1) serotonin-selective reuptake inhibitors (SSRIs); (2) tricyclic antidepressants (TCAs); (3) monoamine oxidase inhibitors (MOAIs); (4) electroconvulsive therapy (ECT); and (5) transcranial magnetic stimulation (TMS). The symptoms that respond best to medication include: psychotic symptoms, somatic symptoms, recurrent depression, a previous history of successful response to medication, a family history of affective illness, and failure to respond to psychotherapy (Hunt et al., 1995). The symptoms that respond best to ECT include: psychotic symptoms, somatic symptoms, a previous history of successful response to ECT, a previous history of treatment failure following drug and combined therapy, the need for rapid response, and medical contraindications to medication. ECT is often considered to be the most effective form of treatment when psychotic symptoms are present (Hunt et al., 1995). TMS is a treatment emerging as a very promising modality for the treatment of depression but still requires considerable research and investigation to determine its most effective application (Holtzheimer & Nemeroff, 2006).

Treating depression with TCAs, SSRIs, and MAOIs, all of which are monoamine agonists, has lead to the mono-amine hypothesis of depression. As the syndrome does not respond to dopamine agonists, most investigators have concentrated on noradrenaline (NA) and serotonin (5HT), although other targets including corticotrophin releasing factor, glucocorticoid receptor agonists, substance P receptor agonists, and N-methyl-D-aspartate (NMDA) glutamate receptor antagonists have each been under intensive study (Holtzheimer & Nemeroff, 2006). As yet the data regarding the monoamine hypothesis are weak, but the hypothesis is still useful as it continues to guide new drug design. The receptor adaptation model (Shelton, 2000) better explains the issue (i.e., 5HT receptors are up regulated causing increased sensitivity of α-adrenoceptors and a decreased sensitivity of the ß adrenoceptors to available levels of serotonin and or noradrenaline) and is thought to account for the fact that it often takes two to three weeks for these agents to have their therapeutic effect, since if they were directly affecting the levels of these transmitters, the changes should be much more rapid.

Cognitive theories of depression contend that the thinking of the individual in the depressed state is biased towards the negative triad of mentation including negative views of the self, the world, and the future. These biases are accompanied by a series of biases in cognition including: arbitrary inference (I am worthless because it is raining), selective abstraction (I voted therefore I am responsible), overgeneralization (one bad day equals a worthless life), and magnification and minimization of day-to-day experiences and achievements.

As a result of these various issues, the depressed individual develops a learned helplessness regarding his or her situation. Passivity occurs due to a history of unpleasant experiences or events that the individual had previously tried to control and could not (c.f., Seligman's dogs). This model has been redefined to focus on hopelessness due to the failure to reliably predict clinical phenomena, although support for the theory remains equivocal (Davison & Neale, 2004).

In the social context, the depressed individual is also subject to the effects of the social environment. The social learning explanation of depression contends that there is often poor social support among depressed individuals and that the symptoms of depression cause rejection and marital hostility, further contributing to maladaptation (Davison & Neale, 2004).

Methodological issues

A number of problems emerge in the use of standardized criteria such as the *DSM-IV* or self-reported inventories such as Minnesota Multiphasic Personality Inventory (MMPI) or the Beck Depression Scale to classify psychopathology in individuals who have suffered TBI. One of the principal problems is the extent to which the depressive symptoms noted following TBI are attributable to the brain injury.

Kreutzer, Seel, and Gourley (2001) for example, noted in their extensive review of the literature that the most frequently endorsed depressive symptoms after TBI were tiredness (46%), frustration (41%), and poor concentration (38%). As noted above, these symptoms are core symptoms of postconcussional syndrome (PCS) discussed in chapter 2. Kreutzer et al. (2001) further noted that the symptoms of irritability, lack of interest, slowness of movement, fatigue, and forgetfulness were the most common symptoms observed after TBI irrespective of the presence or absence of depression. Clearly, once again these types of symptoms are affected by the presence of either depression or TBI, but are not specific to either.

TBI, along with its damage to the brain, comes with a variety of other medical, psychological, and social complications that can make it difficult to specify the source of the depressive symptoms as they pertain to the applied diagnostic criteria. Symptoms commonly encountered in depression including changes to neurovegetative functions such as sleep, motivation, eating, and sexual changes may also occur as a direct consequence of the brain injury associated with the TBI, but may also be attributable to the effects of the acute medical condition from which these individuals also suffer. As all TBI sufferers could also feature a variety of medical problems that accompany the injury (e.g., pain, sensory changes, orthopaedic or other injuries) this may result in a tendency to over diagnose depression subsequent to the injury. On the other hand, TBI sufferers may, as a result of lack of insight or due to denial of injury, fail to report true depression even when it is actually present (Robinson & Jorge, 1994, 2005). Adding to this issue is the compounding effect of the reactive versus endogenous issue adverted to above with regard to the numerous life stresses that must transpire for an individual in the wake of the TBI (Robinson & Jorge, 1994).

One of the most important issues in diagnosis following an injury is to ascertain what degree of the changes noted are reactive to the loss of function associated with the injury itself and how much is attributable to the depressive state, and at what point do the reactions become the basis on which a major endogenous depression is built?

Guze and Gitlin (1994) have drawn a distinction in the way in which affective disorders relate to brain disorder. They contend that the relationship between the neurological condition and the affective state presents three possible aetiologies: integral, reactive, and independent. In the case of Parkinson's disease (PD) for example, they contend that depression is an integral component of the disease (presumably as a consequence of the effect of the disease on the neuromodulatory mechanisms of dopaminergic, noradrenergic, and serotonergic functioning). Patients with PD-related affective disorders are thus considered to show a "true" secondary mood disorder. These individuals often show a negative family and personal history of affective disorders and they have usually been euthymic up until the onset of their PD.

On the other hand, some patients may feature depression as a reaction to the PD (Guze & Gitlin, 1994). These individuals usually lack the defining features of major endogenous depression and do not respond well to antidepressant medication. The third group is made up of individuals who may have an independent affective disorder that has developed separately from the PD. These individuals often have a positive family or personal history of affective disorder, and there is usually lack of a direct association between the organic disease process (e.g., PD) and its severity and the severity of the affective state.

Guze and Gitlin (1994) have proposed a series of criteria that must be met for cerebral dysfunction (such as the neuroanatomical effects of a TBI) to be responsible for the depression. These are:

(1) The dysfunction should be similar in bipolar and unipolar depressions of equivalent severity and should differ significantly from the functioning observed in normal control subjects.
(2) The dysfunction should occur in neurologic conditions with secondary depressions and not in those same conditions without depression.
(3) It should distinguish bipolar mania from bipolar depression.

> The degree of metabolic deficit should correlate with a standard measure of depression severity and should change significantly in the direction of normal values on resolution of the depressed state. (p. 118)

Phenomenology and nosology of secondary affective disorders

The *DSM-IV-TR* (APA, 2000) diagnoses affective disorders following brain injury primarily by their associated syndromic presentation (i.e., major depression, dysthymia, or bipolar disorder) or as a consequence of their association with a particular medical illness (i.e., secondary to the organic disorder such as 293.83 Mood Disorder Due to a General Medical Condition) with the predominant symptom type indicated by subtypes, such as with depressive features, with major depressive-like episode, with manic features or with mixed features. The general medical condition is specified by an Axis III diagnosis (e.g., 850.9 Concussion or 851.80 Contusion, cerebral). The differential diagnosis of this condition could include the following conditions: adjustment disorder with depressed mood, emotional lability, apathy and posttraumatic stress disorder (Robinson & Jorge, 1994, 2005).

One further issue that seems worthy of discussion within the context of the differential diagnosis of mood disorder is the degree to which the diagnosis of pathological laughing or crying might be made. This presentation is characterized by the presence of sudden and uncontrolled outbursts of either laughing or crying that may be either congruent or incongruent with the patient's mood. The patient recognises the state as being excessive and these responses are generally triggered by minor episodes of provocation. The presentation lacks both the persistence of a state characteristic of the mood disorders as well as the neurovegetative features. These patients also tend to be more impaired in their social functioning and feature higher levels of aggression. This condition tends to occur more commonly with focal frontal lesions (Robinson & Jorge, 2005).

The diagnosis of adjustment disorder is also commonly used in the context of TBI. This diagnosis identifies "a psychological response to an identifiable stressor or stressors that results in the development of clinically significant emotional or behavioral symptoms" (APA, 2000, p. 679). These symptoms must develop within three months of the stressor, and must be accompanied by a response that is in excess of what would ordinarily be expected by such a stressor, or which culminates in significant impairment of social or occupational functioning. The adjustment disorder can occur with depressed mood, with anxiety, with mixed anxiety and depressed mood, with disturbance of conduct, with a mixed disturbance of emotions or conduct, or in an unspecified manner and may be either acute (i.e., less than six months) or chronic (greater than six months) in duration (APA, 2000). Clearly disentangling the diagnostic entities of adjustment disorder, major psychiatric diagnosis, PCS, and the clinical symptoms associated with the neurological changes consequent upon the brain injury is no mean feat.

A further problem for the application of the various phenomenological entities associated with mood disorders with TBI is exacerbated by the way in which they are described by the various treating specialties associated with each condition. For example, for the psychiatrist, apathy could be attributable to depression, while to a neuropsychiatrist, neuropsychologists, or behavioural neurologist apathy could signal lesions of the frontal circuitry resulting in the so-called "pseudodepressed syndrome" as described by Blumer and Benson (1975) or the abulic syndrome as described by Mesulam (2000a).

Similarly, manic-like behaviours are described differently by the neurological and psychiatric fields. While the neurological literature refers to disinhibition, "pseudopsychopathic" (Blumer & Benson, 1975) behaviour or acquired sociopathy, psychiatry refers to these states as mania or manic-like states. See chapter 3 for a more complete discussion of the organic personality syndromes associated with TBI.

As was the case with the depressive states, mania subsequent to TBI has been variously described as "secondary mania" (Krauthammer & Klerman, 1978; Starkstein & Robinson, 1997) or in the terms of the *DSM-IV* as a bipolar disorder (Bipolar I Disorder, Bipolar II Disorder, Cyclothymia, and Bipolar Disorder not otherwise specified); personality change due to a general medical condition with manic or with mixed features, which can be further classified into disinhibited or aggressive subtypes, or as impulse control disorders not elsewhere classified. The presence of the TBI would again be noted with the Axis III diagnosis (Robinson & Jorge, 2005). Clearly the terminology for these disorders varies considerably and specific criteria that transcend the boundaries of the involved medical specialties have yet to be developed.

Further complicating this area are the techniques by which the diagnosis of depression is made. Diagnoses of depression in the published research and epidemiological studies in the psychological literature are often ascertained by self-reported scales such as the Beck Depression Inventory or the Minnesota Multiphasic Personality Inventory or by the reports of relatives. Such techniques are fraught with difficulties not least of which include: (1) diminished awareness on the part of the injured individual resulting in inaccurate reporting of symptoms; (2) the presence of medico-legal disputation issues that might produce an exaggerated report of symptoms; (3) the presence of some signs and symptoms (e.g., headache, diminished concentration, memory loss) that may not hold the same affective diagnostic meaning that they do in neurologically unimpaired individuals (Woessner & Caplan, 1995). As Miller, Green, and Meaghes (1979) noted:

> Even a well-designed psychiatric instrument provides information that is either irrelevant or distorted when applied to a medical population. Problems arise because of the unsuitability of the norms, the questionable relevance of clinical signs and the consequent inapplicability of interpretations. (p. 529)

With regard to this latter point, a number of investigators have found that TBI can inflate the level of psychopathology noted on MMPI profiles (including combinations of scales 1, 2, 3, 7, and 8). Removing items that address those issues commonly noted in TBI resulted in normalization of the profiles to nonpathological levels. Alfano, Paniak and Finlayson (1993), using their "neurocorrective approach," noted that the removal of 24 of the MMPI items produced reductions both in group means and in individual profiles of individuals with TBI. Gass (1991) noted a similar effect in the removal of the 14-item MMPI-2 neurological complaints factor.

Woessner and Caplan (1995) noted a similar effect in using the Symptom Checklist-90-Revised (SCL-90-R) (Derogatis, Lipman, & Covi, 1973). These investigators noted that a substantial proportion of the self-reported psychopathology observed in a sample of 23 mild to moderate TBI patients derived from endorsement of the 15.5% of the SCL-90-R that was identified by expert raters to be frequent consequences of TBI. They quite correctly note: "Clinicians cannot allow themselves to be misled by the factor names assigned by an instrument's developer, especially when the measure is applied to a neurological patient" (Woessner & Caplan, 1995, p. 86).

According to Woessner and Caplan (1995), the cure for this problem is for clinicians to carefully review individual responses on self-report questionnaires to ensure their veracity and to integrate this data with information from other sources such as direct observation, interviews, and reports from third parties. This latter approach, although laudable, must also be cautiously applied.

McKenzie, Robiner, and Knopman (1989) noted, for example, that interviewing patients with Dementia of the Alzheimer Type yielded a depression rate of 13.9% using *DSM-III* (APA, 1980) criteria, whereas using information obtained from relatives and carers indicated a rate of 50%. Inflation of scores both from the choice of instrument and by the nature of informant requires exquisite clinical skill.

A further issue is the degree to which self-report can be considered a sound means by which to identify depression, particularly in the context of TBI. This issue also pertains to the relationship between depressive mentation and neurocognitive compromise. An interesting example arises from the study conducted by Rohling, Green, Allen, and Iverson (2002) who conducted a survey of 420 patients with self-reported depression who had been referred for neuropsychological assessment in the context of compensation-related disability claims.

The referral source of the patients was varied but about half of the cases reported suffering a TBI and the remainder were of various neurological presentations. The participants undertook a comprehensive neuropsychological assessment using a flexible battery approach and all participants passed the two symptom validity measures (Computerized Assessment of Response Bias [CARB] and the Word Memory Test [WMT]).

The results of the study indicated that the greater the self-reported depression, the greater the level of emotional, somatic, and cognitive problems reported. However, there were no differences with regard to objective neurocognitive problems. This led the investigators to suggest that depression has no impact on objective cognitive functioning.

The findings of Rohling et al. (2002) echo those of Bieliauskas (1993) in his discussions of depressive pseudodementing syndromes. Bieliauskas noted: "depressive-like symptoms have little or no impact on cognitive functions....these are more likely disease-based rather than the result of emotional factors such as depression" (p. 119). Bieliauskas adds, however, that compromise in cognitive function may occur in cases in which a psychiatric history of primary depression together with a sufficient loss of self-esteem co-occur.

Reitan and Wolfson (1997), in a manner reminiscent of the model proposed by Guze and Gitlin (1994) above, proposed a number of guidelines for determining the respective contribution of the TBI and the associated affective state. Reitan and Wolfson note that individuals who have suffered a TBI and feature significant neuropsychological impairment and who also have elevations on the MMPI have emotional problems caused by the injury. Individuals with TBI who have normal neuropsychological findings (especially several months after the injury) but who have deviant MMPI performances have emotional problems of a neurotic nature. Individuals with TBI who have normal neuropsychological functioning (several months after the injury) and who have normal MMPIs demonstrate the expected pattern of recovery following mild traumatic brain injury (MTBI).

Clearly many issues impinge upon the diagnosis of secondary affective disorder in the context of TBI. These include the degree to which the changes occur as a direct effect of the injury itself rather than as a second effect of the injury (i.e., psychosocial compromise, pain, loss of status and income, etc.), the degree to which various treating professionals view the state in the same way, and the biasing that may occur as a consequence of self-report measures or significant other reports, which may inflate the likelihood of a diagnosis of affective disorder in a TBI-affected individual. Robinson and Jorge (2005) advocate the safest course of action by their statement that "standard *DSM-IV-TR* criteria are the most logical criteria to use for the diagnosis of major depression in the TBI population" (p. 203). Clearly there is no substitute for clinical skill in the context of these complex issues and appropriate reappraisal of the patient on a regular basis will facilitate more concise diagnostic formulation.

Prevalence and incidence of secondary affective disorders including demographic and psychiatric correlates

Probably as a consequence of the inconsistencies in the diagnosis of depression in association with TBI, the prevalence rates of this diagnosis vary from as low as 24% (Guth, 2000) to as high as 70% (Kersel, Marsh, Havill, & Sleigh, 2001; Kreutzer et al., 2001) in traumatically brain-injured individuals. McKinlay, Brooks, and Bond (1981) reported evidence of depressed mood in nearly half of their patients in the 3 to 12 months following injury. Glynda Kinsella and colleagues (Kinsella, Moran, Ford, & Ponsford, 1988) reported a rate of 33% within two years, a similar rate to that noted by Jorge et al. (2004). Gualtieri and Cox (1991) estimated the frequency to be between 25 and 50% and Robinson and Jorge (1994) noted in the follow-up study of 66 patients (GCS 3–15) that 42% developed *DSM-III-R* diagnosed major depression and 9% minor depression at some time during the 12-month follow-up.

In their subsequent study, Robinson and Jorge (2005) used a new sample of 89 TBI patients and noted that 49% (44 of the 89) developed mood disorders during the first year after TBI with major depression occurring in 40% of those patients followed up for one-year postinjury. Of the 30 patients with major depressive disorder, 23 (76.7%) also met *DSM-IV* criteria for anxiety disorder, and aggressive disorder was diagnosed in 33.7%. Almost one third of the patients had a history of substance abuse and 17% had a past psychiatric history.

Hibbard, Uysal, Kepler, Bogdany, and Silver (1998) noted a prevalence of major depression in 61% of their sample of 100 TBI patients evaluated on average 8 years after trauma, as determined using a structured interview and *DSM-IV* criteria. Koponen, Taiminen, Portin, and colleagues (2002), reported a 26.7% lifetime prevalence of major depression in a group of 60 patients followed up for an average of 30 years.

Other early studies of open head injuries, most notably those that studied patients with penetrating missile wounds, vary considerably in their estimation of the frequency of postinjury depression. Feutchwanger (1923) noted that mood symptoms were commonly noted in their sample of 400 subjects who had sustained frontal lobe injuries as a consequence of gunshot wounds. The diagnosis for these patients was most commonly mania. This harks back to the previous discussion of the degree to which a frontal lobe injury with a disinhibited presentation could be inappropriately classified as mania.

Older studies (e.g., Merskey & Woodforde, 1961; Miller, 1961) of closed-head injuries also vary considerably with regard to the reported frequency of postinjury depression. Miller (1961) noted that of the 200 patients referred for medico-legal assessment 14 months on average after suffering a minor TBI, only 9 cases (4.5%) of depression were found, while an overwhelming 47 cases (23.5%) were noted to suffer from "indubitable psychoneurotic complaints" presumably in the manner of the postconcussion syndrome discussed in chapter 2.

Merskey and Woodforde (1961) noted that of their 27 cases of minor TBI referred for assessment in the absence of medico-legal considerations, 7 cases (25.9%) had endogenous depression while 9 cases (33.3%) featured a diagnosis of mixed anxiety and depression. Both Schoenhuber and Gentilini (1988) and Diamond, Barth, and Zillmer (1988) noted similar rates of depression with their respective MTBI samples. Schoenhuber et al. (1988) studied 103 patients with MTBI and noted that 39% of these complained of depression at 1 year following the injury. Using the MMPI, Diamond and colleagues (1988) studied 50 patients 3 months after injury and noted that 26% had scores consistent with a diagnosis of depression.

Varney, Martzke, and Roberts (1987) used a sample of 120 individuals diagnosed using the *DSM-III*, ranging in duration of coma from a few minutes to 8 days, who were interviewed at least two years (mean 3.4 years, range 2 to 8 years) following the injury. Ninety-two of the 120 (77%) reported at least 6 of a list of depressive symptoms (i.e., poor memory or concentration: 96%; anergia: 96%; low libido: 91%; indifference: 90%; irritability: 87%; insomnia: 87%; dysphoria: 85%; anorexia: 77%; crying spells: 67%; suicidal ideation: 51%; social withdrawal: 37%) in contrast to a control group of back-injured subjects only 38% (23/60) of whom reported 6 symptoms. Of the subjects with depression, 46% (42/92) reported that their depressive symptoms did not commence until at least six months after the injury (an observation reported by the investigators and verified by the families of origin).

Varney et al. (1987) also intriguingly noted:

> The National Safety Council estimates that there are 1.9 million head injuries in the United States every year. If current data are correct, then it could be predicted that there are about 1.4 million new cases of depression each year which are a direct result of head trauma; a quite sizable public health problem. (p. 9)

One cannot help but concur.

Van Reekum and colleagues (1996) assessed 18 subjects (10 with severe TBI and 8 with mild or moderate TBI) an average of 4.9 years following the TBI and subjected them to a structured diagnostic interview (the Schedule for Affective Disorders and Schizophrenia (SADS-L) (Endicott & Spitzer, 1978), which gives a *DSM-III* Axis I diagnosis. Of the sample, 11 (58%) received a post-TBI diagnosis of major depression, although two of these also experienced a manic episode. Of these nine subjects, five had their first episode of major depression after the TBI, while the remainder had had another episode prior to the injury. Bipolar affective disorder was found in three subjects (16%) and cyclothymia in a further two subjects. Four of these five subjects featured onset after the injury. Seven subjects (37%) received a diagnosis of anxiety disorder, with five of the seven featuring generalized anxiety disorder. The remaining subject had panic disorder (1), with the others having mixed phobias and obsessive compulsive disorder. Four of the seven developed their anxiety states following the injury. Other diagnoses noted in the sample included anorexia nervosa and alcohol abuse. In all, of the 18 patients, 15 (83%) received an Axis I diagnosis after their TBI, with 10 of the subjects having two or more Axis I disorders after the injury.

Jorge, Robinson, Arndt et al. (1993) have produced perhaps the most comprehensive analysis of the effects of TBI on affective state. This group examined 66 consecutively admitted patients who were psychiatrically assessed within one month of admission and subsequently at 3, 6, and 12 months. Twenty-six percent of the sample was diagnosed with major depression and 3% with minor depression as determined using the observer-rated Hamilton Depression Rating Scale (HDRS) at one month following injury and these rates were maintained over the follow-up.

This group undertook a similar follow-up study (Jorge et al., 2004) with 91 patients examined at baseline and once again assessed again 3, 6, and 12 months after the injury. Using a structured clinical interview based on the *DSM-IV* they observed major depressive disorders in 30 (33%) of patients in the first year postinjury. The depressed patients were more likely to have a personal history of mood and anxiety disorders than the nonmajor depressed patients. The patients with major depression also showed high levels of comorbid anxiety (76.7%) and aggressive behaviour (56.7%) and also had greater deficits in executive functions as assessed using neuropsychological measures than did the nondepressed participants. The changes were also associated with poorer social functioning and decreased left prefrontal volumes particularly of the ventrolateral and dorsolateral prefrontal cortices.

Considerable interest has emerged in the degree to which MTBI can lead to the development of the affective disorders. These issues are discussed at some length in chapter 2. Rapoport, McCullagh, Streiner, and Feinstein (2003) assessed 170 consecutive patients with MTBI and noted major depression in 15.3% of the sample and the diagnosis was invariably associated with poorer outcome. In a related study, Rapoport, McCauley et al. (2002) assessed neurobehavioural outcome using the

Neurobehavioral Rating Scale (Revised) developed by Levin, High, Goethe et al. (1987) to assess the spectrum of TBI-affected individuals including 102 MTBI, 41 moderate, and 139 severe TBIs as measured three months after injury. A principal components analysis of the data indicated that three factors—a cognitive factor, an emotional factor, and a hyperarousal factor—were consistently observed. The severe patients showed more difficulties with the cognitive and hyperarousal factors than did the mild or moderate TBIs. Over one-third of the sample in all severity groups demonstrated evidence of anxiety, depression, irritability, mental fatigability, and memory function.

Levin, Brown, Song et al. (2001) compared 69 mild to moderate TBI patients with 52 general trauma patients at 3 months postinjury. They noted that there were no significant differences in the proportion of major depressive disorders between the two groups. They then combined the groups and noted that across the sample the only association between major depression noted in the sample was with female gender.

Based on these data it seems clear that depression is a common complication of TBI. It is a little more difficult to be definitive about how frequently this occurs, however, due to the variety of methodological issues adverted to earlier in this chapter. A conservative estimate would place the incidence at about 20–40% affected during the first year following the injury, and about 50% experience depression at some stage following injury (Fleminger, Oliver, Williams, & Evans, 2003).

A similar pattern of incidence occurs at the more severe end of the spectrum of injury severity. Oddy, Coughlan, Tyerman, and Jenkins (1985) observed that in their 33 patients with self-reported depression, 10% were depressed at 2 years following the injury. The same level of depression was noted at 7 years following the injury. Van Zomeren and Van Den Berg (1985) noted that 19% of their 57 patients complained of depression 2 years postinjury. Levin and Grossman (1978), using the Brief Psychiatric Rating Scale (BPRS) noted that 35% of their 50 patients were depressed. Tyerman and Humphrey (1984) found that 60% of their 26 severe TBIs were depressed during the period 2 to 15 months following the injury as assessed on a self-report measure. Brooks, Campsie, Symington, Beattie and McKinlay (1986) noted that 57% of their 42 patients were depressed 5 years after the injury according to relatives' reports.

The data with regard to the onset of bipolar disorders after TBI are somewhat more sparse than the data on depression. In their original description of the concept of secondary mania, Krauthammer and Klerman (1978) noted cases of secondary mania occurring as a consequence of drug effects (corticosteroids, isoniazid, procarbazine, bromide), metabolic disturbances (haemodialysis, postoperative states); infections (influenza, Q fever, Post-St Louis type A encephalitis), neoplasm (parasagittal menigioma, diencephalic glioma, 9 various other tumours, suprasellar diencephalic tumour, benign spheno-occipital tumour) and right temporal lobe epilepsy. Interestingly they did not note any case of secondary mania as a consequence of TBI. This absence probably occurs as a consequence of the criteria that they applied in selecting their cases for review. They examined all cases reported in the literature, but excluded the following: (1) those with a clear previous history of manic depressive or other affective disease, and (2) the coexistence of the manic syndrome with any symptomatology of confusional states (acute brain syndromes such as disorientation, confusion, clouding of consciousness or delirium). As a result of this latter preclusion, any instance of secondary mania that occurred in the context of a TBI may have been excluded from the review.

Early reports of the frequency of manic syndromes following TBI vary widely in their reported effects. Achte, Hillbom and Aalberg (1969) noted in their group of 3552 brain-injured war veterans that affective psychoses occurred in 37 patients (1%), of whom only three were diagnosed with manic depression. Lishman (1968) noted euphoric mood in 10 (6.9%) of his 144 patients with TBI.

A number of single case studies have also been reported in this area. Parker (1957) was one of the first investigators to observe the absence of family history in a patient who developed marked mood swings following head trauma. Cohn, Wright, and DeVaul (1977) reported similar results in an adolescent patient with a TBI. In the single case study reported by Sinanan (1984) and in Stewart and Hemsath's (1988) report of a 22-year-old woman who developed bipolar disorder following TBI, once again no family history was noted.

Pope, McElroy, and Satlin (1988) reviewed the charts of 56 patients with a diagnosis of bipolar affective disorder or schizoaffective disorder and noted that of these patients eight (14.3%) had had a TBI (although one patient without loss of consciousness). Varney et al. (1987) in the study discussed above noted that of their 120 patients assessed at least 2 years after injury, only four (3.3%) patients met the diagnostic criteria (*DSM-III*) for mania. Of these, three had a family history of bipolar affective disorder, suggesting that only one patient may have developed the condition in the wake of the TBI.

Shukla, Cook, Mukherjee, Godwin, and Miller (1987) used the Schedule for Affective Disorders and Schizophrenia-Lifetime Version (SADS-L) to diagnose the *DSM-III* and Research Diagnostic Criteria for diagnosis of bipolar disorders following TBI. They prospectively followed up a sample of 20 patients referred to a neuropsychiatry centre following TBI who had features of associated psychiatric disorders. Of these patients, 13 of the 20 (65%) met the criteria for bipolar affective disorder (BAD) type 1; 3 of the 20 for Type 2; 3 met the criteria for schizoaffective mania; and 1 had a history of hypomania. The breakdown of the manic symptoms that they featured revealed a predominance of irritable (85%) rather than euphoric (15%) mood states. Assaultive behaviour (70%) was frequent. The other typical manic features of these patients included: impaired judgement (100%), sleeplessness (100%), grandiosity (90%), pressured speech (80%), flight of ideas (75%), hyperactivity (65%), and hypersexuality (50%). Some caution needs to be exercised in the interpretation of the frequency counts with this study due to the fact that they came from an already selected population who featured psychiatric disturbances subsequent to their brain injury.

Jorge, Robinson, Starkstein et al. (1993) conducted the most comprehensive study of secondary mania following TBI. This study further developed a number of themes raised in their earlier studies (Robinson, Boston, Starkstein, & Price, 1988; Starkstein, Pearlson, Boston, & Robinson, 1987) that observed secondary mania in 17 (Robinson et al., 1988) and 11 (Starkstein et al., 1987) patients following stroke. The authors contended that an interaction between injury to certain regions of the right hemisphere (i.e., orbitofrontal, thalamic, caudate, and basotemporal regions) and genetic or other neuropathological factors may culminate in secondary mania.

Jorge, Robinson, Starkstein et al. (1993) followed a consecutive series of 66 patients with TBI who were evaluated in the hospital and at 3, 6, and 12 months following the injury. Six patients (9%) met the criteria for mania at some point during follow-up. While the presence of mania was not related to severity of injury, degree of cognitive or physical impairment, level of social functioning or previous personal or family history of psychiatric disorder, it was associated with the presence of temporal/basal lesions. The duration of mania in these cases tended to be relatively brief, lasting approximately 2 months.

Of the six patients with the diagnosis, four acknowledged the presence of the elevated mood, while in the other two the mood state was noted by the examining psychiatrist. In all cases, the mood had persisted for the 2 weeks preceding the examination. The patients met the *DSM-III* criteria for diagnosis on only one evaluation (five patients at 3 months and one at the 6-month assessment), indicating that the duration of the mania was short-lived. The presence of an abnormally elevated mood was noted in all six patients on at least two of the four evaluations and the estimated duration of mood elevation was 5.7 months.

Recent literature reviews both by Jorge and Robinson (2002) and van Reekum, Cohen and Wong (2000) have restated the suggestion of a causal association between TBI and bipolar disorders. Van Reekum and colleagues (2000) reviewed literature on 354 subjects drawn from five studies and estimated the relative risk of bipolar disorder following TBI to be 5.3%, based on a presumed prevalence of the disorder of 0.8%. Goldney (2004) in his critique of this literature has raised significant concern regarding this figure and contends that the more recent literature cites a higher incidence rate of bipolar disorder. For example, he cites a number of recent sources (e.g., Angst et al., 2003; Hirschfeld et al., 2003; Keck, McElroy, & Arnold, 2001) that indicate that the frequency of this diagnosis may be as high as 1–3% of the U.S. population. Bennazi (2003), for example, notes that as many as 6.3% of a sample of young adults had probable manic and hypomanic syndromes.

The data emerging from more methodologically sound studies such as the Danish Psychiatric Case and Population Register (Mortensen, Mors, Frydenberg, & Ewald, 2003) found only a small but significantly increased risk of bipolar disorder (BPD) following TBI (Increased relative risk = 1.55, CI 1.36-1.77), but only to those injuries occurring five years prior to admission.

These data taken together caused Goldney (2004) to urge caution in the assumption that all bipolar disorders emerging following TBI are causally related to those injuries: "While the studies reviewed cannot preclude the possibility of such a causal relationship, early clinical reports are now being replaced by more methodologically rigourous studies which shed doubt on the hitherto presumed causal association" (Goldney, 2004, p. 52).

In an interesting collateral examination of the relationship between TBI and secondary mania, DelBello et al. (1999) examined the occurrence of TBI in a group of individuals convicted of sexual offences with and without bipolar disorder and a comparison group of patients with BPD but without a history of sexual offences. Individuals convicted of sexual offences and diagnosed with BPD (i.e., 25 cases) had greater rates of TBI (i.e., 9 of 25; 36%) than individuals convicted of sexual offences with BPD or those with BPD alone. The patients with TBI tended to have mild and moderate rather than severe TBIs and, in most of these subjects, the TBI occurred prior to the first sexual offence and/or the onset of BPD.

In summary, it is clear that TBI can culminate in increased incidence of secondary mania, the level of which is hard to ascertain. It is difficult to be definitive regarding the frequency with which this diagnosis occurs due to the higher likelihood that these patients will be diagnosed through tertiary referral settings and also with regard to the developing data regarding incidence of this diagnosis in the wider community, which increasingly calls into question the likelihood that the emergent diagnosis may well have predated the injury in many cases.

Evolution of secondary affective disorders following TBI

TBI does appear to be an important factor in post-closed head injury (CHI) depression (Busch & Alpern, 1998; Jorge, 2005; McCleary et al., 1998) with most depression emerging some months after injury. Jorge, Robinson, Starkstein et al. (1993) examined 66 consecutively admitted patients who were psychiatrically assessed within one month of admission and subsequently at 3, 6, and 12 months. Twenty-six percent of the sample was diagnosed with major depression and 3% with minor depression as determined using the observer-rated Hamilton Depression Rating Scale (HDRS) at one month following injury. These rates were maintained over the follow-up with 22.2% with major depression at 3 months, 23.2% at 6 months, and 18.6% at 12 months after injury. The group's subsequent study of this phenomenon (Jorge et al., 2004) indicated that of the 30 patients (30/91) who developed major depression following their TBI, 15 (50%) were diagnosed with the condition at initial assessment, 9 (30%) were so diagnosed at the 3-month follow-up, and 6 (20%) at the 6-month follow-up.

In a more in-depth analysis of the course of depression following injury Jorge, Robinson, Starkstein et al. (1993) noted that of the 17 patients diagnosed with major depression at one month following the injury, the depression persisted for 4.7 months on average with a minimum duration of six weeks and a maximal measured duration of 12 months.

A similar set of findings to those of Jorge et al. (Jorge, Robinson, Starkstein et al., 1993; Jorge et al., 2004) were reported in the studies of Kersel, Marsh, Havill and Sleigh (2001a, 2001b) and by Bowen, Chamberlain, Tennant, Neumann, and Conner (1999). At 6 months following injury, 24% of the sample studied by Kersel et al. were reported as showing clinical depression with 9% in the mild and 16% in the severe range, while at 12 months a similar level was observed with 14% rated as mild and 10% as severe.

However, there are some reservations about this finding due to the fact that these levels were based upon self-reports on a short form of the Beck Depression Inventory (BDI), a methodology with a strong likelihood of producing over endorsement. Satz, Forney et al. (1998) reported a similar level of endorsement and further note that there was a considerable discrepancy between the levels of depression noted using self-report as compared to those determined using examiner-rated scales.

Bowen et al. (1999) indicated a higher level of prevalence (35% at 6 months, 39% at 12 months). However, these estimates were based upon the presence of mood disorder rather than depression per se. Much of this evidence led Fleminger et al. (2003) to note that "depression is no more common in the acute phase than the latter stages of recovery during the first year after TBI" (p. 69).

The longer-term follow-up of these patients indicates a somewhat different pattern. Perino, Rago, Cicolini, Torta, and Monaco (2001) noted that depression may be more likely to have its onset after an initial phase of recovery. Goldstein and colleagues (1999) found that post-CHI emotional factors (in this case a geriatric population) often showed gradual increased feelings of "hopelessness and worthlessness as well as a lack of optimism about the future" (p. 42). They suggest post-CHI depression in the elderly generally emerges three months postinjury. Interestingly, Goldstein and colleagues also note that "higher scores on the Geriatric Depression Scale, indicative of greater depression, predict attentional and memory functioning an average of 7 and 13 months postinjury, but not at initial assessment" (p. 43). This suggests attentional deficits associated with post-CHI depression may be significantly influenced by TBI. Karzmark (1992) also noted the importance of TBI in influencing depression status.

Wallace (2000) contended that this effect may be attributable to the development of awareness of the losses following the injury. However, this suggestion has not been without its challenges and the obverse proposal has been made by Ownsworth and Oei (1998) who found that depression following the injury is due to patients' poor insight into their difficulties rather than the reverse. Moore and Stambrook (1995), for example, contend that as the patient begins to understand the changes that have occurred as a result of the injury at the cognitive, behavioural, and emotional levels, learned helplessness, deficits in coping, and alteration in locus of control emerge. These changes in world view create a belief system that extends to many aspects of daily life causing a panoply of effects for the individual. This explanation constitutes the basis for intervention based upon cognitive behaviour therapy with these clients (See Khan-Bourne & Brown, 2003, for an excellent review on this topic).

Clearly the data do indicate that there is a high and persisting level of depression immediately following injury that may be further exacerbated by losses related to individual situations in the period following the injury culminating in later morbidity.

The secondary affective disorders and suicidal ideation and acts

There appears to be a higher likelihood of suicidal thoughts and acts following TBI. Vaukhonen (1959) noted higher rates of suicide in soldiers with TBIs. Brooks (1990) in his long follow-up study of 42 patients with severe TBIs noted that after one year 10% had mentioned suicide, and 2% had made suicide attempts. After the 5-year follow-up, 15% had made suicide attempts and expressed the view that their condition was hopeless and life was not worth living.

In their 25-year follow-up study of 6500 brain-injured individuals who served in the Finnish-Russian War of the 1940s, Achte et al. (1969) noted that 107 (1.65%) had committed suicide. Teasdale and Engberg (2001) noted in their large population study of patients with concussion, cranial fracture, and cerebral contusion or traumatic haemorrhage that the mortality rates from suicide were 3.0, 2.7, and 4.12 times the rate of the general population. Silver, Kramer, and colleagues (2001) noted a similar increase in suicide attempts (i.e., 361 of a sample of 5034 patients). Oquendo and colleagues (2004) noted that of their sample of 325 patients hospitalized with mood disorders, those patents with mild TBIs (n = 109) were more likely to attempt suicide than those without injury. The best predictors of likelihood of suicide attempt in the TBI-affected individuals were feelings of hostility and aggression.

Fleminger et al. (2003) conducted an analysis of the expected suicide rate in brain-injured populations based upon a standardized mortality ratio (SMR), which compares the rate of suicide in the sample of brain-injured individuals with that expected for the population from which the sample was drawn, taking into account the contribution of other demographic factors that contribute to the explanation of the frequency of suicide such as age, gender, and sociocultural background. In particular, Fleminger et al. cite the meta-analysis of Harris and Barraclough (1997) and note that in the study of Achte et al. (1969) discussed above, 107 committed suicide, whereas only 32 would have been expected to do so on the basis of the population estimates.

In a further analysis of five studies of civilian brain injuries, Harris and Barraclough (1997) noted an incidence of five suicides in the total sample of 650 patients; three times more than the expected rate of 1.4. They stated that the SMR for suicide after brain injury was 350, thus indicating that the presence of head injury raised the risk for suicide by three times the national rate.

Tate and colleagues (Tate, Simpson, Flanagan, & Coffey, 1997) noted that in their sample of 896 patients admitted to a rehabilitation unit, 8 committed suicide. As noted above, Teasdale and Engberg (2001) in a major epidemiological study in Denmark with a follow-up period of 15 years noted that the SMRs in the case of concussion were 3.0, 2.7 for skull fracture, and 4.1 for intracerebral haemorrhage. In interpreting this evidence, Fleminger et al. (2003) note: "over a 15 year period following head injury the suicide rate is approximately 1%, which is at least three times the standard suicide rate" (p. 78).

Lesion location and mechanism of secondary affective disorders

If the depression noted following TBI was significantly determined by the neuroanatomical effects of the brain injury as opposed to the sociocultural and clinical phenomena arising as a result of the injury (such as loss of self-esteem, pain, psychological reactions, etc.), then it would be anticipated that there would be a distinct pattern of impairment seen in depression in association with brain injury as opposed to depression independent of the injury. There would also be expected to be a strong association of clinical symptom with lesion site (Fleminger et al., 2003) as well as the demonstration of the "biologic gradient" (i.e., one would expect to see an increased risk of the affective disorders with increased severity of TBI).

Perhaps to begin with a discussion of the relationships between lesion site and postinjury depression it is best to indicate what the condition has not been associated with. Whilst the issue is by no means clear-cut, post-TBI depression has not been found to be related in any meaningful way to duration of loss of consciousness (Bornstein, Miller, & Van Schoor, 1989; Levin & Grossman, 1978), to the duration of PTA (Bornstein et al., 1989) or to the presence of skull fracture (Bornstein et al., 1989). Some relationships have been noted, however, with the level of neuropsychological sequelae (e.g., Bornstein et al., 1989; Dikmen & Reitan, 1977).

These findings are not too surprising in the context of the realization that we still do not have a very good understanding as to how the neuropsychological effects of the affective disorders may manifest in the absence of TBI. It is thus worthwhile to begin at the beginning and then see how this conundrum might be resolved.

As noted in the discussion of the phenomena associated with depression in the absence of TBI discussed above, research into the neurobiology of depression has been pursued at various levels of discourse (e.g., molecular, endocrine, neural, neuroimaging, phenomenological), but as yet this enquiry has failed to provide a definitive account of the causal mechanism of the condition. One of the principal reasons for this is that both biological and psychological systems act in a series of feedback loops, making it difficult to identify which biochemical/behavioural/psychological/social changes preceded the others and thus eventually culminated in the pathology.

The "diathesis stress" model of depression (Nemeroff, 1998) provides an excellent means by which to integrate this evidence. This model proposes that individuals vary in terms of their sensitivity to stress-induced biological responses, due to their genetic endowment. Stressful experiences alter endocrine processes to the extent that normal homeostatic processes are compromised and depression ensues. A stressful experience may thus exhaust psychological coping by compromising underlying biological/motivation processes, while on the other hand (as recent evidence suggests), "stressed" glial cells may contribute to frontal lobe functional pathology via gradual atrophic changes (Drevets, 1999).

Duman, Heninger, and Nestler (1997) further develop this notion suggesting

> One possibility is that many individuals who become depressed may have had a prior exposure to stress that causes a small amount of neuronal damage, but not enough to precipitate a behavioral change. If additional damage occurs as a result of normal aging or further stressful stimuli, these effects may then be manifested in the symptoms of mood disorder. These types of events could explain the decreased volume of specific brain structures in depression. (p. 604)

As discussed in chapter 3, it is clear that the frontal lobes play a crucial role in the perceptual interpretation of the emotional significance of external stimuli and a regulatory role over more primal (subcortical) brain structures such as the amygdala (Le Doux, 1998). Frontal lobe involvement in depression implicates the left and medial prefrontal cortex (PFC) (Elliott, Baker et al., 1997), the left dorsolateral PFC (Busch & Alpern, 1998), as well as the anterior cingulate (Devinsky, Morrell, & Vogt, 1995).

Abnormalities in brain structure and function have been consistently observed in patients with affective disorders and computed tomography (CT) scanning of these patients has revealed ventricular enlargement in bipolar disorders, unipolar depression, and mixed affective disorders (Post, 2000). Numerous studies have shown that elderly depressed individuals possess values more similar to those with irreversible dementia than to normals (Post, 2000). The best replicated finding across various depressed populations (young versus old, drug-naive and medication refractory disease and in patient subgroups) is a decrease in frontal lobe activity during resting-state functional imaging studies (Post, 2000). The changes involve the dorsolateral

(Brodmann's areas (BA) 9, 10, 46) as well as ventral and orbitofrontal cortex (BA 10, 11, 47). Most studies report bilateral changes although asymmetries have also been reported. In addition, limbic (amygdala), paralimbic (anterior temporal, cingulate), and subcortical (basal ganglia, thalamus) loci have been inconsistently identified.

Numerous positron emission tomography (PET) and single-photon emission computed tomography (SPECT) studies have demonstrated an inverse relationship between frontal activity and depression severity (Post, 2000) and significant correlations have been demonstrated with psychomotor speed, anxiety, and cognitive performance (e.g., Austin et al., 1992). The level of frontal hypometabolism noted is comparable in patients with depression of varying types (unipolar, bipolar, and with obsessive-compulsive disorder [OCD]) (Post, 2000) and there have been consistent findings of a negative correlations between HDRS and cerebral activity in depression (Post, 2000).

Mayberg's (1997, 2001, 2006) intriguing work proposes a working neuroanatomical model of depression that proposes that depression comes about as a consequence of three neuroanatomical spheres of activity: (1) the dorsal compartment, which includes both neocortical and superior limbic components and is postulated to mediate cognitive aspects (apathy, psychomotor slowing, impaired attention, and executive functioning); (2) the ventral compartment including limbic, paralimbic, and subcortical regions, which mediate the circadian and vegetative components including sleep, appetite, libido, and endocrine disturbances; and (3) the rostral cingulate, which is distinct from both the dorsal and ventral components that may mediate interactions between the two. Support for the model comes from functional neuroimaging data as well as from event-related activity, electroencephalographic data, and neuropsychological measures. This earlier work is further supported by the very encouraging results arising from the application of deep brain stimulation of the subgenual cingulate area (Mayberg, 2006) in intractable depression.

Considerable dispute has raged in the earlier literature regarding lesion site and side and their effects on post-TBI depression. This arose from the early work of Pierre Flor Henry (e.g., 1974, 1976) who proposed that right hemisphere lesions culminated in affective disorders while left hemisphere lesions resulted in psychosis. In their influential early study of penetrating missile wounds following the Vietnam War discussed above, Grafman, Vance et al. (1986) reported that depressive symptoms were more commonly associated with penetrating missile wounds of the right hemisphere (particularly the right orbitofrontal cortex).

In his series of papers on 670 patients suffering from a variety of penetrating missile wounds Lishman (1966, 1968, 1978, 1997) noted that depression was also most commonly found with lesions of the right frontal lobe. This finding stands in contrast to subsequent studies on the poststroke depression literature (see Robinson, 2000 for a comprehensive review) that suggests that during the acute poststroke period, patients with left frontal lesions had a significantly higher frequency (i.e., 60% left frontal versus 0% right frontal; 13% left posterior versus 17% right posterior) of major depression than individuals with other lesion location.

More recent data has suggested that the left hemisphere is most likely implicated in post-TBI depression. Fedoroff et al. (1992) observed that in their 66 consecutive patients with CHI but no spinal cord or other organ system injury, interviewed one month postinjury using a structured clinical interview (PSE), an observer-rated symptom checklist (HDRS) and the mini-mental status examination (MMSE), 17 subjects (26%) met the *DSM-III* symptom and duration criteria for major depression and a further two patients had dysthymia. There was a significantly higher frequency of previous psychiatric disorder and alcohol abuse in the depressed subjects.

The presence of a left anterior lesions (i.e., left dorsolateral frontal and/or left basal ganglia lesions and, to a lesser degree, parietal-occipital and right hemisphere lesions) was the strongest correlate of those examined of major depression. These results lead the authors to speculate: "this finding suggests that the left dorsolateral frontal cortex and the left basal ganglia are critical structures in the left hemisphere as far as mood is concerned, and they may represent strategic locations for the initiation of major depression" (p. 922). They went on to suggest that this might be due to the lesions interrupting biogenic amine-containing neurons as they pass through the basal ganglia or frontal subcortical white matter.

While these views are interesting in themselves, it is perhaps more probative to have an oversight of the various studies undertaken in this complex issue to determine if any overarching trends emerge. In the comprehensive meta-analysis undertaken by Carson et al. (2000), 143 studies were identified that addressed this question and 48 of these met the criteria for inclusion. Of these 48 studies, 38 showed no association with lesion location, 2 showed increases with left-sided lesions, and 8 showed increases with right-sided lesions. The subsequent meta-analytic investigation indicated no evidence to support increased prevalence of depression with left as compared to right hemisphere strokes. The data also indicated no evidence for selective risk for depression following damage to the anterior regions of the brain (after taking into account that anterior strokes are the most common form of stroke).

There has, however, been some criticism of the review by Carson et al. (2000). The methodology of the review and, most notably the exclusion of some studies, has been a particular focus of concern (Dilley & Fleminger, 2006). A subsequent meta-analysis has suggested that the proximity of the lesion to the left frontal pole does predict depressive illness (Narushima, Kosier, & Robinson, 2003) and this observation has been further supported by a subsequent analysis from Finland (Vataja et al. 2004). Thus, while the possibility of a sided contribution to the emergence of depression is an interesting one, the veracity of this suggestion remains in contention.

One possible means of saving the hypothesis of a specific lesion prompting depression may be to make the assumption of "non-imaging detectable" neural damage as indicated by neuropsychological deficit. The lack of detailed injury data is a significant limitation, however, and lead Nelson, Drebing, Satz, and Uchiyama (1998) to observe: "More problematic is the inherent assumption that all CHI patients are alike. We know from the pathophysiology of head injury that different subtypes emerge involving, for example, orbitofrontal and dorsolateral areas of the brain" (p. 559).

While there are some doubts about the directness of the relationship between neuroimaging evidence and functional evidence (e.g., Anderson et al., 1995), there is considerable debate in the literature as to whether, where, how, or why neuropsychological deficits occur in depression (Caine, 1986; Elliott, Baker et al., 1997; Rohling et al., 2002). Various methodological and theoretical anomalies have prevented the emergence of any cohesive account of research findings thus far (Rosenstein, 1998).

As noted above, some authors (e.g., Reitan & Wolfson, 1997; Veiel, 1997) go so far as to suggest few, if any, intrinsic depressive deficits exist. Others, taking a more moderate view, concede that where deficits do occur, they are either "replete with inconsistencies" (Rosenstein, 1998, p. 139) or are very difficult to define. Dolan, Bench, Brown, Scott, and Frackowiak (1994) note "the underlying nature of depression related cognitive deficits has been a source of extensive theoretical debate. Psychological theories include motivational deficits, lack of effort, poor encoding strategies or defective processing resources" (p. 849).

McAllister-Williams, Ferrier, and Young (1998) also cogently observe "if neuropsychological deficits were secondary to low mood, one would expect the degree of neuropsychological dysfunction to reflect this. Early studies support this but it has been challenged by recent studies" (p. 573).

Most authors agree that neuropsychological deficits are associated with depressive illness in some way or another. The central point of concern, as hinted above, is whether these deficits are "primary" (i.e., intrinsic to the condition) or "secondary" (i.e., the result of otherwise intact cognitive capacities failing due to lack of functional opportunity, such as via lowered subcortical arousal).

In both TBI and non-TBI affected individuals, depression exacerbates CHI-induced cognitive impairment (Brooks, 1984) and leads to poor social functioning (Busch & Alpern, 1998; Jorge, Robinson, Starkstein, & Arndt, 1994). Perhaps one of the best means of addressing these problems presented by the sometimes contradictory literature is to use meta-analysis.

One of the most useful studies along this line of enquiry is the analysis conducted by Hans Veiel (1997). Veiel's analysis only examined depressed young or middle aged individuals with clearly defined major depression. Using these exclusion criteria, he developed a database of 13 studies. He notes that the results of the studies can be classified into three levels of effect. He notes low levels of effect on studies that measure attention and concentration issues. He notes a moderate level of effect of depression on visuo-motor tracking, visual/spatial functions, and verbal fluency. He observes high levels of effect on measures of mental flexibility and control and composite indicators of brain impairment (i.e., the pathognomonic index of the Luria Nebraska Battery).

Veiel notes that 50% of patients with major depression will score two or more SDs below normals on the Trail Making Test—Part B (TMT[B]) or on the Colour-word form of the Stroop Task as well as on composite indicators (e.g., the pathognomonic indicator of Luria Nebraska Neuropsychological Battery [LNRB]), 15% will score in this range on tests of memory, visuomotor tracking/scanning, visual spatial functions and verbal fluency. On tests of simple attention, they will perform in a manner similar to normals. He notes that the level of disruption of cognition is of a severity comparable to that of severe TBI.

Conclusion

It is clear that pervasive deficits in emotional status occur in the wake of a TBI. Problems have emerged in the specification of this deficit due to issues associated with the nature of the relationship between the injury, the substrate upon which the injury acts, and the effects of the injury on the individual's life and circumstance in the wake of the blow. It is clear that approximately 20–30% of individuals will have a diagnosable affective disorder following the injury and that this level of deficit will persist for a number of years. The literature on the relationship of the side and site of the blow has been less than conclusive and it now seems most likely that there is no direct relationship between the site or side of the injury and the subsequent affective state.

6 Reality distortion following TBI (1): *Psychosis, denial, and deficits in the social perception of emotion*

In the next two chapters, I will embark on an unusual approach to the issues of postaccident behavioural and emotional disorders and concentrate on the issue of reality distortion following TBI. The distortion of reality can take a number of forms outlined in the design matrix below:

	ORGANIC ILLNESS	
REALITY	Present	Absent
Distorted	Schizophrenia or post-traumatic psychosis	Somatoform disorder, factitious disorder or malingering
Not distorted	Denial of deficit and impairment in the social perception of emotion	Unimpaired

Figure 6.1 The relationship between reality orientation and organicity.

Following a traumatic brain injury (TBI), individuals can develop a number of reality distortions. The condition can be associated with hallucinations and delusions either as a result of an existing schizophrenia or due to the development of a posttraumatic psychosis, denial of symptoms, or an inability (as a consequence of the injury) to recognize and comprehend their own emotional states or those of their significant others, or recognition of a condition as real when most examiners would not consider it to be so (i.e., abnormal illness behaviour) including factitious disorders, conversion disorders, and malingering. In this chapter I will review the literature on the psychoses and denial of impairment, and in chapter 7, I will focus on abnormal illness behaviour, factitious disorders, and malingering.

There are relatively few studies of the emergence of secondary psychosis following TBI, and it is clear that the relationship between the brain injury and the development of the psychotic condition is one that has not been easy to disentangle. As I have previously noted, the effects of the TBI on psychosocial aspects of the individual's life are by no means irrelevant in the subsequent development of any psychopathology and this is as applicable in the more severe psychiatric conditions as it is in the less severe ones.

Psychosis represents a relatively low frequency but high impact complication of TBI that causes enormous stress to the individual and his or her family (McAllister & Ferrell, 2002). It also provides the possibility of fascinating insights into the mechanism of action of both psychosis and TBI that can act to further inform the study of both conditions.

Background

The study of schizophrenia has had a long and tortuous history. The distinction between *dementia paranoides* and *catatonia* was made by Kahlbaum in 1863. Kahlbaum noted that with *dementia paranoides* there was a clear pattern of prominent delusions in association with the gross disorganisation of behaviour and paranoia, characterised by systematised delusions, whilst there was an overall preservation of intellect and behaviour. The notion of *catatonia*, on the other hand, was used to describe a pattern associated with the patient's tendency to remain mute and motionless.

In 1896, Emil Kraepelin noted the similarities between these various syndromes and manic depressive psychosis and applied the term *dementia praecox* to all three forms. He subsequently accepted the notion of a fourth form, *dementia praecox simplex* characterised by a gradual onset and lack of initiative. For Kraepelin, the defining features of his "dementia" were the onset early in life and the irreversible progression of the state to a permanent dementia. The system of disorders under the umbrella of *dementia praecox* Kraepelin proposed was well accepted and was preserved as a part of the official nomenclature of the disorder in the United States until 1950.

The more recently used term *schizophrenia* can be attributed to the Swiss psychiatrist Eugen Bleuler who proposed the term in his classic text *Dementia Praecox or the Group of Schizophrenias* in 1911. Bleuler differed from Kraepelin in that he did not believe that the irreversible decline in function observed in these states was an essential or even defining feature of the disorder. Bleuler maintained that the illness was characterised by a particular type of thinking and feeling in response to the outside world, rather than merely a degenerative pattern.

Such a split in the perceptions of the disorder between Bleuler and Kraepelin underlines an oft-visited issue regarding the nature of these disorders: Do these conditions represent a degenerative state or a particular set of defining behavioural aberrations? As recently as the theories of Crow (1980) in dividing the disorder into positive (Bleulerian) and negative (Kraepelinian) symptoms, the issue has still not been settled and, as with most disputes in psychology and psychiatry, the truth probably lies somewhere between the two competing opinions.

The term schizophrenia, which has generally been interpreted as a splitting of the mind, actually refers to the fragmentation of the psyche into its component parts. Thus, there is a split within the individual between his or her cognition and his or her emotional responses or motor behaviours. Bleuler (1911) divided the symptoms of schizophrenia into those that were fundamental to the condition (i.e., present in every case of the disorder, such as disorders of affect, attention, and volition) and those that were accessory (i.e., not considered to be permanent features, such as hallucination and delusion).

In 1952 and 1953 a new chapter began in the management and perception of these conditions with Delay and Deniker's introduction of the agent chlorpromazine in France for the treatment of various psychiatric conditions. This was followed closely by the agent reserpine that had a similar application (Delay & Deniker, 1956).

Simultaneously, numerous clinical reports appeared in the literature describing the efficacy of these treatments in symptomatic relief of the schizophrenias. This new chapter also caused a further challenge to Kraepelin's concept of schizophrenia. The new agents had their exclusive effects on hallucination, delusion, and thought disorder, while having virtually no effect on the disorders of affect, attention, and volition. It thus seemed that there were at least two groups of symptoms within the spectrum of schizophrenia, those that responded to the new antipsychotic medications and those that did not.

Kurt Schneider (1959), having noted the effect of these agents on what were to become known as the positive symptoms of schizophrenia, began to categorise these symptoms. In contrast to Kraepelin's earlier work (1896), which contended that the negative symptoms were the defining nature of schizophrenia, Schneider maintained that a series of symptoms observed only in schizophrenia and in no other condition could be developed. The list of his ten first-rank symptoms of schizophrenia (Schneider, 1959) included:

(1) Hearing one's own voice spoken aloud.
(2) A hallucinatory voice talking about the patient in the third person.
(3) Hallucinatory voices making a running commentary on the patient's actions.
(4) Somatic hallucinations that the patient blames on external agencies.
(5) Thought withdrawal, such that the subject feels that the thought have been taken from his head, as if a person or some external force were removing them.
(6) Thought insertion, such that the subject believes that thoughts that are not his own and are being put into his head in some way.
(7) Thought broadcasting, such that the subject feels that his thoughts are being broadcast, so that other people can hear and know what he or she is thinking.
(8) Thought blocking, such that the stream of though becomes disordered and gaps or lapses in the continuity of the thought appear.
(9) Delusional perception, the patient sees or hears things that are not there.
(10) All experiences of feeling, drive, or volition that are judged to be made or influenced by others.

Schneider (1959) also proposed the existence of a series of second-rank symptoms, which were not diagnostic of schizophrenia of themselves but nonetheless contributed to the diagnosis. While Schneider's first-rank symptoms have been very influential in the formulation of the diagnostic criteria of schizophrenia, a number of investigators have criticised his approach in neglecting the core negative symptoms (e.g., Andreasen, 1983). There is also significant variability regarding the prevalence of first-rank symptoms in different cultures that may indicate that culture significantly contributes to the emergence of these symptoms in these patients (Ndetei & Vadher, 1984).

Based on the differential effects noted with the antipsychotic medications, Crow (1980) proposed that schizophrenia consisted of two semi-independent syndromes. He described these syndromes in a manner originally proposed by the father of English neurology, John Hughlings Jackson, as comprising positive (symptoms that were additional to those seen in the normal state) and negative (features that are present in the normal state but which are absent in the condition). We have previously visited this dichotomy in the discussion of the symptoms of damage to the frontal lobe in chapter 3.

Nancy Andreasen's (Andreasen, 1983, 1984; Andreasen & Olsen, 1982) work also supported the suggestion of two types of schizophrenia. Andreasen provided a more comprehensive definition of the two syndromes and a more reliable means of measuring them in the form of the Scales for the Assessment of Positive and Negative Symptoms (SAPS and SANS). The positive symptoms included (Andreasen, 1984):

Hallucination: Sensory experiences in the absence of any stimulation from the environment (e.g., audible thoughts/voices arguing/voices commenting).

Delusion: Holding a belief that the rest of society would generally disagree with or view as a misinterpretation of reality.

Bizarre behaviour: The practice of unusual or uncharacteristic behaviours or rituals such as aggressiveness or saving body products.

Thought disorder: Problem with the form of thought including incoherence, neologism (generation of nonwords), loosening of association, clang associations, poverty of speech, perseveration, and thought blocking.

These are clearly quite consistent with Schneider's (1959) earlier descriptions of the behaviour of these patients. The positive symptoms are relatively responsive to the actions of the antipsychotic agents, which it was later established worked by blocking dopamine receptors. Crow (1980) suggested that these symptoms were thus attributable to dopamine uptake. In contrast, the negative symptoms that are not amenable to the actions of these agents must be attributable to some other cause.

The negative symptoms are much in line with Kraepelin's (1896) original formulation and include (Andreasen, 1984):

Flattening of affect: Virtually no stimulus can elicit an emotional response (i.e., blunting and apathy). These individuals may also show inappropriate affect where their response is out of context with the usually accepted response.

Alogia: Decrease in the flow and spontaneity of speech.

Avolition: Decrease in the ability to motivate oneself or get things started.

Anhedonia: Inability to feel pleasure in any activity.

Attention deficit: Inability to attend and track mental operations.

As the symptoms were considered to be chronic and irreversible, Crow (1980) proposed that they must be attributable to structural changes to the brain itself in the form of ventricular dilatation.

The typology proposed by Andreasen (1983, 1984) and Crow (1980) has proven very fruitful and has resulted in numerous papers, conference presentations, and books on this topic. It is fair to say that Crow's original speculations led to a renaissance of the inquiry into the nature and causes of the schizophrenias. However, the simple dichotomous approach to the classification of schizophrenia has been questioned due to its failure to comfortably fit with the data. This doubt, or perhaps more appropriately refinement, of Crow's original typology comes from factor analytic approaches to the domains of symptoms within the spectrum of the schizophrenias. While the original factor analytic approaches advocated by Andreasen (Andreasen & Olsen, 1982) appeared to support the notion of the positive and negative dichotomy, more recent work by Liddle and colleagues (Liddle, 1987) indicated that the puzzle was slightly more complex.

Using scales based upon the SAPS and SANS, Liddle's (1987) factor analyses revealed three syndromes: (1) a psychomotor poverty syndrome much like Andreasen's negative symptoms; (2) a disorganisation syndrome consisting of formal thought disorder, inappropriate affect and poverty of content of speech; and (3) a reality distortion syndrome consisting of delusional and hallucinatory symptoms. A review of the clinical heterogeneity of schizophrenia by Buchanan and Carpenter (1994) noted that no less than 15 studies have arrived at a three-factor solution to the number of syndromes under the umbrella of schizophrenia using a range of different diagnostic scales.

Andreasen and Carpenter (1993) sounded a cautionary note on the rush to yet another series of symptom profiles in schizophrenia. They observed that the three clusters must be recognised as dimensions of the psychopathology determined by the artificial statistical technique of factor analysis rather than as subtypes of the disorder. A subtype by its definition is a unitary individual phenomenon, while a dimension of psychopathology can have magnitude that may overlap and/or be additive within the given individual. Thus the statistical existence of a particular syndrome cluster does not necessarily mean that the next individual who walks into your office will feature any such thing.

DSM-IV-TR (APA, 2000) lists six criteria on which the diagnosis of schizophrenia can be made. The most salient of these are: (1) the presence of two or more characteristic symptoms that must be present for a significant proportion of time during a one-month period. These symptoms include delusions, hallucinations, disorganised speech, disorganised or catatonic behaviour, and negative symptoms including flattening of affect, alogia, or avolition; (2) social or occupational dysfunction; and (3) a continuous duration of the disturbance for a period of six months. (Readers should consult *DSM-IV-TR* the full listing of the criteria.)

The *DSM-IV-TR* also lists five subtypes of schizophrenia: (1) the paranoid type, characterised by delusion and frequent auditory hallucinations and a relative absence of negative symptoms; (2) the disorganised type, characterised by disorganised speech, behaviour and affect; (3) the catatonic type, characterised by motor symptoms including immobility or hyperactivity in association with posturing; and (4) the undifferentiated type, which includes the features listed in one of the other categories but does not meet the criteria for the other subtypes; and (5) the residual type, characterised by features that are largely of the negative state.

Posttraumatic psychosis is a generic term commonly used in the literature but which has no formal status in the *DSM* and describes a psychotic illness in a person who has experienced brain trauma. The definition is unclear as it can be quite difficult to definitively ensure that the psychosis was caused by the TBI rather than occurring as a result of genetic predisposition or some other cause (Corcoran, McAllister, & Malaspina, 2005).

Methodological issues

Smeltzer, Nasrallah, and Miller (1994) identified a number of methodological difficulties associated with the published descriptions of posttraumatic psychosis. These include: imprecise descriptive terminology, variations in diagnostic definition, failure to use reliable diagnostic criteria, differences of effect as a function of different populations (e.g., soldiers versus civilians, adults versus children, psychiatric versus general hospital patients), difference in the aetiology of the head injury (i.e., open versus closed, severe versus minor, blunt versus penetrating), varying durations of follow-up and the frequent use of retrospective data. Each of these could have a significant effect in the observed psychiatric state.

The condition can be considered to be independent of the injury if the injury is not considered to be aetiologically relevant. This might occur if the clinician were unaware of the history of injury, if a large amount of time has elapsed since the injury and the individual had been free from symptoms for a long time, if the individual experienced psychotic symptoms before the onset of the injury or the degree of the trauma was minor rendering the likelihood of the condition emerging as a result of the injury relatively low (Smeltzer et al., 1994).

Phenomenology and nosology of secondary psychotic disorders

The *DSM-IV-TR* (APA, 2000) classifies posttraumatic psychosis as a psychotic disorder due to a general medical condition (i.e., concussion or cerebral contusion), which can occur either with delusions (293.81) or with hallucinations (293.82). The Manual states:

> Although there are no infallible guidelines for determining whether the relationship between the psychotic disturbance and the general medical condition is etiological, several considerations provide some guidance in this area. One consideration is the presence of a temporal association between the onset, exacerbation, or remission of the general medical condition and that of the psychotic disturbance. A second consideration is the presence of features that are atypical for a primary Psychotic Disorder (e.g., atypical age of onset or presence of visual or olfactory hallucinations). (p. 335)

The condition must feature prominent hallucination or delusion, there should be evidence from the history, examination, or other clinical findings that the condition is a direct effect of the medical condition, and that the disturbance is not better accounted for by some other condition and also that the condition does not occur in the context of a delirium (APA, 2000).

In the previous edition of the Manual (*DSM-III-R*, 1987) this condition was referred to as an organic delusional disorder or an organic hallucinosis, dependent upon the relative prominence of these symptoms in the clinical picture (Smeltzer et al., 1994).

The term posttraumatic psychosis is a general term that describes a psychotic illness that emerges in the wake of brain trauma. Smeltzer and colleagues (1994) propose that as the association between the injury and the psychosis is a temporal one, it should include all forms of psychotic disorder. While the term *psychosis* is often equated with the diagnosis of schizophrenia, it is more accurately viewed as a nonspecific presentation of many conditions including depression, bipolar disorders, delirium, and dementia amongst other conditions (McAllister & Ferrell, 2002).

Sachdev, Smith, and Cathcart (2001) noted one or more delusions in all 45 of their patients who were diagnosed with a schizophrenia-like psychosis following TBI and they observed that the psychosis was characterized by on overwhelming presentation of the positive symptoms of schizophrenia rather than a negative symptom presentation. Only 22.2% of the patients demonstrated negative symptoms including flattening of affect, avolition, and asociality, although agitated and aggressive behaviour occurred in 40%.

All of the subjects featured delusions with the most common being persecutory delusions (55.5%), but 22.2% featured referential delusions, 22.2% featured delusions of control, 20% featured delusions of grandiosity and 15.4% featured religious delusions. Delusions of thought alienation (i.e., thought broadcasting, thoughts being inserted or withdrawn from the mind as described by Schneider above) were less common (13.3%) and somatic passivity was less common still (6.7%). The so-called organic delusions (Capgras, misidentification, erotomania, people stealing, or hiding) were not seen at all in these patients. Hallucinations were predominantly auditory in form (84.4%) with voices commenting on the person being most commonly reported (55.5%). Visual hallucinations were much less common (20%) and tactile hallucinations rarer still (4.4%).

Lishman (1997) described another psychotic condition associated with TBI that occurs in the early stages following the injury. This is a phase that he contends is incorporated within the posttraumatic amnesia (PTA), but can be distinguished from it. The presentation of acute posttraumatic psychosis (APTP) covers a wide range of clinical pictures in the early postinjury phase. Some patients feature little change other than increased lethargy and cognitive deficits. These patients are often perplexed and prone to irritability and restlessness, which gives way to a more somnolent state until the patient passes back into a state of ongoing consciousness.

However, Lishman (1997) found that in some cases there is a more florid presentation:

> Some patients pass through an excitable and overactive phase with florid disturbance of behaviour which can be long continued and pose serious problems of management. Sometimes this is attributable to the abnormal experiences and delusional misinterpretations of post-traumatic delirium, but sometimes it proves to foreshadow enduring changes of temperament and behaviour occasioned by the injury. The patient may be abusive, aggressive, and markedly uncooperative. Very occasionally crimes of violence are committed at the height of such disturbance, and afterwards the patient has no knowledge of their occurrence. (p. 168)

Prevalence and incidence of psychosis following TBI

One of the interesting things about the available literature on this presentation is the number of times that it has been reviewed and re-reviewed. A large number of the studies in the area represent evaluative reviews of various assemblies of the available published cases (e.g., Davison & Bagley, 1969; Fujii & Ahmed, 2002; Zhang & Sachdev, 2003), and in each review (probably because slightly different studies are used) marginally different emphases and findings have emerged.

The rate of emergence of psychosis reported in the earlier literature (i.e., involving eight studies describing 12,385 patients between 1917 and 1964) were reviewed by Davison and Bagley (1969). They reported that the rate of the development of psychosis following TBI ranged from 0.07 to 9.8% with a median rate of 1.35%. They estimated the lifetime prevalence of posttraumatic psychosis over a 10- to 20-year period following the injury to be two to three times the expected incidence in the noninjured population.

Goldney (2005) noted that both schizophrenia and TBI are relatively common clinical phenomena, with the lifetime risk of schizophrenia being 0.8% (Jablensky, 1995) and with as many as 5.7% of the population having a TBI with a loss of consciousness of more than 15 minutes (Anstey et al., 2004). As a result, the likelihood that these two diagnoses may co-occur, particularly as the peak incidence time for both conditions is in early adulthood, is not insubstantial.

Lishman (1973) reviewed the histories of 670 British soldiers who had sustained penetrating missile wounds during the Second World War and noted that 0.7% of these demonstrated unequivocal psychosis. The subsequent studies of Brown et al. (Brown, Chadwick, Shaffer, Rutter, & Traub, 1981) and that of Thomsen (1984) reported higher incidence rates ranging from 3.2 to 20%. Thomsen (1984, 1987) noted that in the 40 patients reviewed 10 to 15 years following a severe TBI, the incidence of posttraumatic psychosis was 20% (i.e., 8 of the 40) with six of these eight patients having a delayed onset. Some questions have been raised with regard to the nature of the sample identified by Thomson and the diagnostic formulations regarding their presentations.

The description of these patients by Thomsen (1984, 1987) at 2.5 (early) and at 10 to 15 years (late) following injury indicated that 80% displayed changes in personality early as compared to 65% at the late follow-up; 60% (early) and 68% (late) showed decrease in social contact; 43% (early) and 53% (late) showed aspontaneity; 23% (early) and 68% (late) showed increased sensitivity to distress; and 20% (early) and 55% (late) showed lack of interests. Clearly, these descriptions are not identical to the negative symptoms of schizophrenia but are reminiscent of them, and it could be argued that such a presentation could be accommodated within the spectrum of schizophrenia. Alternatively, it could be argued that the presentation of these features is consistent with the notion of compromise of the dorsolateral and medial prefrontal cortex (Crowe, 1992) presenting a subcortical pattern of dementia in the wake of the injury (see the discussion of the organic personality syndromes in chapter 3).

Ota (1969) studied 1,168 adults admitted to the hospital following their TBI and noted functional or organic psychosis in 2.7%. Miller and Stern (1965) did a long-term follow-up of 100 patients following TBI and noted that 10 of them featured psychosis, all of whom featured dementia. Violon and De Mol (1987) noted that in their 503 patients, 3.4% developed psychosis in the 1 to 10 years following injury.

In their review of six cases of posttraumatic psychosis De Mol, Violon, and Brihaye (1982) noted that the presentation of psychosis following injury principally consisted of delusion, hallucination, the presence of paranoid and mystical ideas, autism, psychomotor instability, and fugues. They noted that the demography of the condition indicated that it occurred mostly in young men before the age of 30. The severity of the TBI did not predict the likelihood of the condition and the temporal lobes were implicated in one third of their sample.

In a subsequent study (Violon & De Mol, 1987) these investigators observed 18 cases of regressive or chronic acquired delusional states amongst the 530 unselected case histories of patients at a neurosurgical unit in Belgium. They identified 6 cases (1.1%) who featured posttraumatic schizophrenia, with the remaining 12 cases displaying paranoid or mood disorders.

In their retrospective review on the characteristics of psychotic disorder due to brain injury, Fujii and Ahmed (2002) reanalyzed 69 of the published case studies from 39 articles reporting the condition and observed that in the majority of cases the patients were male with an onset of the condition within the first two years following either a moderate or severe injury. The majority of the cases showed computed tomography/magnetic resonance imaging (CT/MRI) and electroencephalogram (EEG) scan abnormalities, most of these located in the frontal and temporal lobes. The majority of cases also presented with the positive (i.e., delusions and hallucinations) rather than the negative symptoms of schizophrenia.

Monosymptomatic psychoses also occur following TBI, but they do so only rarely. Reduplicative paramnesia is a syndrome originally described by Arnold Pick (1903). It is characterized by the delusional belief that a familiar place exists in two places at the same time. The condition is one of a family of delusional presentations including delusions of passivity (the thought that one is controlled by some external agent), Capgras (the delusion of the substitution of a significant other with an impostor), the Cotard's delusion (the delusion that one is dead), and the Fregoli delusion (the delusion of a persecutor who is able to change appearances and appear as different people).

Each of these conditions has been reported following TBI although admittedly such syndromes are quite rare (e.g., paranoid delusions: Prigatano, O'Brien, & Klonoff, 1988; reduplicative paramnesias: Filley & Jarvis, 1987; Marshall, Halligan, & Wade, 1995; Murai, Toichi, Sengoku, Miyoshi, & Morimune, 1997; Rogers & Franzen, 1992; Capgras: Bienenfeld & Brott, 1989; Hayman & Abrams, 1977; Silva, Leong, & Luong, 1989; Weston, & Whitlock, 1971; and the Cotard delusion: Young, Robertson, Hellawell, de Pauw, & Pentland, 1992).

De Clérambault's syndrome has also been noted as a possible complication of TBI. This syndrome is characterised by, generally, a woman having the conviction that she is involved in amorous communication with a person of higher social rank. This person was the first to make advances towards her and to fall in love with her. This may be associated with the view that the object can never find happiness without her, that his overt attachments or marriage are invalid, that contact is made indirectly by means of his immense resources, his conduct may be outwardly paradoxical, and that their relationship is universally acknowledged and socially approved. The onset of the delusion is precise and sudden, it has a strong affective colouration, a strong tendency towards action to further the relationship, and a lack of themes not related to the principal object of the delusion (Enoch & Trethowan, 1979; Signer & Cummings, 1987).

Filley and Jarvis (1987) report a case of reduplicative paramnesia in which the delusion appeared more than three years after the injury and was associated with pathology of the right hemisphere and bifrontal compromise. This long lag between the injury and the emergence of the delusion is similar to that noted in eight patients who demonstrated the emergence of a delayed psychosis following right temporoparietal stroke or trauma reported by Levine and Finkelstein (1982). The precise location of the lesion proved difficult to confirm, nonetheless, the authors contended that right hemisphere structures were critical in the emergence of the delusion.

Loyd and Tsuang (1981) reported a single case study of a 37-year-old woman who presented with the visual hallucination of snakes 10 months following a mild traumatic brain injury (MTBI). They contended that this presentation could not be explained by other factors and was a manifestation of the postconcussion syndrome.

In Fujii and Ahmed's (2002) review the most common types of delusions observed following TBI were persecutory delusions, followed in decreasing order by grandiose, somatic, Capgras, reduplicative paramnesia, religious, reference, stealing, erotomanic, Cotard's, and jealousy. Half of the patients featured hallucinations and the most common form was auditory followed by visual. Only 8 of the 55 patients reported negative symptoms.

Cummings (1985, 1986) raises a very interesting point about the nature of the delusional framework following any type of brain impairment:

> The most common variety of delusion manifested by patients with neuromedical illnesses involves ideas of reference, false beliefs of persecution and fears of death or injury. The delusions may be highly complex, intricately structured belief systems involving complicated plots and dependent upon many confirmatory observations, or they may be transient, loosely held, and poorly structured beliefs such as fears that one's house may be broken into or one's possessions taken. Complex delusions are manifested only by patients with preserved intellectual function, whereas simple delusional syndromes may occur in patients with compromised neuropsychologic abilities. (p. 299)

Cummings's observation is an interesting one and reinforces the notion that the ability to develop a delusion framework is contingent upon the integrity as well as the disintegration of the cerebral systems. A delusion that requires lots of confirmation, internal consistency, and elaboration indicates the overall integrity of many aspects of the brain that is producing the delusion system and underscoring how much processing is going right while only some is going wrong.

The literature (e.g., Wilcox & Nasrallah, 1987a, 1987b, 1987c) suggests that there are a number of risk factors that predispose an individual to the development of posttraumatic psychosis. These include: (1) early age of injury (Wilcox & Nasrallah); (2) genetic or other forms of environmental vulnerability to the condition; (3) the severity of the injury and whether it was a closed rather than open head injury (Lishman, 1968); and (4) the site of the brain lesions, particularly if they are in the left hemisphere (Buckley et al., 1993). A comprehensive discussion of the location of lesions follows.

With regard to the early age of injury, Wilcox and Nasrallah (1987a, 1987b, 1987c) undertook a comprehensive chart review of 659 hospitalized patients admitted between 1934 and 1944. Four patient groups were established based on the research diagnostic criteria of Feighner and colleagues (1972): schizophrenia (200 patients), mania (122 patients), depressive illness (203 patients), and surgical patient controls (134 patients). Blind rating of the patients for the presence of head injury (i.e., head trauma before age 10 that either resulted in loss of consciousness (LOC) of at least one hour or that caused vomiting, confusion, or visual changes sufficient to warrant medical intervention) indicated the presence of head injury in 11% of the schizophrenia patients, 4.9% of the manic patients, 1.5% of the depressive patients, and 1.5% of the surgical controls.

Nasrallah, Fowler, and Judd (1981) also noted that up to 15% of patients with a diagnosis of schizophrenia present with a history of head injury and proposed that head injury may serve to trigger the emergence of a schizophrenia-like psychosis, but only in appropriately predisposed individuals.

However, this view is by no means universally held. In perhaps the most comprehensive examination of this phenomenon, Nielsen, Mortensen, O'Callaghan, Mors and Ewald (2002) undertook a study employing 5179 male and 3109 female patients (i.e., all patients admitted to Danish psychiatric hospitals between January 1, 1978 and December 31, 1993 with a diagnosis of schizophrenia) and compared these to 51,790 male and 31,090 female controls. With regard to the effects of concussion on the later development of schizophrenia, the odds ratios for patients with a diagnosis of schizophrenia did not differ from the controls and, surprisingly, male patients with schizophrenia had significantly fewer concussions than did controls, while females had significantly more.

On balance the study indicates that male patients with schizophrenia had suffered fewer head injuries as well as fewer other forms of fracture than did controls, while the opposite was the case for the females. On this basis it is clear that if head injury did have any role in the development of subsequent schizophrenia it is at best a modest one, with only 8.5% of male patients and 3.1% of female patients with schizophrenia previously hospitalized for TBI.

The differential diagnosis of Psychotic Disorder due to Traumatic Brain Injury and schizophrenia often centres upon the degree to which the conditions exist in the context of a positive family history of the schizophrenia spectrum disorders. Surprisingly, in those studies where it has been possible to investigate the family history of the schizophrenia spectrum, the incidence of schizophrenia in the relatives of patients with psychosis did not exceed the level observed in the general population, and was considerably lower than that observed in relatives of patients with a diagnosis of schizophrenia without a history of brain injury (McAllister & Ferrell, 2002).

This finding has not been noted in all studies and the study by Sachdev et al. (2001) using regression analysis observed that the best predictors of the development of the schizophrenia-like psychosis was a positive family history for the condition and the duration of the loss of consciousness, supporting the notion of a genetic predisposition to the condition. However, this finding was noted in only a small percentage of the sample.

Evolution of the secondary psychosis following TBI

The duration of the period following the injury that results in the emergence of a posttraumatic psychosis has been reported throughout the literature and can last as little as one month (Levine & Finkelstein, 1982), 12 months (Delahunty, Morice, Frost, & Lambert, 1991), three years (Barnhill & Gaultieri, 1989; Filley & Jarvis, 1987), 10 years (Barnhill & Gaultieri, 1989) or more (i.e., 11 years: Levine & Finkelstein, 1982). Slater, Beard and Glithero (1963) also noted a prolonged lag of between 10 and 14 years from the onset of temporal lobe epilepsy to the appearance of the schizophrenia-like psychosis (Crowe & Kuttner, 1991).

Fujii and Ahmed (2002) noted in their review that the period of delay before onset of the psychosis ranged from zero to 34 years with the mean number of years post-trauma to onset being 4.1±6.6. The mode of onset was less than one year (38%) and the median was one year, with 72% of the cases reporting an onset before the mean. Twenty of the 59 cases (34%) reported a history of seizures, a level that the authors observed was much higher than that noted in TBI populations (12%).

The relationship between the emergence of posttraumatic psychosis and TBI is not a simple one. Possible aetiological factors include: the presence of seizure and possibly "subclinical" seizure activity (e.g., Parnas, Korsgaard, Krautwald, & Jensen, 1982; Ferguson & Rayport, 1984), disruption of subcortical monaminergic systems (Van Woerkom, Minderhaud, Gootschal, & Nicholai, 1982), possible early neurodegenerative effects (Mortimer, French, Hutton, & Schuman, 1985), or some combination of these and possibly additional factors.

Lishman (1997) noted a similar list of factors contributing to psychiatric disability following TBI including: the mental constitution of the individual, the premorbid personality; the emotional impact of the injury; circumstances, setting, and the emotional repercussions of the injury; iatrogenic factors; environmental factors; compensation and litigation; the response of the patient to the intellectual impairments sustained; the development of epilepsy; the amount of brain injury sustained; and the location of that injury.

Smeltzer and colleagues (1994) expanded this list further and included other factors, such as interaction of the effects of the current injury with previous brain insults, expansion of the variety of environmental factors, the presence of legal issues, and the response to the psychical as well as the mental impairments.

What does seem clear is that the organic psychoses including organic delusional disorders are a product at the very least of disordered subcortical-limbic functioning and these are probably closely related to the disturbances thought to responsible for idiopathic schizophrenia (Cummings, 1986; Lichter & Cummings, 2001).

Lesion location and the mechanism of secondary psychotic disorders

Hilbom's (1960) study which we have discussed previously undertook a retrospective review of 3552 Finnish soldiers from World War II. Of these, 33 demonstrated posttraumatic psychosis. Of the 33, 21 (63%) had lesions of the left hemisphere, 9 (26%) to the right hemisphere, and 3 (11%) had damage to both. Forty percent of the soldiers had damage to the temporal lobes. Achte et al. (1969) in a follow-up study of 317 of these patients noted that 23.8% of the localizable lesions were in the frontal lobes while 20.4% were located in the temporal lobes.

Davison and Bagley (1969) reviewed 14 studies that reported posttraumatic psychosis and noted that in a large number of the 40 cases identified, the lesions were diffuse and bilateral (17 cases), nonetheless a still sizable proportion of patients (16) featured left-sided lesions while a smaller proportion (7) had right hemisphere lesions. Fourteen sustained injuries to the temporal lobes while 9 had injuries to the frontal lobes. Davison and Bagley also noted that the onset of the psychosis was more commonly related to diffuse injuries and in those patients who featured coma greater than 24 hours.

Fujii and Ahmed's (1996) study archivally examined the emergence of posttraumatic psychosis in 15 inpatients with histories of delusions and hallucinations following TBI. The majority of these patients (9) featured bilateral abnormalities on imaging studies and of the patients who only featured unilateral lesions, almost twice as many (4) featured left hemisphere lesions as compared to the two patients who featured unilateral right-sided lesions. The modal lesions were of the right temporal region, followed closely by lesions in the left temporal, and then left frontal areas. The majority of the patients surveyed were male (14 male to 1 female) and one third of the sample had a history of documented history of seizures and/or EEG abnormalities of the temporal lobes.

In integrating their data with the available literature, Fujii and Ahmed (1996) noted that their data in association with that of the previous studies indicates that posttraumatic psychosis suggests a preponderance of left-sided lesions, most commonly those associated with the temporal lobe followed by a high percentage of pathology associated with the frontal lobe. However, laterality has been an inconsistent explanatory variable in this literature (as was noted with both anxiety and affective states), although some have suggested that left temporal lesions may more commonly be associated with the schizophrenia-like psychosis of temporal lobe epilepsy (TLE) (Sachdev et al., 2001).

Fujii and Ahmed (2002) noted that the location of the lesions noted on EEG were 16 temporal, 5 frontal, 2 parietal, 5 occipital, 1 central, and 6 diffuse. CT and MRI data on the 36 patients with sufficient data to analyze indicated that there were 23 frontal, 15 temporal, 11 with ventricular enlargement, 10 diffuse cortical, 8 parietal, 6 subcortical, 5 cerebellar, 3 central, and 3 brain stem. Males were over represented in the sample even after correcting for the higher base rate of injuries to males in the TBI literature as discussed in chapter 1.

Once again, the lack of support for the notion of a "biological gradient" noted with the affective and anxiety disorders was similarly not observed in the literature regarding posttraumatic psychosis. Nielsen and colleagues (2002) noted that there was no biologic gradient with regard to the association between TBI and posttraumatic psychosis in those patients who had merely been concussed from those who had sustained severe head injuries. This lack of association was also noted in the study by Achte et al. (1969) who observed ironically that MTBI was more commonly associated with posttraumatic psychosis than were more severe injuries.

With regard to the site and side of the lesions implicated in the development of the psychosis, it is useful to consider the sites that have been implicated in schizophrenia as a means of correlating these with the compromised sites noted in TBI. A wealth of CT and MRI studies have identified dilatation of the lateral and third ventricles, reduced volumes of the frontal and temporal lobes (particularly the hippocampi) and the thalamus, and enlargement of the basal ganglia, particularly the caudate and the globus pallidus. Other regions including the anterior cingulate and the cerebellar vermices have also been implicated (Crowe, 1998; McAllister, 1998; McAllister & Ferrell, 2002).

Functional imaging studies including positron emission tomography (PET), functional magnetic resonance imaging (fMRI), and single-photon emission computed tomography (SPECT) have indicated reduced metabolism in the anterior cingulate (Yücel et al., 2002), the dorsolateral prefrontal cortex (DLPFC) (Buchsbaum, 1995a; Buchsbaum et al., 1992; Weinberger, Berman, & Zec, 1986), the hippocampus and amygdala (Tamminga et al., 1992, Velakoulis et al., 2006) and reduced metabolism in the basal ganglia (Buchsbaum et al., 1992).

Koufen and Hagel (1987) assessed 100 patients who had demonstrated psychosis within the first month following the TBI. Of these, 95 demonstrated EEG abnormalities: 70 were bilateral, 12 patients left sided, and 13 with right-sided foci. The majority of the disturbances were noted in the temporal lobes. The authors concluded that bilateral cerebral compromise was most likely to lead to psychosis following TBI.

However, Smeltzer et al. (1994) questioned this interpretation on a number of grounds, including the fact that the "psychosis" was neither defined nor the mechanism of diagnosis explained, leading Smeltzer and colleagues to conclude that the patients should be more appropriately diagnosed as demonstrating delirium or amnesic syndromes according to the *DSM*.

Summary

It is clear on the basis of the review of the available literature that TBI is a risk factor for the development of psychosis. The frequency of the condition however continues to be rare, and the coincidence of these two diagnoses (i.e., TBI and psychosis) that increase in frequency at the same development period, should suggest further caution with regard to the causative rather than correlational association between the two entities (David & Prince, 2005).

The associations gleaned from the literature suggest that the presentation of the condition would usually occur early following the injury (i.e., within the first two years), and that it is commonly associated with lesions in the frontal and temporal lobes. Males are affected more than females and the presentation more commonly features positive symptoms (hallucinations and delusions) rather than negative ones possibly as the negative symptoms are more likely to be viewed as the chronic effects of a TBI rather than as a part of the schizophrenia spectrum. There does not appear to be a preponderance of evidence to support a genetic predisposition in these patients, although some minor inflation of the propensity has been noted in some studies.

Numerous other complex and interacting factors also influence the development of this condition and the psychosocial effects of the injury cannot be underestimated.

Impaired self-awareness following TBI

It has been clear for quite some time to researchers and clinicians who work in the rehabilitation of individuals following brain injuries including TBI that these individuals have some difficulty in adequately perceiving the changes in cognition, emotion, and personality that may have occurred as a consequence of their injuries (Kendall & Terry, 1996; Levin, 1995; Prigatano, 1991, 1992). For example, Freeland (1996) has observed that up to 45% of individuals with moderate to severe TBI demonstrate deficits in awareness. This section examines the processes involved in these changes.

Background

It has long been known that individuals do not function socially in the same way subsequent to the injury as they did before. Lezak (1978), for example, has spoken of the psychological "death" of the injured subject following the trauma. Not infrequently in clinical practice, the spouse of the injured individual reports that "on the morning of the accident my husband went off to work and he never came home again." These changes in the most subtle aspects of interpersonal exchange probably constitute the fundamental aspect of the change for the family and loved ones following the injury.

McDonald, Flanagan, Rollins, and Kinch (2003) noted that poor social behaviour and communication is a common concomitant of severe TBI and can be characterized by "self-focused conversation without interest in other people, immature and inappropriate humour, frequent interruptions and sudden topic shifts, blunt manner, overly familiar and disinhibited remarks or advances, inappropriate levels of self disclosure, difficulty shifting from a topic and slowness of comprehension" (p. 219). They have also noted problems with social perspective taking in these subjects, as well as difficulties in picking up social inferences despite their normal capacity to interpret sincere conversational interchanges.

Patients with impaired self-awareness (ISA) following injury tend to overestimate their behavioural competencies, particularly with regard to social and emotional functioning (McKinlay & Brooks, 1984), as measured both by self-report and in comparison to the reports of relatives and treaters (Prigatano, 1996; Prigatano, Altman, & O'Brien, 1990). This deficit has been consistently associated with poor treatment motivation and outcome (Lam, McMahon, Priddy, & Gehred-Schultz, 1988; Malec & Moessner, 2000) and long-term employability (Ezrachi, Ben-Yishay, Kay, Diller, & Rattock, 1991; Sherer, Bergloff, Levin et al., 1998; Sherer et al., 2003).

Individuals with TBI are also less likely to complain of changes in judgment, personality, or behaviour following the injury and are reported to be less likely to acknowledge problems with executive functioning (Flashman, Amador, & McAllister, 2005).

The self-reports of these patients with regard to their competencies do not correlate well with their levels of neuropsychological test performance, whereas the reports of relatives and treatment teams do (Prigatano, 1996; Prigatano & Leathem, 1993). Noting a similar result, Allen and Ruff (1990) observed that unimpaired controls tended to overestimate their abilities on some cognitive tasks but not others, while patients with TBI did so consistently and did so to a greater extent on virtually all tasks.

It has also been noted that the consistency of reporting of ISA noted following the injury differs as a function of domain of activity. McKinlay and Brooks (1984) noted that in their sample of 55 patients measured 3, 6, and 12 months postinjury, the patient and family showed concordance in their reporting of sensory impairments, poorer concordance on measures of cognitive functioning, and poorer concordance still on measures of emotional responding with the patients consistently reporting fewer and less severe emotional concerns than did the family. This effect was also noted by Sherer and colleagues (2003) who observed that the patient's self-rating did not correlate well with family, clinician, or significant other rating, although the family and significant other ratings did correlate well with one another. Once again the concordance in the reporting changes between the patients and the significant other or clinician was better for sensory as opposed to cognitive or emotional functioning.

A similar finding was made by Sbordone, Seyranian, and Ruff (1998) who noted that while 58.8% of significant others observed emotional lability or mood swings, only 5.9% of the mild to moderate TBIs reported such changes in themselves. Similarly, 29.4% of the significant others observed circumstantial thinking or loss of train of thought while none of the patients did so. The authors contend that these changes were most likely due to poor awareness on the part of the patients rather than due to psychological denial as they were all engaged in worker's compensation claims, indicating that they would be more likely to endorse impairment for the purpose of compensation seeking.

Prigatano and colleagues (Prigatano & Leathem, 1993; Prigatano, Bruna et al., 1998; Prigatano, Ogano, & Amakusa, 1997) have noted that this result applies across a number of different cultural contexts indicating that the compromise is most likely attributable to an organic rather than to a sociocultural effect. In a cross-cultural study of patients from New Zealand, Prigatano and Leathem (1993) noted that patients with an English ancestry performed in a manner similar to the levels of ISA noted in American samples (Prigatano, 1992; Prigatano & Altman, 1990; Prigatano, Altman, & O'Brien, 1990; Prigatano & Klonoff, 1997) with the patients consistently overestimating their ability to control their emotions as compared to the reports of their relatives. New Zealand patients of Maori origin on the other hand, reported levels of competency far below their relatives' reports or those of their English comparators.

In a subsequent study using Japanese TBI patients, Prigatano and colleagues (Prigatano et al., 1997) noted that these patients overestimated their behavioural competencies as compared to therapist ratings, but not those of relatives. The patients tended to overestimate their self-care skills but not their abilities to interact in socio-emotional situations. The authors also noted that the speed with which the patients performed the Finger Tapping task related to their impaired self-awareness, possibly implicating diffuse axonal injury as the substrate for these behavioural changes. The authors concluded that "patients across cultures with brain dysfunction seem to have reduced insight into their actual level of neuropsychological functioning" (p. 135).

In a further study working with patients with TBI in Spain, Prigatano and colleagues (Prigatano et al., 1998) noted a similar finding to those noted with their North American patients with individuals with TBI rated both by themselves and by significant others as being less competent than controls. The Spanish patients with TBI consistently overestimated their behavioural competency, and the severity of the injury was related to the deficits in self-awareness, supporting the notion that across cultures, self-awareness several months after injury is consistently impaired, possibly indicating that this disturbance may represent a residual effect of the initial disturbance in consciousness associated with the injury.

Prigatano et al. (1997) also noted another interesting clinical finding in the context of the study. The authors noted that "relatives often accurately rate the degree of impairment in other brain dysfunctional patients. However, when asked to make judgments about their own children, they find the task more difficult, at least from the perspective of the rehabilitation staff. When relatives are asked to make specific ratings about their own children, many seem to underestimate the patients' degree of impairment, at least in the neuropsychological rehabilitation setting" (p. 141).

These changes have significant implications to the employment situations that TBI patients may pursue subsequent to the injury often with profound consequence to these individuals and further impact upon their often tenuous postaccident self-esteem. These problems also affect the personal relationships of these individuals, and they often do not recognize how their impulsiveness, capriciousness, irritability, and their angry or childish responses in certain situations may adversely affect their significant others. This culminates in a situation in which they may alienate family or friends and then appear bewildered by how they are so unfairly misjudged and misunderstood (Prigatano, 1991) by them.

Methodological issues

Clearly since changes in emotional and self-awareness behaviours subsequent to injury are more ephemeral and less easily quantified, more exquisite methods for the assessment of these in behaviour are needed to quantify the changes noted for measurement and rehabilitation focus. Skye McDonald (McDonald et al., 2003) and her colleagues, for example, developed a more comprehensive means of assessing impairment in social interaction in TBI patients with their Awareness of Social Inference Test (TASIT).

This battery involves three subtasks: (1) the emotional evaluation test that assesses recognition of spontaneous emotional expression (i.e., happy, surprised, sad, anxious, angry, disgusted, and neutral); and two social inference tasks (2) minimal and (3) enriched. The former assesses the patient's ability to comprehend videotaped exchanges of sincere versus sarcastic communications, and the enriched task assesses the ability of the patient to identify lying versus sarcasm. Their preliminary study with 12 patients with severe TBI noted that the patients were poorer at judging emotions versus controls, and had particular difficulty recognizing the emotions of neutral, fearful, and disgusted items. The patients proved as capable as the controls in understanding lying and sincere exchanges, but had greater difficulty with the sarcasm items.

A number of other more ecologically based approaches to assessment of these deficits have also been pursued. Hart, Giovannetti, Montgomery, and Schwartz (1998) have used tests of naturalistic action (e.g., making toast and wrapping a gift) to evaluate the ability of TBI patients to monitor and self-correct their actions. They noted that their TBI participants showed awareness of proportionally fewer of their errors on these tasks than did the controls. Despite displaying poorer performances on the tasks, the TBI participants did not rate themselves as performing more poorly. The authors noted that the TBI may affect error detection and correction by interfering with the allocation of attentional resources for successfully completing simultaneous monitoring and execution of these tasks.

Questionnaire measures have also been commonly used in this area of study, with the Patient Competency Rating Scale developed by Prigatano and colleagues (Prigatano, Fordyce, Zeiner et al., 1986) the most studied. The more recently developed Awareness Questionnaire (Sherer, Bergloff, Levin et al., 1998) has also been used in a number of studies. Comparison between the two (Sherer et al., 2003) indicates that while the two measures only correlate moderately with each other, they both performed comparably as measures of ISA after TBI. The authors contend that patient/clinician discrepancies appear a more valid measure of ISA early after TBI than do patient/family discrepancies echoing the issue identified by Prigatano (1997) above.

Phenomenology and nosology of impaired self-awareness following TBI

Impaired self-awareness after TBI includes at least two types of reality distortion for the injured individual. The first of these is the impaired awareness of the self following injury. This process is defined by Prigatano (1991) as follows: "This experience of normality despite brain damage, coupled with the simultaneous perception of an altered sense of self, is the clinical definition and manifestation of what is referred to as a disturbance in self-awareness of deficit after traumatic brain injury" (p. 112).

The second and related process that is associated with the disturbance of self-awareness following TBI is unawareness of deficit. This presentation was originally termed anosognosia, which describes the clinical presentation of individuals who as a consequence of nondominant hemisphere injury (usually as a consequence of stroke) may disown or fail to recognize an affected limb, usually on the left side of the body (Lishman, 1997), although a less severe presentation can also be noted with lesions of the left hemisphere (Lebrun, 1987).

In its mildest form, the patient may only show a lack of concern for the disability, attaching little importance to the hemiplegia. When confronted by the change, the patient may minimize the problem and respond in a facetious or flattened manner (anosodiaphoria). In the more compete presentation, the patient may ignore the compromise completely, making no complaint about the disability and ignoring the implications of the change (Lishman, 1997).

Prigatano and Johnson (2003) have taken these observations a step further in their description of the three vectors of consciousness. Developing on the original work of Zeman (2001) they describe three meanings of the word consciousness. The first of these refers to the waking state spanning from being alert through drowsiness and then on to sleep. The second meaning is the concept of "consciousness of experience" (Prigatano & Johnson, 2003, p. 14) and by this they mean the content of personal experience from moment to moment. The third meaning is "consciousness of mind" (Prigatano & Johnson, 2003, p. 14) by which they mean any mental state with a propositional content.

Prigatano and Johnson (2003) contend that each of these aspects of consciousness can be affected by TBI. In the first sense, it affects arousal and alertness and when this aspect is disturbed, the individual can become hyperaroused, confused, and unable to respond meaningfully to the world. Compromise in the second vector is consistent with frank anosognosia as discussed above. Compromise of the third vector culminates in compromise in "the patient's 'insight' and judgment" of other people's mental states as their own. This is the third dimension of consciousness that Zeman (2001) identifies. It touches on what is *not* being discussed as the "theory of mind" (Prigatano & Johnson, 2003, p. 16). The authors conclude that each of the disturbances of consciousness can and does occur as a result of TBI including speculations about how these might be distinguished neuroanatomically as well as in having important implications for interventions with these individuals. This model represents an excellent synthesis of the various constructs of altered awareness following injury and how these might be sensibly integrated.

Prevalence and incidence of impaired self-awareness following TBI

The first paper that appeared in the literature on the presentation of impairment in the social perception of emotion in other people was by Prigatano and Pribram (1982). In this study, the authors noted that using the Ekman and Friesen (1976) stimulus pictures that greater misperceptions of facial affect was associated with posterior as compared to anterior lesions. Both bilateral and unilateral frontal lesions were associated with deficits in the memory of facial affect, but there did not seem to be any effect for side of lesion associated with perception or memory of facial affect. However, right frontal lesions seemed to particularly disrupt the recall of facial emotion.

The study also divided the patients based on having either a closed head injury (10 patients) or cerebrovascular accident (CVA) and tumour (7 and 3 respectively). The head-injured participants performed less accurately than the other clinical group indicating that closed head injury (CHI) patients were inferior to controls and other brain injured patients in their perception of facial affect. All clinical groups could determine the affect of happy and angry faces more easily than sad or fearful ones.

Prigatano and Pribram's (1982) study was subsequently replicated and expanded by Jackson and Moffat (1987) using 15 patients who had suffered severe head injuries and comparing these to 15 age- and IQ-matched controls. They noted that head-injured patients were impaired in their recognition of mood as presented in visual static images. The authors noted that head-injured patients may feature disproportionate impairment on tasks that measure emotional recognition from facial expression that was not specific to the mood conveyed by facial or postural cues.

Interestingly, as well as showing impaired performance relative to controls on the number of items correct, the TBI-affected patients also proved less able to identify negative as compared to positive emotions. The authors noted that TBI is associated with an impairment in the ability to accurately recognize social cues as portrayed by facial emotion and that this impairment may "promote the maintenance and possibly the genesis, of poor social skills and antisocial behavior commonly found following severe closed head injury" (p. 298).

On the related function of empathy, Grattan and Eslinger (1989) note that their patients with brain injury scored lower on an empathy scale than did the controls and at six months following the TBI, the patients reported fewer empathic responses as compared to preinjury levels, a behavioral change that was confirmed by their relatives. Milders, Fuchs, and Crawford (2003) have interpreted this failure as signaling possible deficits in theory of mind, "the ability to recognize and make inferences about other people's intentions and mental states" (p. 159), the third vector of consciousness described by Prigatano and Johnson (2003) above.

Spell and Frank (2000) examined the ability of TBI patients to recognize facial emotion and vocal prosody in 24 patients and matched controls and once again noted deficits in the perception of facial emotion in the clinical group. However, the two groups were not matched on neutral facial processing tasks leaving open the possibility, although an unlikely one, that the effect may have been due to task difficulty (Green, Turner, & Thompson, 2004).

Milders et al. (2003) noted that TBI patients were impaired in their ability to recognize expression in the face and voice, in detecting social faux pas, and on a single measure of cognitive flexibility, the Ruff Figural Fluency Test (Ruff, 1996). The TBI patients also demonstrated increased levels of unusual and inappropriate behaviours, increased depression, apathy, withdrawal, and diminution of communicative ability.

These researchers proposed a framework for interpreting social behavior disturbances following TBI that they drew from the schizophrenia literature (Corrigan, 1997). They contend that "inadequate social behaviour could result from: (1) insensitivity to important social cues, such as emotional expressions; (2) impaired understanding of social situations and other people's intentions; and (3) failures to adjust one's behaviour in accordance with social rules and demands" (p. 169). They note that in their own study of this issue the problem underlying the deficits was most closely associated with impairment of the ability to understand social situations and the intentions of others, consistent with much of the literature reviewed above.

Evolution of impaired self-awareness following TBI

In a recent study, Green et al. (2004) investigated the effects of acute rather than chronic effects of TBI were considered in 30 TBI participants and 30 age-matched controls on a task measuring accuracy of neutral and emotional face perception (i.e., from the Florida Affect Battery of Bowers) (Blonder & Heilman, 1989). The TBI group performed less accurately than the controls on the facial emotion perception tasks but equivalently on the nonemotional component of the task. Nonfocally injured subjects (i.e., patients with diffuse white matter lesions) were as impaired on the tasks as those with lesions in the cortical regions considered to be implicated in facial emotions deficits (i.e., posterior right hemisphere). The authors concluded that diffuse axonal injury of itself could be a sufficient lesion to produce impairment in facial emotion processing, supporting the notion that the function is subserved by a modular representation that could be disrupted by damage to processing centres or to the interaction of the various centres responsible for the complex behavioural function.

Lesion location and mechanism of action of impaired self-awareness following TBI

Many of the studies of emotional processing subsequent to brain injuries have focused on the issue of the location of a lesion necessary to produce disorders in this function. A number of studies in the non-TBI literature have implicated the posterior parts of the right hemisphere (e.g., Adolphs, Damasio, Tranel, & Damasio, 1996; Borod, 1996; Strauss & Moscovitch, 1981) and advocate a critical role particularly for the right somatosensory cortices (Adolphs, Damasio, Tranel, Cooper, & Damasio, 2000) and the right mesial anterior infracalcarine cortex (Adolphs et al., 1996).

A number of studies have also implicated the amygdala (Adolphs, Tranel, Damasio, & Damasio, 1994; Calder, Young et al., 1996) based on the model of Le Doux (1996). However, studies have produced equivocal findings on the role of the frontal cortex. Those tasks that have shown a strong loading on the frontal lobes tend to be the ones that have an explicit verbal encoding requirement such as verbal labeling (Adolphs et al., 2000; Kawasaki et al., 2001; Keane, Calder, Hodges, & Young, 2002) but not for more conceptual tasks of emotional evaluation (Adolphs et al., 2000).

Hornak, Rolls, and Wade (1996) noted that patients with lesions of the ventral prefrontal area who had been rated by nursing staff as showing poor ability to recognize other people's moods demonstrated impairment on a recognition test of emotional expressions. The association between the task performance and the functional ability was significantly correlated. Other investigators (Adolphs et al., 2000; Kawasaki et al., 2001; Keane et al., 2002) observed similar results implicating the orbitofrontal region, the operculum, and the superior medial and anterior regions of the cingulate.

Not too surprisingly, given the role of the frontal lobes in planning, anticipation, and error utilization as well as the role of the ventromedial prefrontal lobes in emotional and cognitive integration as adverted to by the somatic marker hypothesis (Damasio, 1994), the tasks that best predict social reintegration following injury are those that tap into frontal executive functioning.

Villki et al. (1994) noted that performance of patients with TBI on tasks of cognitive flexibility predict their return to work and social activity following the injury. Tate (1999) noted that rule breaking errors on tests of verbal fluency (Crowe, 1992) proved a good indicator of impulsive behaviour and restlessness both as rated behaviorally as well as the levels endorsed by relatives. Patients who were rated as less empathic towards others were also those who performed worst on tests of cognitive flexibility, however, there was no relationship with performance on tests of intelligence or memory (Grattan & Eslinger, 1989).

The fact that TBI is often associated with compromise in white matter integrity as discussed in chapter 2, has implicated this process in the mechanism of emotional processing (e.g., Adolphs et al., 1996, 2000; Green et al., 2004), particularly those regions that surround and connect the occipital and somatosensory cortices implicated in facial emotion processing.

Conclusion

Disorders of self-awareness have a number of implications for the rehabilitation of the individual following the TBI. If the patient does not recognize his or her altered cerebral function as a result of the injury, he or she may continue to produce inappropriate responses, without any modification in these behaviours contingent upon feedback. Whilst insight is not essential for ameliorating these behavioural responses (e.g., Sohlberg, Mateer, Penkman, Glang, & Todis, 1998), the deeper and more integrated the understanding of the behaviour one achieves the greater the likelihood that it will be generalized to other situations (Kent, 1999). Similarly if he or she is not capable of empathically and sympathetically responding to the emotional and social cues provided by significant others this will result in miscommunication and resentment on the part of the interlocutor. These changes will significantly affect both the work situation that they choose following the injury (if they are capable of assuming such a role), but also in continuing in socially inappropriate and ineffective behaviours leading to further loneliness, stigmatization, and opprobrium in social situations.

A second implication of these disorders is their impact upon the integration of cognitive and emotional components of experience (Prigatano, 1991; Prigatano & Johnson, 2003). It is clear that the ability to be able to recognize postinjury changes is not unitary and these patients are often more aware of their physical and sensory changes subsequent to the injury as well as their ability to perform activities of daily living rather than of their cognitive, social, emotional, or behavioural functioning. Lack of awareness is not an all or nothing thing, so injury-related problems may persist due to the underestimation or minimization of their implications (Hart et al., 1998). The collection of changes for the TBI patient thus presents a complex set of interactive social and emotional forces operating on an individual whose social and emotional repertoire is already depleted as a direct and pervasive effect of the injury.

7 Reality distortion following TBI (2):

Abnormal illness behaviour including the factitious disorders, the somatoform disorders, and malingering

At some point in the evaluation of every individual who has sustained a traumatic brain injury (TBI) the question arises: Are the responses and the behaviour of this individual in this circumstance consistent with an actual emotional or behavioural disorder as a consequence of the injury, or are the observed deficits due to some other cause? In the context of the almost inevitable medico-legal disputation that ensues following a head injury (in which sizeable sums of money may be at stake) the degree to which the individual may be either consciously or unconsciously faking brain damage or, more euphemistically, not performing to the best of his or her ability, must be entertained.

This issue has been succinctly put by Miller (1983) who observes:

> If damage in structure X is known to produce a decline on test T it is tempting to argue that any new subject, or group of subjects, having a relatively poor performance on T must have a lesion at X. In fact the logical status of this argument is the same as reasoning that because a horse meets the test of being a large animal with four legs then any newly encountered large animal with four legs must be a horse. The newly encountered specimen could of course be a cow or a hippopotamus and still meet the same test. Similarly new subjects who do badly on T may do so for reasons other than having a lesion at X. (p. 131)

Failure on tests of psychological functioning may occur as a consequence of a number of factors, and the clinician must be constantly alert to the various possible causes of poor performance. In patients with behavioural or emotional disorders this caution is doubly appropriate due to the effects of medication, compliance, motivation and preoccupation.

Any suggestion that such a concern may be one relegated to the "bad old days" before neuropsychology was forced to reexamine itself in the context of the seminal work of Ziskin, Rodgers, and Faust is demonstrated by the very concern raised by Miller (1983) in the recent paper of Sterr, Herron, Hayward, and Montaldi (2006). In discussing the possibility of persisting deficit in mild traumatic brain injury (MTBI) patients with and without postconcussional syndrome (PCS), Sterr et al. note:

> It therefore appears plausible to assume that microstructural damage can persist, and that this tissue damage may form the pathophysiological foundation of the

> persisting sequelae some MTBI patients' experience. This assumption gives rise to the hypothesis that the neural damage affects information processing, and henceforth the prediction that only those MTBI patients who suffer chronic PCS symptoms show neurobehavioral deficits. (p. 2)

Regarding the summary of their findings Sterr et al. (2006) also note:

> A correlation was found between PCS symptom severity and test performance suggesting that participants with more pronounced PCS symptoms performed worse in cognitive tasks. In contrast, MTBI patients with no PCS showed performance similar to matched controls. We further found that loss of consciousness, a key criterion for PCS diagnosis, was not predictive of sustained PCS.
>
> Conclusion: The results support the idea that MTBI can have sustained consequences, and that the subjectively experienced symptoms and difficulties in everyday situations are related to objectively measurable parameters in cognitive function. (p. 1)

It seems that once again, unfortunately, the cow and the hippopotamus are being mistaken for the horse!

Methodological issues

Assessment in patients with a psychiatric diagnosis is a difficult task even for well-experienced clinicians (Crowe, 1998b). However, this problem is quadrupled if there are extramural forces at work in the form of compensation seeking, lack of motivation, or the attempted evasion of criminal responsibility. Let us now examine some of the issues underlying this difficult clinical conundrum.

Phenomenology and nosology of abnormal illness behaviour following TBI

A number of definitional issues surround this area and it seems worthwhile to clarify some of these before we go further. *DSM-IV-TR* (APA, 2000) defines somatoform disorders as "a pattern of recurring multiple, clinically significant somatic complaints" (p. 486). This description is reserved for those conditions in which the physical symptoms suggest a general medical condition but are not fully explained by that general medical condition. The Manual draws a distinction between somatoform disorders and factitious disorders and malingering in that, in the former case, the symptoms are not intentional or under voluntary control.

The Manual indicates that the common features of the somatoform disorders include: (1) the presence of subjective physical symptoms that suggest a medical illness or syndrome that is not fully explained by or attributable to a general medical condition, substance abuse, or other type of mental disorder; and (2) the absence of voluntary control over symptomatology (APA, 2000).

The Manual suggests that there are a number of entities under the umbrella of somatoform disorders including somatisation disorder, undifferentiated somatoform disorder, conversion disorder, pain disorder, hypochondriasis, body dysmorphic disorder, and those somatoform disorders not otherwise specified. Readers should consult *DSM-IV-TR* (APA, 2000) for a full description of these conditions.

Somatisation disorder features a history of multiple unexplained symptoms and complaints beginning before the age of 25 that can often be traced to events and circumstances that emerge in childhood and adolescence (APA, 2000). The symptoms of the condition can mimic other syndromes such as PCS or posttraumatic stress disorder (PTSD) or may be more florid with an atypical or bizarre pattern of quality, location, or duration (Miller, 2001). Insofar as it is possible to ascertain the underlying motivation for this presentation, the behaviour is frequently inferred to be a plea for support and reassurance, manipulation of the affection of a significant other, or a quest for the satisfaction of dependency needs by reliance on caretakers (Miller, 2001).

The coincidence of a TBI with somatoform disorder may result in a pattern of presentation on the part of the individual that may indicate a pattern of malingering and somatoform disorders—most notably somatisation disorder, conversion disorder, and pain disorders—should be considered in the differential diagnosis of these patients following TBI.

Conversion disorder is of particular interest in the context of a past history of TBI as the conditions affect voluntary motor or sensory functions that suggest a neurological or other general medical condition. Miller (2001) contends that the unconscious motivation underlying this presentation involves the attempt to resolve intrapsychic conflicts such as dependency issues by channelling them into physical impairment. There may also be an actual symbolic "conversion" of an intrapsychic conflict that is represented by the somatic expression: for example, the paralysis of an arm in a patient who fears acting upon a hostile impulse (Miller, 2001) or hysterical aphonia in a patient who fears the outcome of what may come from the mouth.

Conversion disorder can be difficult to discern from actual illness and common misdiagnoses may emerge in conditions that are relatively ambiguous on presentation such as myasthenia gravis, idiopathic dystonia, or multiple sclerosis (APA, 2000). Typically, the presence of actual neurological disorder does not preclude the diagnosis of conversion disorder and up to one third of individuals with conversion symptoms have a previous diagnosis of a neurological condition. The distinction between conversion disorder and malingering may merely be the absence of intentional production of the symptoms.

One of the interesting features of conversion disorder is that the symptoms typically do not conform to the usual anatomical or physiological patterns. For example, a paralysis may be in the form or a glove or stocking distribution and may be delimited by perceived boundaries rather than anatomical ones (the wrist for example) whilst the distribution of the anaesthesia and their responsivity to particular forms of sensory stimulation do not accord with anatomical reality. The patient may also show little apparent anxiety or concern about the apparently massively debilitating nature of his or her presented problems, a situation that Charcot (1825–1893) originally referred to as "la belle indifference" (beautiful indifference).

Factitious disorders are characterized by either psychological or physical symptoms that are intentionally produced with the view of fulfilling a sick role. The *DSM-IV-TR*

(APA, 2000) divides the factitious disorders into (1) factitious disorder with predominantly physical signs and symptoms, and (2) factitious disorder with predominantly psychological signs and symptoms. The former category includes chronic factitious disorder with physical symptoms that has been historically referred to as Munchausen Syndrome, a presentation named after the legendary Baron Munchausen, who undertook fantastic travels and celebrated extravagant tales of his own prowess as described in the book by Rudolf Raspe (1859). This condition is characterised by an "illness" that revolves around a lifestyle focussing on hospitalization, surgeries, and contentious battles with physicians (Cunnien, 1997). Factitious PCS can be noted in the differential diagnosis of individuals with TBI (Cunnien, 1997).

The diagnosis of factitious disorder with psychological symptoms denotes a presentation of intentionally produced psychological symptoms without any identifiable external incentive (APA, 2000). It is the issue of "external incentive" that is used to differentiate the condition from malingering, however, as noted by Cunnien (1997, p. 25): "The mere presence of external gains cannot negate the primacy of psychological motives." Clearly, both psychological and other incentives can co-exist and behaviours can be motivated by both external and internal gain.

Chronic factitious disorder with psychological symptoms has been historically referred to as Ganser Syndrome, a mixture of organic, affective, and psychotic symptoms (Miller, 2001) that includes clouding of consciousness, hallucination, hysterical conversion, and a strange pattern of cognitive impairment featuring "approximate answers" (e.g., 2 + 2 = 5). Nowadays the full spectrum of the presentation is rarely seen, and the diagnosis is made based largely on the presence of the approximate answers alone (Miller, 2001).

Ganser Syndrome was originally described in 1898 by Sigbert Ganser after attending three patients who featured the characteristic "Ganser" response. These are sometimes referred to as answers past the point or approximate answers. The patient's responses to questions are markedly inaccurate and often absurdly so. However, they betray knowledge of purpose of the question by their close approximation to the correct answer and imply that this, too, is available at some level.

To prevent massive overdiagnosis, the proviso was added that the false response although wrong is never far wrong and bears a definite and obvious relationship to the correct answer, indicating clearly that the patient has grasped the question. The apparent dementia that accompanies the approximate answers is usually incomplete, inconsistent, and often self-contradictory. Disorientation is invariably present, but the apparently gross disturbance of intellect is not reflected in the patient's overall behaviour.

Prevalence and incidence of abnormal illness behaviour following TBI

The factitious disorders are rarely seen and are diagnosed in less than one percent of referrals to psychiatric services (Cunnien, 1997). The lifetime prevalence for somatisation disorder ranges between 0.2 and 2% among women and less than 0.2% among men (APA, 2000), while conversion disorder occurs in about 1–3% of outpatient referrals to metal health clinics. These figures compare very unfavourably with the frequency with which a diagnosis of malingering is made (see below) and the number of cases of the various factitious and somatisation disorders is a literal drop in the ocean when compared to the estimated and guesstimated numbers of cases of malingering.

Evolution of abnormal illness behaviour following TBI

The factitious disorders are distinguished from malingering by the fact that with malingering the individual is producing the symptoms intentionally and he or she has a clear goal in mind (i.e., financial gain, evading imprisonment) whereas overt incentives are absent in factitious disorders.

Cullum, Heaton, and Grant (1991) proposed that the distinction between primary and secondary gain is somewhat artificial and they prefer the notion of gain of itself, irrespective of whether the benefit is conscious or unconscious. It follows from their suggestion that all psychologically determined symptoms involve gain. In somatoform disorders this involves anxiety reduction and a symbolic statement of the disorder that is unconsciously determined. In the case of factitious disorders there is a conscious attempt to adopt the sick role to avoid an emotional conflict. In malingering the activity is again under conscious control and is directed towards a demonstrable and tangible benefit.

These conditions are characterized by the fact that they do not have a biological origin. The malady is, by definition, a misinterpretation or embellishment of the usually observed pattern of disorder associated with a given diagnosis. The tendency to invoke the notion of the subconscious or the unconscious is popular in explanations of these phenomena. It is difficult to ascertain how informative these approaches actually are, as rarely does this area result in extensive research, exploration, or theory generation. This problem has not prevented a huge explosion of studies reported in the literature on the issue of malingering and impaired effort, but much of this literature focuses upon the identification of nongenuine response sets rather than in trying to come to grips with the mechanism or underlying cause of the behaviour other than the completely obvious. This problem is exacerbated as the gold standard for identification of malingering, for example, can only occur based on self-report, and the number of individuals prepared to "crack" under Perry Mason's incisive interrogation on the witness stand is relatively low.

In these types of cases, the evidence obtained from neuropathology and structural and functional imaging results in a diagnosis by exclusion. It is the X-ray or computed tomography (CT), magnetic resonance imaging (MRI), or single-photon emission computed tomography (SPECT) scans that indicate *no abnormality* in the examinee who is to all intents and purposes severely impaired that raises the index of concern.

One matter on which all investigators who study these conditions do agree is that conversion symptoms occur much more frequently in women than they do in men (Boffeli & Guze, 1992). Whether this observation occurs as a consequence of sex differences at a biological, psychological, or social level is difficult to ascertain.

Due to the fact that the somatoform, factitious, and dissociative disorders are each due to an interpretation on the part of the patient of what neurological and neuropsychological symptoms *should* look like, they do not conform in any consistent way to the usual patterns of *actual* behavioural and emotional disorder. Description in the literature has indicated a tendency by patients to focus on particular aspects of cognitive or psychological functioning, an approach that is usually based upon their previous knowledge and understanding of what a particular neurological or neuropsychological disorder should look like.

Lesion location and mechanism of the abnormal illness behaviour following TBI

To understand the mechanism of the action of these disorders, it is necessary to understand the knowledge and the sophistication of the subject who suffers from them. Clearly the more experienced and knowledgeable the subject is, the more likely that their symptomatology will look real. The subject who has had previous exposure to a friend or relative with Broca's aphasia, for example, is likely to present with agrammatism and halting speech; the client who has seen Alzheimer's disease at close quarters is more likely to present with amnesia, aphasia, apraxia, and agnosia.

This is not to gainsay the fact that even relatively naïve individuals with relatively little motivation can manufacture convincing evidence of psychiatric disorder at least on self-report measures. As noted in the discussion of PTSD in chapter 4, Lees-Haley and Dunn (1994) found that 99% of untutored undergraduates could achieve a performance satisfying *DSM-IV* criteria for PTSD on a symptom checklist. Burges and McMillan (2001) noted a similar level of endorsement and observed that 94% of their sample of 136 night class college students could satisfy the criteria of PTSD after being read a vignette. Clearly it is possible for relatively untrained individuals with little or no knowledge of PTSD to fake responses on symptom checklists sufficient to achieve the diagnosis. It is anybody's guess how convincing a highly motivated individual facing a large financial settlement or the avoidance of prison or military duty might be capable of appearing.

With regard to the issue of the tendency of clients to embroider their clinical symptomatology, the technique of assessment, reassessment, and assessment yet again that is characteristic of our adversarial legal system almost begs the client to overpresent and embroider his or her symptoms. Most assessors ask the same set of questions and generally, since the assessor has asked the question so often before, the answers are virtually written down before the client has even responded.

The traumatically brain-injured subject invariably complains of problems with memory, attention, irritability, tiredness, and vague depressive and anxious mentation. The assessor is astounded if the subject does not complain of these and if he or she does not, the assessor will invariably ask why not. In this context it is quite easy for the injured subject to learn how to play the game and present the most "convincing" set of symptoms to achieve the desired outcome.

As noted above, the likelihood of an increase in the presentation of psychologically based factitious disorders is a growing clinical reality. If we consider these symptoms a cry for help, then the fact that a glove or stocking anaesthesia can be immediately dismissed by the general practitioner (GP) as a clear attempt at attention seeking, will result in the lessened likelihood of the presentation of such a symptom in the future due to its ineffectiveness in eliciting the desired outcome. The presence of ongoing compromise following mild traumatic brain injury (MTBI), chronic unremitting tiredness, ongoing pain, prolonged reactions to commonly encountered products and chemicals, or the presence of migrainous headaches may result in a more sympathetic hearing on the part of the GP and, as a consequence, validation of the problems by the world.

Dissociative disorders are characterized by the disruption of the flow of consciousness, memory, identity, or perception of the environment, including such patterns of disorder as dissociative amnesia, dissociative fugue, dissociative identity disorder, and depersonalization disorder. (Readers should consult *DSM-IV-TR* for a full description of these conditions.) This symptom occurs most commonly in the context of the anxiety disorders, most notably PTSD, and is considered in the discussion of this condition in chapter 4.

Malingering

As Rogers (1997) has cogently noted

> Diagnoses of the mental disorders and the evaluation of psychopathology rely heavily on the honesty, accuracy, and completeness of patients' self-reporting. Most symptoms of disorders are not directly observable by others. Therefore each patient's presentation becomes a critical component of the clinical assessment. Distortions, both intentional and unintentional, complicate the assessment process. (p. 1)

Mankind has been interested in the notion of malingering from our earliest history and reports of malingering go back at least as far as the ancient Greeks (Brussel & Hitch, 1943) and the ancient rabbis of the second century BCE (Nies & Sweet, 1994). The word "malingering" was first defined in Grove's *Dictionary of the Vulgar Tongue* in 1785 (Brussel & Hitch, 1943) in the military context as "one who under the pretence of illness evades his duty." Bailey (1998) contends that the word malingerer derives from the term *malingroux*, a word used to describe the practices of eighteenth century French beggars who injured themselves for financial gain.

The *DSM-IV-TR* (APA, 2000) includes malingering as a V-Code under the category of Other Conditions which may be a Focus of Clinical Attention. Thus, while the condition is considered to be worthy of clinical attention, it is not considered a mental disorder per se (Slick, Sherman, & Iverson, 1999).

The Manual (APA, 2000) defines malingering as "the intentional production of false or grossly exaggerated physical or psychological symptoms, motivated by external incentives such as avoiding military duty, avoiding work, obtaining financial compensation, evading criminal prosecution, or obtaining drugs.... Malingering should be strongly suspected if any combination of the following is noted:

(1) Medico-legal context of presentation (e.g., the person is referred by an attorney for examination).
(2) Marked discrepancy between the person's claimed stress or disability and the objective findings.
(3) Lack of cooperation during the diagnostic evaluation and in complying with the prescribed treatment regimen.
(4) The presence of Antisocial Personality disorder.

> Malingering differs from Factitious Disorders in that the motivation for the symptom production in Malingering is an external incentive, whereas with the factitious disorders the external incentive is absent. Evidence of an intrapsychic need to maintain the sick role suggests Factitious Disorder. Malingering is differentiated from Conversion Disorder and other Somatoform Disorders by the intentional production of symptoms and by the obvious, external incentives associated with it. (pp. 739–740)

Thus, the notion of malingering refers to a voluntary production or exaggeration of symptoms with a view to presenting oneself as worse than one actually is to achieve a demonstrable and predictable gain. In the psychoanalytic tradition, gain has generally been divided into primary versus secondary gain. Primary gain is considered to represent the reduction in anxiety and relief generated by the unconscious emotional conflict. Secondary gain describes the psychosocial benefit of the sick role including such things as release from unpleasant responsibility, increased personal attention and sympathy, and financial reward. As noted above (Cullum et al., 1991), the actual basis on which determination of the source of the conflict is made is at best tenuous, so acceptance of the fact that motivation to achieve a particular outcome by illness behaviour is probably the most economical account of the behaviour.

There have, however, been a number of problems identified with regard to the criteria proposed by the Manual. These include: difficulty with judging the difference between external versus psychological incentives and volitional versus unconscious behaviours; the specification that if the client presents with one of the other somatoform disorders (e.g., conversion or factitious disorder) this precludes the dual diagnosis of somatoform disorder and malingering; and the fact that the criteria were developed in the context of psychiatric presentations, thus making the application of these in nonpsychiatric patients (i.e., patients with TBI) more difficult to apply (Slick et al., 1999).

Most clinicians would agree that malingering can be regarded as unlikely if data from a variety of sources (i.e., serial testing/consistency with actual behaviour) confirm the test findings. Inconsistent results in the examination, evidence of lying or exaggeration during the interview, poor performance on tests of an autobiographical nature, and a level of performance below that usually expected given the nature of the injury can be viewed as warning signs but must, of themselves, be regarded as inconclusive.

Price and Stevens (1997, p. 79) prepared a list of ten signs and symptoms that they consider indicate increased likelihood of malingering in traumatically brain-injured subjects. These include:

(1) An eagerness to discuss or call attention to symptoms in an overly dramatic manner.
(2) Making false imputations about valid symptoms.
(3) Endorsing symptoms rarely found in credible patients with head trauma and reporting improbable numbers of symptoms.
(4) Simulating positive symptoms more often than negative symptoms.
(5) Endorsing more blatant than subtle brain injury symptoms.
(6) Endorsing symptoms that are of unusually extreme severity, even if bizarre and ridiculous.
(7) Reporting symptoms, performing tasks, or failing to perform tasks that are inconsistent with their own previous reports, reports from others or observations of their behaviour in other situations.
(8) Presenting a constellation of signs and symptoms that are inconsistent with a recognizable brain injury and demonstrating a course of the alleged injury that is contrary to the development of actual injuries.
(9) An eagerness to endorse new symptoms suggested by the neuropsychologist.
(10) Focusing on his or her perceived disability rather than the alleged injury and rarely mentioning or acknowledging his or her abilities or capacity (p. 79).

Mittenberg, Patton, Canyock, and Condit (2002) noted similar diagnostic impressions that support a diagnosis of probable malingering or symptom exaggeration including: a severity or pattern of cognitive impairment that is inconsistent with the condition; scores below cut-off on forced choice or other forms of malingering tests; discrepancies between records, self-report, and observed behaviour; implausible symptoms reported in the interview; implausible changes in test scores over repeated examinations; scores above validity scale cut-offs on objective personality tests; and scores below chance on forced choice tests.

In an attempt to expand and formalize these criteria Slick et al. (1999, pp. 552–555) proposed a set of research diagnostic criteria on which they contend a diagnosis of malingering can be made. For a diagnosis of definite Malingering Neurocognitive Deficit (MND) the authors propose:

(1) The presence of a substantial external incentive [Criterion A].
(2) Definite negative response bias [Criterion B].
(3) Behaviors meeting necessary criteria for group B are not fully accounted for by Psychiatric, Neurological or Developmental Factors [Criterion D] (p. 552).

For Probable MND:

(1) The presence of a substantial external incentive [Criterion A].
(2) Two or more types of evidence from neuropsychological evidence from neuropsychological testing, excluding definite negative response bias [two or more of Criteria B2-B6].

Or

(1) One type of evidence from neuropsychological testing, excluding definite negative response bias, and one or more types of evidence from Self-Report [one of Criteria B2-B6 and one or more of Criteria C1-C5].
(2) Behaviors meeting necessary criteria for group B and C are not fully accounted for by Psychiatric, Neurological, or Developmental Factors [Criterion D] (pp. 552–553).

For Possible MND:

(1) The presence of a substantial external incentive [Criterion A].
(2) Evidence from Self-Report [one of more of Criteria C1-C5].
(3) Behaviors meeting necessary criteria for group C are not fully accounted for by Psychiatric, Neurological or Developmental Factors [Criterion D].

Or

(1) Criteria for Definite or Probable MND are met except for Criterion D (i.e., primary psychiatric, neurological or developmental etiologies cannot be ruled out). In such cases, the alternate etiologies that cannot be rules out should be specified (p. 553).

For Criterion A there must be evidence for at least one clear and identifiable incentive for exaggeration or fabrication, for example a personal injury settlement, disability pension, evasion of criminal prosecution or release from military service. For Criterion B there must be evidence of exaggeration or fabrication on neuropsychological testing as demonstrated by: (1) definite negative response; (2) probable negative responses bias; (3) a discrepancy between the test data and known patterns of brain functioning; (4) observed behaviour; (5) reliable collateral reports; or (6) documented background history. Criterion C focuses on evidence from self-report that is noted to be discrepant from (1) documented history, (2) known patterns of brain functioning, (3) behavioural observations, (4) information obtained from collateral informants or (5) evidence of exaggerated or fabricated psychological dysfunction. Criterion D indicates that the observed behaviours are not otherwise explained by intercurrent psychiatric, neurological, or developmental factors.

Two possible means of identifying exaggeration or fabrication of cognitive dysfunction have been discussed in the literature. The first set of techniques involves the evaluation of exaggeration of the reporting of symptoms most commonly by using questionnaire measures such as the MMPI, and the second by identifying poor motivation and/or effort on tests of neuropsychological functioning (Larrabee, 2000, 2005).

The MMPI has long been regarded as a sensitive measure for the detection of deviant response sets. The F Scale, F-K index, the Gough Dissimulation Index, and the Fake Bad Scale, as well as checking the 16 repeated items all represent reasonable means of detecting exaggerated symptomatology, malingering, and random or feigned responses (Etcoff & Kampfer, 1996; Shores & Carstairs, 1998).

A rich literature has developed on the use of the MMPI and MMPI-2 as a means of assessing malingering in forensic and brain-injury settings (e.g., Arbisi & Ben-Porath,

1995; Berry, 1998; Berry, Baer, & Harris, 1991; Berry & Butcher, 1998; Berry, Wetter et al., 1995; Gandolfo, 1995; Larrabee, 1998, 2005; Lees-Haley, 1992, 1997; Lees-Haley, English, & Glenn, 1991; Rogers, Sewell, & Salekin, 1994; Rogers, Sewell, & Ustad, 1995; Tsushima & Tsushima, 2001; Wetter, Baer, Berry, Smith, & Larsen, 1992) Readers should consult this literature for more detailed discussions of the malingering issues.

Exaggeration of symptom reporting on the MMPI-2 can be assessed using the following scales F, Back F, Variable Response Inconsistency (VRIN), True Response Inconsistency (TRIN), Infrequency Psychopathology Scale and exaggerated somatic symptomatology can be assessed by noting elevations over T 79 on Scales 1 and 3, plus elevated Lees-Haley Fake Bad Scale (Larrabee, 2000, 2001, 2005).

Exaggerated psychopathology can be evaluated using the F, F-K, Back F, and the Arbisi and Ben-Porath (1995) F (p). VRIN is considered useful for ruling out random responding as a cause of elevated F (Wetter et al., 1992). Psychopathology tends to be exaggerated more commonly in settings where malingering obviates responsibility for mandatory duties such as military service or the consequences of prosecution for alleged crimes (Larrabee, 2000, 2001, 2005).

Although exaggerated psychopathology does occur in personal injury settings, it is more typical for these patients to exaggerate their somatic, affective, and cognitive complaints, producing significant elevations on MMPI-2 scales 1, 2, and 3 with secondary elevations on 7 and 8 (Larrabee, 2000, 2001, 2005). The F scale and related measures are not sensitive to this type of malingering (Larrabee, 1998; Millis & Kler, 1995) and detecting this type of exaggeration is most effective using the Lees-Haley Fake Bad Scale (Lees-Haley, 1992).

Evaluating poor motivation and/or effort on neuropsychological testing is determined by three means: observation of poor performance on tasks that are easily performed by injured individuals who are not litigating, evaluation of patterns of responding characteristic of malingering, and symptom validity testing using a forced choice methodology (Larrabee, 2000, 2005).

The typical example of tasks that are easily performed by nonlitigating persons who have bonafide neurological disorder include the early malingering tests developed by the French neurologist André Rey (1964), including the Rey 15 Item Test and the Dot Counting Test. These tasks were developed to appear as if they measured an actual cognitive function such as memory, but are consistently performed in an unimpaired fashion by nonlitigating patients who have brain impairment, making impaired performance appear highly suspicious. Whilst the principle underlying their development is sound, their sensitivity and specificity to malingering tends to be low as compared to other procedures (e.g., Greiffenstein, Baker, & Gola, 1996; Schretlen, Brandt, Krafft, & Van Gorp, 1991; Spreen & Strauss, 1998; Vallabhajosula & Van Gorp, 2001).

The second technique involves the application of pattern analysis. This approach determines impaired motivation by detecting score patterns that are atypical for the neurological disorder in question (Larrabee, 2000, 2005). Walsh (1991), for example, has outlined a number of strategies to determine faking by his inferential technique of syndrome analysis. The examinee's performance is evaluated not so much as a deviation from statistical normality as in terms of conformity with a recognised syndrome of cognitive deficit. This results in a series of error types that are inconsistent with organic dysfunction. The error types include frequent additions or omissions in digit span sequences (often involving the last number in a series), answering a question by simply restating the question, incorporating factual elements of a question in an answer, failure of performance level to vary with difficulty level of the test (the sin of summation), regular omissions from the serial additions test, and gross distortions in the reproductions of designs from memory. Rawling and Brooks (1990) continued this work and noted a number of error types specific to dissimulation in head-injured groups. Unfortunately, the precision with which techniques such as those advocated by Walsh can be applied is notoriously unreliable, thus a number of investigators have developed more concise formulations of these behaviours.

Malingerers frequently show impairment on motor function tasks that is out of keeping with the nature of the injury and may perform more poorly on gross as compared to the fine motor tasks (Binder & Willis, 1991; Greiffenstein et al., 1996; Heaton, Smith, Lehman, & Vogt, 1978; Mittenberg, Rotholc, Russell, & Heilbronner, 1996; Rapport, Farchione, Coleman, & Axelrod, 1998). They also will frequently show disproportionate impairment on measures of attention relative to other problem-solving and memory tasks, in particular, very impaired performance on Digit Span sequencing (Binder & Willis, 1991; Greiffenstein, Baker, & Gola, 1994; Heaton et al., 1978; Iverson & Tulsky, 2003; Millis, Ross, & Ricker, 1998; Mittenberg, Azrin, Millsaps, & Heilbronnner, 1993; Mittenberg, Theroux-Fichera, Zielinski, & Heilbronner, 1995; Mittenberg, Rotholc et al., 1996), often display marked impairment in recognition memory (Binder, Villanueva, Howieson, & Moore, 1993; Millis, 1992; Millis & Kler, 1995; Sweet et al., 2000), and may also demonstrate atypical error patterns on measures of problem solving, such as the Category Test (DiCarlo, Gfeller, & Oliveri, 2000; Tenhula & Sweet, 1996), the Wisconsin Card Sorting Test (Bernard, McGrath, & Houston, 1996), and a higher ratio of loss-of-set to categories achieved (Suhr & Boyer, 1999) than seen in nonlitigating closed-head injury patients.

Mittenberg and colleagues (Mittenberg et al., 1993, 1995; Mittenberg, Rotholc et al., 1996) have reported discriminant function equations on the Wechsler Adult Intelligence Scale-Revised (WAIS-R), the Wechsler Memory Scale-Revised (WMS-R) and the Halstead Reitan Battery (HRB) that have proven capable of differentiating noninjured simulators from bonafide head-injured patients with a hit rate of 91% of subjects based upon the discriminant function score derived from the WMS-R; 79% with the WAIS-R, and 88.8% using the HRB. This approach using the WAIS received further support in a subsequent validation study conducted by Greve, Bianchini, Mathias, Houston and Crouch (2003).

Another example of this type of approach is afforded by the technique developed by Killgore and DellaPietra (2000). Using a number of items from the recognition trail of Logical Memory Delayed Recognition items from the WMS-III, these authors have developed a Rarely Missed Index (RMI). This represents the items that were correctly answered by participants who had not previously heard the passages and, as a result, had determined the correct response by the context of the questions. Using a cut-off score of less than 136, the RMI achieved a sensitivity of 97% and specificity of 100%. While the RMI technique is a promising approach, no further validation study has as yet taken place to determine its reliability. The necessity to infer the correct answer from the context of the other questions on the recognition format relies upon relatively intact levels of intellectual functioning and this could raise some concern about its validity, hence, at this point in time the method should be viewed as worthwhile but not definitive. The fact that nearly 40% of the total score relies on the response to a single question (question 18) also raises some concerns about the psychometric properties of the technique.

Modern symptom validity testing was developed by Pankratz (Pankratz, 1979; Pankratz, Fausti, & Peed, 1975). These techniques invariably use a forced-choice recognition test format. The key assumption underlying this form of symptom validity testing is that a person who performs at a level significantly worse than chance (i.e., performs outside the confidence interval for chance performance) must at some level have the correct answer available to them in order to perform so poorly and, consequently, must be malingering (Larrabee, 1992). Choosing by chance alone, the examinee would be expected to be correct about 50% of the time. A simulator overestimating the degree of impairment may thus be induced to score below chance (Larrabee, 2000).

These procedures involve presenting a very large series of items such as multi-digit numbers (e.g., Portland Digit Recognition Test [PDRT], Binder & Kelly, 1996; Computerized Assessment of Response Bias [CARB], Allen, Conder, Green, & Cox, 1997; Conder, Allen, & Cox, 1992; Victoria Symptom Validity Test [VSVT], Slick, Hopp, Strauss, Hunter, & Pinch, 1994), words (Recognition Memory Test, [RMT], Warrington, 1984; Word Memory Test [WMT], Green, Allen, & Astner, 1996) or pictures (Test of Memory Malingering [TOMM], Tombaugh, 1996, 1997; RMT, Warrington, 1984; Faces WMS-III; Wechsler, 1997) that are evaluated by two-alternative forced-choice testing.

These tasks are scored in two ways: First, is the obtained performance significantly worse-than-chance? The frequency with which such a response set occurs tends to be quite rare and as a result this tends not to be a very discriminating technique for identification. For example, in the comparison between the WMT, the CARB, and the TOMM undertaken by Gervais, Rohling, Green, and Ford (2004) the authors noted that only four TOMM protocols of the total 519 (i.e., 0.07% of cases) contained scores below chance (i.e., less than 18 on Trials 1, 2, or the recognition trial) on any trial of the TOMM. They noted only 9 worse than chance performances on the CARB and only six on the WMT. Certainly when such a performance does occur it is so compelling as to be tantamount to confession, however, on balance the frequency with which it would occur tends to be very low (i.e., in less than 2% of cases). Mittenberg and colleagues (Mittenberg et al., 2002) noted a similarly rare rate of identification of this response set (i.e., with such a score only observed by 30.04% of their assessor respondents, the lowest level of endorsement noted in their list of 9 possible indicators of probable malingering or symptom exaggeration).

Second, the responses are scored by determining an objective cut-off that minimizes false positive identification in nonlitigating patients with moderate to severe brain disease (Larrabee, 2000, 2005). In these instances, the sensitivity of the task will contribute to the degree to which it is capable of determining failure rate. For example, in the study of Gervais et al. (2004) just discussed, the investigators noted that failure rates varied from 11% of claimants on the TOMM, to 17% on the CARB, to 32% on the WMT. Clearly these tasks are not equally sensitive to response bias or suboptimal effort.

In their review, Etcoff and Kampfer (1996) evaluated a number of symptom validity tests and indicators and classified them according to their ability to reliably identify dissimulation in neuropsychological assessment. The instruments were classified according to a scheme developed by Rogers (1988) that postulates five levels of certainty as to whether a given test measures a characteristic reliably. These range from definite (accurately classifies 90% or more of individuals based on extensive cross-validated research), probable (research studies consistently established statistically significant results that accurately differentiate at least 75% of the criterion groups), tentative (shows statistically significance in expected direction but has little or no practical value in classifying subjects), little practical value, or no practical value at all.

Etcoff and Kampfer (1996) classified six tests as meeting the criterion of a definite certainty of identifying malingering: (1) the Hiscock Digit Recognition Test (72- and 36-item versions), (2) the Portland Digit Recognition Test (72-item version and 54-item version with conservative scoring), (3) the F Scale and (4) the F-K Index on the MMPI, (5) a WAIS Digit-Span age corrected scale score less than 4, and (6) an error score of 24 or more on the Speech Sounds Perception Test.

Tests given a probable rating included the Hiscock Digit Recognition Test (48-item Victoria version), the Portland Digit Recognition Test (the 54- item version with liberal scoring), the Rey 15-item test with a score of 7 or less, the Fake Bad Scale on the MMPI, Recognition Memory Score on the California Verbal Learning Test, a WAIS Digit-Span age corrected scale score less than 7, and an error score of 17 or more on the Speech Sounds Perception Test (Etcoff and Kampfer, 1996).

Clearly, the base rate with which such a response set occurs is a crucial aspect of the nature of this presentation and one of which the clinician must constantly be aware of. A sample of some of the frequency data presented in the literature to date as summarised by Larrabee (2001), who indicates that a weighted total for eight studies reporting frequency counts indicating the base rate of response bias and malingering in litigating and compensation-seeking subjects, was 41% of the 1,177 subjects assessed.

Mittenberg and colleagues (2002) surveyed 131 neuropsychologists in an attempt to determine how frequently they encountered malingering in their practices. An incidence of probable malingering was noted in 29% of personal injury cases, 19% of criminal cases, 30% of disability cases, and 8% of medical cases. These figures compare favourably to similar studies (e.g., Binder, 1993; Green, Rohling, Lees-Haley, & Allen, 2001; Greiffenstein et al., 1994).

In their survey of expert's practices Slick, Tan, Strauss, and Hultsch (2004) noted that in their respective practices half of the experts indicated a base rate of possible malingering of at least 10% and one-third of 20% or higher. Definite malingering was estimated to occur in at least 10% of the cases in two thirds of the expert sample and in at least 20% by one-third. Part of the explanation for this somewhat lower estimate than that noted by Larrabee's (2001), Mittenberg et al. (2002) or Gervais et al. (2004), may stem from the fact that the experts reported that the Rey 15-item test and the TOMM were the most commonly used measures of malingering.

The 15-item test lacks sensitivity and specificity (e.g., Greiffenstein et al., 1996; Schretlen et al., 1991; Spreen & Strauss, 1998; Vallabhajosula & Van Gorp, 2001), and the TOMM reported the lowest level of detection in comparison to the CARB and the WMT in the Gervais et al. (2004) study. Gervais et al. indicated that the TOMM had the lowest failure rate because it was relatively less sensitive to exaggeration than the other two measures.

Slaker et al. (2004) further noted that when asked how they presented their opinions regarding this diagnosis, most experts (i.e., more than 80%) indicated that in couching their opinion, they tended to indicate that their results were invalid, inconsistent with the severity of the injury, or indicative of exaggeration. They were cautious with the use of the term "malingering" and 12.5% indicated that they never used the term, while 41.7% did so only rarely.

The argument raised by Slick et al. (1999) is of particular interest here and their point that:

> Consistent with APA guidelines, euphemisms or descriptors such as "poorly motivated" or "poor effort" should not be used as synonyms for malingering as persons who malinger may be highly motivated to appear realistically impaired, and expend a significant amount of effort in doing so. Similarly, it is technically incorrect and possibly misleading to refer to symptom validity tests and most other measures of response bias, exaggeration, or fabrication as measures of "effort" or "motivation," as these tests do not directly measure the motivation behind behavior or the level of effort expended. (p. 557)

Clearly this is not an irrelevant clinical problem and, as noted by Green and colleagues (2001), the effects of response bias and malingering are several times more powerful in their disruption of cognition than are the effects even of TBI alone (Green et al., 2001), the condition that most assessments were probably set in train to diagnose. The one concern associated with this argument, however, is that in medico-legal disputes, it is the responsibility of the tribunal to determine the ultimate issue (i.e., is the person injured or not) and as a result calling the behaviour malingering even if it is so, may be encroaching upon the domain of the trier of fact. As a result, it is perhaps most prudent to refer to the behaviour as "demonstrating less than genuine effort" or as "inconsistent with the nature of the injury sustained" to circumvent this problem.

As a general rule, most examiners recommend that at least one and preferably two or more tests of symptom validity be administered (e.g., Gervais et al., 2004; Inman & Berry, 2002; Larrabee, 2005; Slick et al., 2004; Spreen & Strauss, 1998) to ensure as much consistency as possible in observing the behavioural pattern.

Conclusion

The assessment of abnormal illness behaviour including the factitious disorders, the somatoform disorders, and malingering in assessment following a TBI is complex. Passing symptom validity testing does not disprove malingering. Conversely, failing symptom validity testing does not necessarily invalidate the examinee's performance on all other tests used in the evaluation (Larrabee, 1992). The final judgment must, in the end, be a clinical one made by a clinician weighing all of the available evidence gathered in the assessment. Nonetheless, it is essential for clinicians to conduct evaluation of dissimulation within the context of their clinical examination as, particularly in this setting, neuropsychological test performance is crucially dependent on the motivated, cooperative effort of the person being examined. Yet again, Teuber's (1916–1977) dictum that absence of evidence does not equate to evidence of absence, seems most apposite in this context. If the motivation and cooperation of the examinee are not measured, how then can one form any tenable opinion as to the nature of these matters?

8 Disturbances of neurovegetative functioning following TBI

In this chapter I will examine disorders of neurovegetative functioning in the form of the disorders of eating and sleeping, pain, and substance-use issues associated with the injury. Many of these processes are mediated by the deep mesencephalic regions of the brain and, as a result, are much less accessible to the usual behavioural and psychological probes used to investigate changes in the more eloquent regions of the brain.

Neuropathological investigations of patients who have died from cerebral trauma consistently indicate that traumatic brain injury (TBI) can result in severe damage to neuroendocrine function. The studies show a high prevalence of hypothalamic and pituitary lesions, ranging from massive infarction of the anterior pituitary to widespread haemorrhage in the hypothalamus (Clark, Raggatt, & Edwards, 1988). It is probable that the force of the blow to the head is transmitted centripetally, resulting in disruption of these core brain structures. Crompton (1971) noted that pituitary damage was noted in between 40 and 60% of fatal TBI cases at postmortem. A further 42% of these cases featured hypothalamic lesions, which usually occurred as a consequence of tearing of the penetrating arteries. Fractures of the *sella turcica* have also been noted to occur in 20% of fatal head injuries (Young, Olin, & Schmidek, 1980). Clearly the relationship between postmortem studies and studies conducted in those individuals who survive the traumatic brain injury may well be quite different. Nonetheless, the pathomechanical stressors that occur as a result of TBI, including rotational acceleration and shear forces, indicate that the neuroendocrine function following traumatic brain injury may be influenced by a direct lesion effect as well as by shear forces.

These deep brain lesions are also thought to be related to the disruption of a variety of neurohormones including corticotrophin-releasing hormone (CRH), cortisol, vasopressin, and prolactin as well as disrupting other hormone systems including those related to the thyroid and the gonads as well as the hormones that control diuresis and glucose metabolism.

For example, patients followed for 2 to 10 months following TBI demonstrated elevated morning levels of cortisol, absence of diurnal cortisol variation, and non-suppression to dexamethasone challenge (Cohen, Oksenberg, Snir, Stern, & Grosswasser, 1992). Glucose loading in acute TBI patients was associated with increase in growth hormone (King, Knowles, McLaurin et al., 1981), prolactin secretion was noted to be elevated at various stages following severe TBI (Valenta & De Feo, 1980) and it is postulated that this latter disturbance may be attributable to the hypothalamic mechanism that controls the hormone's secretion (Molitch, 1992). Disturbances in the metabolism of thyroidal, gonadal, glucagon/glucose, and antidiuretic hormone secretion have each been reported (Jackson & Mysiw, 1989) subsequent to TBI.

Neurogenic fever resulting from alteration in hypothalamic temperature set point culminating in abnormal increases in body temperature has also been noted following TBI, and this phenomenon is more likely to occur in individuals with diffuse axonal injury or damage to the frontal lobe (Thompson, Pinto-Martin, & Bullock, 2003). Study of cadavers has revealed that 42.5% of brains examined post-TBI reveal hypothalamic injury (Crompton, 1971).

Disorders of eating

Changes in dietary habits following TBI have been noted with regard to decrease in appetite and the emergence of anorexia following the injury (Levin & Summers, 1992) and the sensory disturbances related to the changes of taste and smell associated with the damage to the olfactory apparatus (Schechter & Henkins, 1974). Changes to swallowing have also been noted to have a significant impact upon return to regular feeding routines as well as being a good indicator of recovery in severe injuries (e.g., Dolberg, Barkai, Gross, & Schreiber, 2004; Duong et al., 2004; Formisano et al., 2004; Mackay, Morgan, & Bernstein, 1999).

While the Kluver-Bucy syndrome would not be an unexpected outcome in the context of TBI, it seems to be a relatively rarely reported complication of the injury, although a number of cases have been reported in the more recent literature. Some investigators have claimed to have observed a partial Kluver-Bucy syndrome, the veracity of which has been vigorously debated (Salim et al., 2002; Slaughter, Bobo, & Childers, 1999). The Kluver-Bucy syndrome was originally described by Kluver and Bucy (1937, 1938) after the bilateral removal of the temporal lobes and rhinencephalon in adult monkeys. The syndrome as described by Kluver (1958) has never been observed in man, although an entity strongly resembling it has (Poeck, 1985). Characteristic features of the Kluver-Bucy syndrome in man include: (1) heightened oral tendency; (2) placidity; (3) changes in sexual behaviour; (4) severe disturbance of memory; (5) hypermetamorphosis; and (6) probable visual agnosia. Poeck (1985) has suggested that only those subjects featuring the strong oral tendency be classified as Kluver-Bucy syndrome, either partial or complete. The oral tendency seems to undergo a development course and Lishman (1987) has suggested that the hyperphagia is often a terminal phenomenon progressing to the eating of any material available. The syndrome has been reported in a number of degenerative diseases including herpes simplex encephalitis, surgical amygdalotomy, posttraumatic encephalopathy, paraneoplastic limbic dementia, adrenoleukodystrophy, bilateral temporal infarction and resection, Pick's disease, Alzheimer's disease, hypoglycaemia, and toxoplasmic encephalitis (Lilly, Cummings, Benson, & Frankel, 1983).

Anatomically it has been argued that, as with the monkey, bilateral involvement of the temporal lobes, particularly Ammon's horn, is essential for the production of the full syndrome (Poeck, 1985). While bilateral temporal lobectomy or partial bilateral resection can produce the syndrome (only transiently in the case of bilateral amygdalotomies), it does not do so invariably, with the most notable example of the failure to elicit a Kluver-Bucy syndrome following large mesial bitemporal resection being the much-studied amnesic patient, HM (Scoville & Milner, 1957).

Fujii, Fujita, Hiramatsu, and Miyamoto (1998) also raised the interesting situation in which two individuals who had had food aversions prior to injury. One patient was averse to meat and Spanish paprika prior to the injury and had no such aversion once her appetite had returned to a normal level postinjury, and the second had a similar aversion to Spanish paprika as well as to raw fish, wasabi, and onions, which he willingly ate following the injury. However, at six months postinjury the aversion to wasabi reappeared in association with an aversion to the taste of fish bones. Clearly, although the mechanisms of eating and taste sensation can be affected by TBI, in all it would appear that these sorts of changes are a relatively rare postinjury complication.

Disorders of sleeping

Sleep and wakefulness are two opposite states that compete with each other for the control of consciousness. Wakefulness is maintained by the reticular activating system (RAS) assisted by the activity of the catecholaminergic and cholinergic transmitter systems that convey the activation of the RAS via the thalamus to the cortex. Sleep is promoted by the activity of the dorsal raphe, which acts in accord with other brain stem nuclei to deactivate the RAS. Serotonergic neurons dampen down sensory activity and inhibit motor activity during sleep, promoting slow wave activity in the cortex (Culebras, 1992a, 1992b).

Sleep disorders following TBI may result from a variety of causes. Some may be preexistent while others may occur as a direct result of the brain injury. Sleepiness is a common cause of road fatalities (36%: Leger, 1994) and collisions (42–54%: Leger, 1994). Motor vehicle and industrial accidents are more likely to occur in individuals who have sleep apnoea, and it has been estimated that 90% of men and 98% of women with obstructive sleep apnoea (OSA) remain undiagnosed (Young, Evans, Finn, & Palta, 1997). In the unimpaired middle-aged working population, this condition occurs in 2% of women and 4% of men (Guilleminault, Faull, Miles, & van de Hoed, 1983).

Early studies of the prevalence of sleep disorders following TBI focussed on the use of sleep pattern as an indicator of recovery from coma. Bergamasco, Bergamini, Doriguzzi and Faciani (1968) noted that the return to a more normal sleep pattern, with increase in the prevalence of REM sleep, was a useful predictor of emergence from coma. This measure was also noted to correlate with cognitive recovery (Ron, Algom, Hary, & Cohen, 1980).

Sleep disturbances are common following TBI and the frequency ranges to up to 70% of patients (Keshavan, Channabasavanna, & Reddy, 1981; McLean, Dikmen, Temkin, Wyler, & Gale, 1984). In their preliminary analysis of sleep disorders in a small sample of TBI patients, Castriotta and Lai (2001) noted that sleep disorders, most notably sleep-disordered breathing, were greatly underdiagnosed and largely untreated in this population.

The sleep disorders represent a complex set of conditions. Nonetheless, a number of the conditions in the context of TBI deserve particular consideration. These are: posttraumatic hypersomnia, narcolepsy, central sleep apnoea, obstructive sleep apnoea (OSA: the cessation of breathing with continued effort to breathe), nocturnal seizures, and insomnia (Castriotta & Lai, 2001).

It tends to be the case that immediately following the injury, the subject reports difficulty in falling asleep with associated frequent waking, whereas after several years, the pattern tends to be more consistent with persisting somnolence (Cohen et al., 1992). The most commonly noted sleep disorders following TBI are insomnia, hypersomnia, and sleep-wake schedule disturbances and although the parasomnias (undesirable motor and behavioural events occurring during sleep) do occur, their incidence is fairly rare (Rao & Rollings, 2002). For example, while Webster, Bell, Hussey, Natale and Lakshminarayan (2001) noted that 36% of their participants had sleep apnoea (primarily central although some OSA) three months following TBI, these conditions did not correlate with measures of TBI severity or other demographic measures. The diagnosis of posttraumatic narcolepsy is also quite rare (Bruck & Broughton, 2004; Castriotta & Lai, 2001; Lankford, Wellman, & O'Hara, 1994).

Insomnia reflects a difficulty in initiating or maintaining sleep or of nonrestorative sleep that lasts for at least a month (APA, 2000) and is usually associated with day-time fatigue or impaired functioning. The observation of overwhelming fatigue is a common concomitant of the postconcussional syndrome (PCS) as discussed in chapter 2. Cohen and colleagues (1992), in their study of 22 hospitalised TBI patients who sustained the injury over the preceding 3 to 5 months, noted that 81% complained of difficulty falling to or maintaining sleep. The consecutive study of Mann, Fichtenberg, Putnam, and De Santis (1997) followed 50 patients in postacute settings, and noted a 30% frequency of insomnia.

Fichtenberg, Millis, Mann, Zafonte, and Millard (2000) noted no relationship between insomnia and gender, education, age or time since injury, but did note that the presence of pain doubled the level of insomnia, with the most common complaint being with the maintenance of uninterrupted sleep. Pain has also commonly been associated with sleep problems in mild TBI (Beetar, Guilmette, & Sparadeo, 1996; Clinchot, Bogner, Mysiw, Corrigan, & Fugate, 1996).

In their subsequent study, Fichtenberg, Zafonte, Putnam, Mann, and Millard (2002) noted a 30% frequency of insomnia (with sleep initiation problems twice as common as problems with sleep duration). The investigators observed that the frequency of this condition was also high in the rehabilitation comparison group.

Prigatano, Stahl, Orr, and Zeiner (1982) observed that patients with chronic TBI complained of diminished stage 1 sleep and featured more awakenings as compared to age-matched control participants. The latter measure was also reported to be related to increased ratings of general psychopathology (Prigatano et al., 1982).

Overall, about a 30% incidence of insomnia in TBI subjects is noted across the published literature (36% at 1 month: McLean et al., 1984; 37% at 3 months: Keshavan et al., 1981; 30% at 4 months: Fichtenberg et al., 2002; 27% at 1 year: McLean, Dikmen, & Temkin, 1993) although the figure has ranged from as low as 2–4% (Cohen et al., 1992; Rutherford et al., 1979), to as high as 56% (Beetar et al., 1996). Persisting insomnia following the injury, however, tends to be quite uncommon (Tobe, Schneider, Mrozik, & Lidsky, 1999).

Hypersomnia is defined as excessive sleepiness as demonstrated by prolonged sleep episodes or daytime sleep episodes occurring almost daily for at least one month and causing distress or impairment in functioning (APA, 2000). Cohen and colleagues (1992) observed hypersomnia in 73% of their patients 2 to 3 years following TBI. Guilleminault and colleagues (Guilleminault, Yuen, Gulerick, & Karadeniz, 2000) in their study of 184 patients studied approximately 15 months postinjury, that of the patients who complained of excessive daytime somnolence, 98% also observed impairment of daytime functioning. The predictive variables for sleepiness included coma of greater than 24 hours, head fracture, pain, and neurosurgical intervention following the trauma. Worthington and Melia (2006) noted that 47% of their sample of 135 TBI patients demonstrated disturbance of arousal or sleep pattern up to 10 years postinjury.

The possibility that arousal disturbances may impact in an ongoing way on cognitive and other functioning has been highlighted by Bleiberg, Garmoe, Halpern, Reeves, and Nadler (1997). These investigators were interested to ascertain the cause of variability in the performance of TBI patients on a day-to-day comparison. They noted that TBI patients demonstrate greater performance variability than did unimpaired control subjects and that this variability was proportionate to the overall slowing of performance noted in this group. They further observed:

> In summary, static, single point assessments, whether with standardized neuropsychological tests or with the ANAM [Automated Neuropsychological Assessment Metrics] battery, may fail to reveal potential dynamic abnormalities in patterns of acquisition and maintenance of performance across days. The current data suggest that such dynamic abnormalities may characterise a subgroup of individuals with mild TBI. This subgroup may appear normal during single-point neuropsychological assessments, but shows abnormalities in the acquisition and maintenance of performance across days. (p. 252)

This raises the fascinating possibility that the single-point estimate of cognitive functioning characteristic of most neuropsychological assessments may be diagnostically inadequate in some patients due to the variability in the nature of the condition that may not be static from day to day. Certainly the point that these authors raise must at least urge caution in the conviction with which some of the statements about the permanence of the cognitive deficits noted following TBI can be made.

Circadian rhythm sleep disorder (formerly sleep–wake schedule disorder) represents a disturbance of sleep–wake cycle and also commonly occurs as a consequence of TBI. These patients are subject to a displacement of their sleep patterns from their normal circadian rhythm and as a result are unable to go to sleep or stay awake at a desired time. The architecture of the sleep produced, however, is not disrupted (APA, 2000). While several varieties of the disorder do exist (i.e., delayed sleep phase, jet lag, shift work, and unspecified types), in the context of TBI, the most commonly noted presentation is the delayed sleep-phase type (Quinto, Gellido, & Chokroverty, 2000; Patten & Lauderdale, 1992). In their study of 15 patients, Schreiber and colleagues (Schreiber, Klag, Gross, Segman, & Pick, 1998) noted that more than half of the patients had delayed sleep-phase syndrome with the remainder featuring unspecified (disorganised) type.

The cause of the condition is thought to be related to damage to the suprachiasmatic nucleus of the hypothalamus (thought to be the location of the human circadian clock or zeitgeber) as a result of the damage to the core centres of the brain, including the paraventricular nucleus around the third ventricle, probably as a result of acute alterations in intracranial pressure following the injury.

Frieboes et al. (1999) noted a number of alterations to sleep-endocrine relationships months to years following TBI. These included reduction in non-REM stage 2 sleep in the first half of the night and increased REM sleep in the second sleep cycle. With regard to endocrine functioning the nocturnal growth hormone peak was blunted and the maximal prolactin secretion was increased but the cortisol levels were unchanged.

While a number of neuroendocrine disturbances have been noted to be associated with TBI, as yet the use of pharmacological means to redress these problems with agents such as melatonin has proven relatively unsuccessful. Using a randomized double-blind controlled cross-over trial, Kemp, Biswas, Neumann, and Coughlan (2004) noted no differences between TBI patients with chronic sleep disturbance and their baseline state in sleep latency, duration, quality, or daytime alertness for either melatonin or amitryptiline. However, the effect-size analysis did show some encouraging prospects.

Some benefit has also been noted with the use of cognitive behavioural therapy (CBT) for insomnia with TBI patients. Ouellet and Morin (2004) noted a decrease in sleep onset from 47 to 18 minutes, and a decrease in nocturnal awakening from 85 to 28 minutes on average with eight weekly individual CBT sessions using a variety of approaches including stimulus control, sleep restriction, cognitive therapy, and sleep hygiene education. Sleep efficiency increased from 58% to 83%. The improvements were corroborated by polysomnography and the gains were maintained at the 1- and 3-month follow-ups.

One aspect of sleep that has been relatively infrequently studied within the head-injury literature is the influence of the TBI on the mechanisms associated with dreaming. Prigatano, Monte, William et al. (1982) and Ron et al. (1980) followed traumatically brain-injured patients during periods exceeding 6 months following the injury and reported that these patients gradually recover to an almost normal amount of REM sleep during this period. Prigatano et al. (1982) noted in his series that his patients reported a decrease and even absence of dreams although their sleep cycles (including REM sleep) were almost normal. Benyakar, Tadir, Groswasser, and Stern (1988) assessed 51 married head-injury patients regarding the frequency and content of their dreams before and after injury. The number of patients reporting dreams with threatening content rose from 11.8% in the preinjury phase to 33.3% in the postinjury period. The percentage of patients reporting dreams with sexual content decreased from 39.3% before the head injury to 19.6% at the postinjury period. Whilst this remains an interesting finding, there has not been subsequent replication and the contention that self-reports of pre- versus postinjury introspections regarding behaviour can be viewed as valid data must be carefully scrutinized (Lees-Haley et al., 1997).

Sleep disorders following TBI are quite common, and immediately following the injury the subject tends to report difficulty in falling asleep with associated frequent waking, whereas after several years the pattern tends to be more consistent with persisting somnolence. The incidence of insomnia is about 30% of TBI patients. While a number of other sleep disorders can occur in the context of TBI these tend to be relatively rare. The downstream effects of sleep disturbance including increased tiredness, irritability, and compromise in levels of attention and concentration have profound implications for the day-to-day functioning of individuals following TBI, indicating that restoration of appropriate patterns of sleep is one of the highest rehabilitation priorities for TBI-affected individuals.

Pain following TBI

Inevitably the same traumas that result in brain injury also often result in other forms of physical injury. These two sites of injury can and often do co-exist and, as a result, the impact of pain-related phenomena in tandem with TBI can culminate in chronic pain states compounding cognitive dysfunction, emotional well-being, and functional capacity (Bohnen & Jolles, 1992).

The International Association for the Study of Pain (Merskey & Bogduk, 1994, p. 209) defines pain as "an unpleasant sensory and emotional experience associated with actual or potential tissue damage, or described in terms of such damage." While acute pain invariably indicates injury and or disease, chronic pain lasting beyond the time frame necessary for tissue healing to occur is defined most commonly as featuring six continuous months of pain. Not uncommonly psychopathology and other environmental factors play a prominent role in chronic pain (Jacobson & Mariano, 2001), although a diagnosis of chronic pain does not preclude an underlying tissue injury or disease.

Various forms of pain can arise in the context of the recovery following TBI contingent upon the nature of the initial injury and the subsequent development of the condition over the ensuing period. The most commonly encountered forms of pain syndromes following TBI include dysautonomia, neuropathic pain, spasticity, headache, heterotopic ossification (a nonmalignant overgrowth of bone often occurring after a fracture) (Harris, Nagy, & Vardaxis, 2006), deep vein thrombosis, genitourinary and gastrointestinal pain, and the pain associated with orthopaedic trauma including shoulder pain (see Ivanhoe & Hartman, 2004 for a recent review).

Neuropathic pain has three commonly encountered forms: (1) complex regional pain syndrome (CPRS), (2) central pain syndrome (CPS), and (3) peripheral neuropathy. CPRS Type 1, or reflex sympathetic dystrophy, occurs in 12% of TBI patients with the mean onset within four months of injury (Gellman, Keenan & Botte, 1996). CPS or thalamic pain can occur following any central nervous system (CNS) lesion but especially so after damage to the ascending somatosensory pathways, the thalamus, the thalamocortical connections, and the cortex (Andersen, Vestergaard, Ingeman-Nielsen, & Jensen, 1995). The onset is usually within the first two months following the injury (Beric, 1998; Bowsher, 1996).

The peripheral neuropathies are usually associated with metabolic disorders including diabetes, or nutritional disorders including the long-term effect of alcoholism, but focal compression and heterotrophic ossification can also result in this presentation (Ivanhoe & Hartman, 2004).

Headache is a common complaint following TBI and is often included as one of the most common presenting and persisting symptoms of the chronic PCS (Martelli & Zasler, 2001; Nicholson, 2000) discussed in chapter 2. The International Headache Society employs the term posttraumatic headache (PTHA) to describe the emergence of headaches following head trauma that commence within 14 days of the return of consciousness following the injury (1988).

While there are no pain receptors in the brain itself (i.e., the white matter, the ependymal linings of the ventricles, and the choroid plexus are not pain sensitive and much of the cortex, pia, and arachnoid matter can be electrically stimulated, burned, or cut without pain), certain parts of the dura at the base of the brain and the dural arteries are sensitive to pain (Bonica & Loeser, 2001). Secondary vascular lesions of the brain, particularly of the thalamus, may be a source of central pain (Bonica & Loeser, 2001). The hypothalamus and the limbic structures have an important role in the motivational, emotional, and affective components of the pain experience and these structures are quite commonly implicated in damage arising as a consequence of TBI. Migraine can also be triggered by head trauma often in the context of sporting activities including "heading" the ball in soccer (Bennett, Fuenning, Sullivan, & Weber, 1980).

Headache occurs in as many as 90% of patients during the recovery process following TBI (Keidel & Diener, 1997). The level of chronic PTHA lasting 6 months or longer has been reported to be as high as 44% (De Bendittis & De Santis, 1983; Martelli, Grayson, & Zasler, 1999).

Evans (2004), in his authoritative review on this topic, notes that the percentage of patients who have headache at 1 month posttrauma varies from 31.3% (Lewine, Davis, Sloan, Kodituwakku, & Orrison, 1999) to 90% (Dencker, 1944); at 3 months from 47% (Levin, Mattis, Ruff et al., 1987) to 78% (Rimel et al., 1981); at 12 months from 8.4% (Rutherford, Merrett, & McDonald, 1978) to 35% (Dencker, 1944), and the levels may still be as high as 20–24% at 96 months postinjury (Edna, 1987; Keidel & Diener, 1997). These levels of incidence have lead Martelli and colleagues (1999) to the conclusion that PTHA is the most common postconcussive symptom and is the most frequently noted form of pain associated with mild traumatic brain injury (MTBI).

Numerous possible conditions can contribute to the emergence of headache in the period following trauma (as of course do those occurring in the absence of such an event) and these include a variety of musculoskeletal and neuropathic causes. The former category includes such entities as temporomandibular joint dysfunction and myofascial pain syndrome. Also "depression, level of activity, life stressor, caffeine, hormonal factors, diet, sleep and exercise ability" (Ivanhoe & Hartman, 2004, p. 34) could each alone or in concert contribute to the problem.

Other conditions such as heterotopic ossification are also noted following TBI with up to 33% of patients showing clinically significant effects of the condition. (Bagley, 1979). Deep vein thrombosis is a commonly noted complication of TBI (Stone & Keenan, 1992) with an incidence of 53.8% (Geerts, Code, Jay et al., 1994).

Fractures and dislocations are observed in 71–80% of TBI patients (Bontke, Lehmkuhl, Englander et al., 1993), and 20% of patients complain of limb pain six months or more following the injury (Gellman et al., 1996) Shoulder pain resulting from joint damage, either as a result of the trauma or from the subsequent patient transfer and management postinjury, also commonly occur (Zuckerman, Mirabello, & Newman, 1991). This is not to mention the 11% of undiagnosed fractures and dislocations noted in an adult head injury unit that were missed on initial presentation (Garland & Bailey, 1981). Constipation and urinary retention are also considered to be among the most common preventable causes of patient pain and discomfort (Ivanhoe & Hartman, 2004) postinjury.

The frequency with which the various pain syndromes occur following TBI has been difficult to precisely describe. Kleppel, Lincoln, and Winston (2002) note that 71% of TBI admissions needed narcotic pain medication at the time of discharge and 41% reported postconcussive symptoms. Uomoto and Essleman (1993) noted that 95% of patients with a mild TBI but only 22% of moderate to severe TBIs reported pain following TBI with 89% of the mild and 18% of the moderate to severe patients reporting headache with a lesser frequency of pain at other sites including neck, back, and shoulder. Lahz and Bryant (1996) noted the 52% of moderate to severe and 58% of mild TBIs referred to a tertiary centre reported chronic pain states. Once again, headache was the most commonly reported pain problem (i.e., 47% mild and 34% moderate to severe) with an equivalent level of neck, shoulder, back, and upper and lower limb pain reported independent of TBI severity.

Interestingly, the possibility that cognitive impairment may interact with pain reporting has been noted both by Lahz and Bryant (1996) and Yamaguchi (1992) with severe headaches reported less often by the more cognitively impaired. Hart, Martelli, and Zasler (2000) reviewed the ability of pain itself to impact on the processes of cognition has been reviewed by and noted:

> Numerous studies reviewed here have demonstrated neuropsychological impairment in patients with chronic pain, particularly on measures assessing attentional capacity, processing speed, and psychomotor speed....There is also support for an association between impairment and other symptoms often associated with pain such as mood change, increased somatic awareness, sleep disturbance and fatigue. (p. 147)

Beetar et al. (1996) noted that 59% of their TBI sample reported pain at least once following TBI as compared to only 22% reporting in a neurological sample. This data led Tyrer and Lievesley (2003) to speculate that "about half of patients who sustain a TBI and who are referred to specialist clinicians are likely to have a chronic painful complaint subsequently" (p. 196).

Treatment for post-TBI pain involves the variety of approaches that have proven successful in pain that occurs in the absence of the TBI, with the principal success associated with multidisciplinary pain management approaches (see Tyrer & Lievesley, 2003, for a recent review). Some specific concerns noted for the treatment of pain conditions in the context of TBI include the fact that it can take longer for TBI patients to complete treatment programs than it does for non-TBI affected individuals (Andary et al., 1997; Branca & Lake, 2004). Also many patients who develop pain following TBI engage in a number of the behaviours seen in non-TBI pain populations including avoidance of physical exertion, overdependence on others, and the benefits that accrue as a consequence of the sick role (Tyrer, 1986). Readers should refer to chapter 7 for a discussion of these latter issues.

Substance abuse issues

The issue of substance abuse surrounding TBI presents a complex and interacting web of effects associated with the injury. Substance-abuse issues can be significant either before the injury, at the time of the injury, or during the postinjury response period.

The literature indicates that between 44 and 79% of TBI patients have a positive history for alcohol abuse that predates the injury, while 21–37% report a history of illicit drug abuse (Taylor, Kreutzer, Demm, & Meade, 2003). This history is most commonly associated with the demographic features of failure to complete high school, an aetiology related to violence, male gender, being unmarried, and being unemployed at the time of the injury.

Studies with regard to the likelihood of intoxication at the time of the injury indicate that 25–75% of TBI survivors are likely to be alcohol affected when the injury is sustained. Seventy-eight percent have a positive blood alcohol level (BAL) at the time of hospital admission, and nearly 50% are intoxicated (i.e., BAL greater than 100mg/dl) at the time of hospital admission (Corrigan, 1995; Drubach, Kelly, Winslow, & Flynn, 1993; Galbraith, Murray, Patel, & Krill-Jones, 1976; Rimel, Giordani, Barth, & Jane, 1982; Taylor et al., 2003). A similar level of intoxication (17–62%) has been noted at the time of spinal chord injury (SCI) (Kolakowsky-Hayner et al., 2002) and over 30% of SCI patients test positive for illicit drugs (Heinemann, Mamott, & Schnoll, 1990; O'Donnell, Cooper, Gersner et al., 1981; Young, Rintala, Rossi et al., 1995).

Patients with a positive BAL at the time of admission feature lower Glasgow Coma Scale (GCS) scores (Kelly, Johnson, Knoller, Drubach, & Winslow, 1997) as well as more marked severity of injury (Bigler et al., 1996; Brickley & Shepherd, 1995; Gurney et al., 1992; Kaplan & Corrigan, 1992; Sparadeo, Strauss, & Barth, 1990). They also have higher rates of respiratory complication (Gurney et al., 1992), longer periods of postinjury agitation and tend to have poorer cognitive functioning at the time of discharge (Sparadeo & Gill, 1989).

Kelly and colleagues (1997) observed that there is an additive effect of substance abuse in association with TBI that causes more pronounced neuropsychological impairment, particularly on measures of memory functioning. These patients also feature higher mortality rates although there has not been unequivocal support for this suggestion in the literature (Fuller, 1995; Kaplan & Corrigan, 1992; Ruff et al., 1990), as well as featuring higher levels of neurobehavioural and occupational problems (Sabhesan, Arumugham, Ramasany, & Natarajan, 1987). When substance abuse occurs in association with TBI (after controlling for the effects of head injury severity) the effects of substance abuse in concert with TBI resulted in greater atrophic changes to the brain as measured using quantitative MRI (Barker et al., 1999). The neuropsychological test performances of the two samples demonstrated no differences. A further injury-related issue associated with alcohol abuse is that these individuals are also less likely to use seatbelts, culminating in multiple trauma and increased length of hospitalization (Kaplan & Corrigan, 1992).

A number of studies have attempted to validate self-report inventories of substance abuse in association with TBI and relatively good reliability and validity have been established for the CAGE (Ashman, Schwartz, Cantor, Hibbard, & Gordon, 2004) and the Brief Michigan Alcohol Screening Test (BMAST) (Cherner, Temkin, Machamer, & Dikmen, 2001; Fuller, Fishman, Taylor, & Wood, 1994). Reasonable, although somewhat less powerful, results have been noted using the Substance Abuse Subtle Screening Inventory (SASSI-3) (Arenth, Bogner, Corrigan, & Schmidt, 2001; Ashman et al., 2004).

While it is clear that the association between substance abuse and the injury is an important and a complex one, it is really only in the last 15 years or so that it has been studied in any comprehensive way. Corrigan's review in 1995 represented one of the first attempts to integrate and synthesize this literature. He surveyed 11 research reports (most published in the period from 1990 to 1995) that examined the relationship between intoxication or a history of substance abuse in individuals who had experienced TBI. The results of Corrigan's review were clear:

> Studies showed alcohol intoxication present in one third to one half of hospitalizations; data from other drug intoxication were not available. Nearly two thirds of rehabilitation patients may have a history of substance abuse that preceded their injuries. Intoxication was related to acute complications, longer hospital stays, and poorer discharge status; however, these relationships may have been caused by colinearity with history. History of substance abuse showed the same morbidity, and was further associated with higher mortality rates, poorer neuropsychological outcome and greater likelihood of repeat injuries and later deterioration. The effect of history may be caused by subgroups with more severe substance abuse problems. (p. 302)

Not too surprisingly Corrigan (1995) noted that patients with a history of substance use predating the TBI were more likely to be male, over age 30, with lower education and socioeconomic status, and were commonly intoxicated at the time of the injury.

Since Corrigan's (1995) review there have been a number of further studies contributing to the strength of this association. Dikmen, Machamer, Donovan, Winn, and Temkin (1995) studied a consecutive series of 197 hospitalized TBI survivors followed up over the ensuing year following the injury. Alcohol use was noted to decrease following the injury, but was noted to be on the rise again at the one-year time point, but had not at that stage reached the preinjury levels.

A number of investigators have homed in on this period of postinjury reflection and response as the ideal time at which to institute interventions to curtail alcohol and drug use. Kreutzer, Witol, and Marwitz (1996) view the postinjury period as a "window of opportunity" for substance abuse intervention. They noted that drinking rates amongst young TBIs declined over the initial follow-up, but returned to previous levels following the second follow-up assessment. A similar pattern of resumption of drinking has been noted with SCI patients with 73% resuming drinking within 18 months of injury (Heinemann, Goranson, Ginsburg, & Schnoll, 1989; Heinemann,

Keen, Donohue, & Schnoll, 1988). Bombadier and Rimmele (1998) noted a high index of "readiness to change" in an SCI sample following injury.

Kreutzer, Wehman, Harris, Burns, and Young (1991) noted that there was a significant decrease in the rates of drinking and drug abuse in their TBI sample. Six years following the injury, 95% of the sample was abstinent from illegal drugs and 50% abstinent from alcohol. Twenty-eight percent of the sample were moderate to heavy drinkers following the injury, a rate higher than that noted in the general population.

Kolakowsky-Hayner and colleagues (2002) noted that of individuals classified as heavy drinkers before the injury, only 29.4% remained so in the wake of the injury, with 23.5% decreasing to the moderate level, 5.9% became infrequent drinkers and over 40% became abstinent altogether. With their moderate drinkers, 12% increased to heavy drinking, 62.5% remained moderate, and 25% became abstinent. Half of the light drinkers increased to moderate and the other half gave up alcohol altogether. No person abstinent before the injury took up drinking after the injury. The authors concluded that "rehabilitation professionals have an important window of opportunity to intervene after a traumatic brain injury to address patients' risk for post-injury substance abuse" (p. 590).

More severe TBI (i.e., lower GCS), higher blood alcohol level in the emergency department, and older age at time of injury predicted greater decreases in drinking (Kolakowsky, Hayner et al., 2002). A similar profile of at-risk TBI patients was noted by Bombadier, Rimmele, and Zintel (2002) who noted their at-risk sample was likely to be single, male, and with less than a high school education.

Kreutzer, Witol, Sander et al. (1996) undertook a cross-sectional and longitudinal study of 322 and 73 patients respectively assessed at one to four years following their TBIs. The data indicated that the sample had a similar proportion of moderate to heavy drinkers (22–29%) as the general population, although abstinence rates were higher than in the noninjured population. They noted variability in drinking rates, but a trend towards increasing consumption in the period following the injury. The conclusion of the study indicated that TBI reduces, but does not overcome, preinjury alcohol abuse issues.

Hibbard et al. (1998) used the structured clinical interview for the *DSM-IV* (SCID) in 100 TBI patients living in the community. In the retrospective component of the study they noted that 40% of the sample met the criteria for substance abuse or dependence before their injuries. In fact, the study demonstrated that substance abuse was the most common psychiatric disorder before injury and the second most common (28%) up to the 7-year postinjury follow-up.

Bombadier et al. (2002) noted a similar finding to the previously mentioned three studies with high rates of alcohol-related problems before injury. One third of the group (142 of 156 consecutive admissions to a rehabilitation unit) were intoxicated at the time of the injury. Fifty-nine percent were considered "at-risk" drinkers with high levels of preinjury alcohol use, while 49% self-reported significant alcohol problems. Thirty-four percent reported recent illicit drug use and 37% featured positive toxicological results for illicit drugs. Forty percent of the sample had positive toxicological results for marijuana, cocaine, or amphetamine within three months of their injury, with marijuana accounting for more than half of the illicit drug use.

Cocaine and amphetamine use was noted with 17–22% of the sample but drug use without alcohol use was rare, occurring in only 2% of the sample.

Postinjury alcohol and drug use indicate that individuals who continue to abuse alcohol and drugs following the injury display higher rates of psychiatric disorder and aggressive behaviours. They also feature higher arrest rates, decreased incidence of return to work, and higher rates of referral for supported employment (Edna, 1984; Kreutzer et al., 1991; Kreutzer, Witol, Sander et al., 1996; Sparadeo & Gill, 1989).

In their review of this literature Taylor et al. (2003) came to the following conclusions:

> A history of pre-injury alcohol abuse has been associated with post-injury emotional or cognitive deterioration, military discharge from duty, decreased likelihood of return to work or other productive activity, and lower life satisfaction. Additionally, research revealed an association between a history of alcohol abuse and numerous negative neurological outcomes, including higher mortality rates, increased risk of re-injury, later deterioration, lower probability of good outcome, greater volume of intracranial haemorrhage, weaker quantitative EEG improvement, and local brain atrophy. Intoxication at the time of injury has also been found to be associated with negative neurological outcomes such as acute illness and complications, longer hospital stays, poorer discharge status, increased duration of agitation, and required procedures. (p. 174)

Treatment programs for the substance-abusing subset of individuals affected with TBI has resulted in a number of therapeutic intervention approaches (See Taylor et al., 2003, for a recent review) including individual (Corrigan, Lamb-Hart, & Rust, 1995) and group approaches (Delmonico et al., 1998). Corrigan (1995) also adverts to an interesting side issue regarding attribution and blame associated with the TBI in the context of substance-abuse problems. He notes that many rehabilitation professionals prefer to view the TBI subject as a victim of circumstance rather than as having contributed to their own state. The use of substances in the context of the injury is not consistent with such a view of the injury and, in some sense, makes the individual "responsible" for their injury. This issue is exacerbated if the individual persists with the substance abuse following the injury as a statement of the exertion of less than maximal effort to recover. Clearly many practitioners shy away from such characterizations and take the more innocuous therapeutic route of advising against use (Corrigan, 1995).

Conclusion

Clearly neurovegetative functions subserved by the core areas of the brain including the hypothalamus and its associated areas can be compromised as a consequence of TBI culminating in disorders of eating, sleeping, and pain. These are an omnipresent part of the postinjury state for many individuals who have been affected by TBI. Whilst disruption of eating is relatively rarely observed following TBI, sleep disorders are common both immediately following the injury (when the subject tends to report difficulty in falling asleep) and after several years the pattern tends to be more consistent with persisting somnolence. The incidence of insomnia tends to be about 30% of TBI patients. Pain is also a common concomitant of TBI with headache occurring in as many as 90% of patients during the recovery process following TBI. The level of chronic posttraumatic headache lasting six months or longer has been reported to be as high as 44%. This is not to discount the other pain symptoms associated with TBI including shoulder and other orthopaedic pain and neuropathic pain of various forms. Alcohol and other substance abuse presents as a significant issue both preceding and following the injury. Individuals with a history of alcohol abuse in association with their TBI have a worse outcome on all measures of injury severity and in the quality of their treatment response. Some authors contend that the postinjury period represents an ideal time in which to make significant intervention for the treatment of substance abuse, hopefully to reduce the likelihood of further morbidity associated with the combined neural insult.

9 Disturbances of sexual functioning

One common effect of traumatic brain injury (TBI) that has received only limited investigation to date is the alteration in sexual desire and performance associated with the injury (Elliott & Biever, 1996). It is estimated that TBI affects approximately 7 million people per year throughout the world. These injuries primarily affect men, with over 25% of TBIs occurring prior to age 25 (Ducharme & Gill, 1990). Independence and sexuality are crucial developmental tasks that need to be addressed during these early adult years and TBI, with its complex and interacting sequelae, can have a seriously detrimental effect on the development and nurturance of normal sexual behaviour. The cognitive, behavioural, and physical impairments as well as the hormonal changes and psychological reactions to the cognitive and other deficits can combine to result in a lethal cocktail of sexual and emotional maladaptation. Often in the rehabilitation setting, the only time when the sexuality of the individual with TBI comes to attention is when the treating team are tearing out their hair due to the sexually disinhibited and inappropriate behaviour of that individual (Miller, 1994).

Background

A number of definitions of sexual function and dysfunction seem worthwhile at the outset. Ringman and Cummings (2000) divide sexual behaviour into a scheme that distinguishes the motivational (pertaining to libido, or desire to engage in sexual activity), orientational (concerning the object of sexual desire), and mechanical (pertaining to the ability to engage in actual sexual acts) aspects of sexual behaviour. This seems a useful scheme and will be applied in the discussions of sexual behaviour in this chapter. The principal focus will be on the first two categories of sexual change, as the mechanical aspects of sexual functioning are largely mediated by areas other than the central nervous system (CNS) and are best served by a discussion from a urological, neurological, or orthopaedic point of view. Sexually inappropriate behaviour can be defined as behaviour that is explicitly sexual in nature or the product of an underlying sexual conflict that is harmful physically, mentally, or emotionally to the individual or to someone in his or her environment (Crewe, 1984; Zencius, Weslowski, Bourke, & Hough, 1990).

A second distinction that seems worthwhile is the division of postinjury sexual changes into hyposexuality (a decreased in libido or ability), hypersexuality (an increase in libido or ability), and alteration in the orientation of sexuality (altered sexual preference or the paraphilias). Each of these types of changes has been observed as a consequence of TBI.

The anatomy and physiology of normal sexual behaviour is yet to be precisely delineated. However, the complexity of the neural and hormonal—not to mention the cognitive and emotional systems—involved in normal sexual functioning are significantly perturbed as a result of TBI (Horn & Zasler, 1990). Reflexogenic erection due to direct tactile stimulation of the genitals, prostate, or urethra occurs through activation of the reflex arc at segment S2-S4 in the spinal chord, while psychogenic erection (i.e., arousal as a consequence of mental stimulation) is initiated from higher in the CNS at the thoraco-lumbar segments T12-L4, the subcortex and the cortex. TBI may result in dysfunction at both the genital and psychogenic levels. In the cortex, under the influence of the limbic system and the hypothalamus, psychological stimuli are converted into neuropsychological excitation, which is transmitted to the genitalia resulting in sexual arousal (Kaufmann, 1981).

As a result of TBI, women may experience changes in menstrual cycle, dysfunctional bleeding, decreased amounts of cervical mucous, discharge of breast milk, increased facial or body hair, worsening of acne, change in sex drive, polycystic ovaries, or recurrent spontaneous abortion (Horn & Zasler, 1990). Men often complain of decreased sex drive, impotence, inability to ejaculate, infertility, loss of facial hair, or testicular atrophy. The problems typically reported in sexual function following TBI include: impotence, loss of sensation, poor lubrication, ejaculatory dysfunction, and loss of desire (Horn & Zasler, 1990). Disturbances of body image, sexual identity, and self-esteem issues are very common in those individuals with TBI who have insight into their postinjury state (Ducharme & Gill, 1990; Keppel & Crowe, 2000). The changes in self-concept, cognitive function, and social judgment brought about by TBI place the patient at increased risk for sexuality related problems, including unsuccessful interpersonal relationships, disease, and abuse or exploitation (Medlar & Medlar, 1990).

It is worthwhile to address the issue of the neuroanatomical and neurophysiological changes as a consequence of TBI at a number of levels in the hierarchy between the sensory receptors and the cortical representation of sexual function. Much of the data pertaining to localisation of sexual functioning in humans has been gathered from experimentation with primates, and a direct demonstration of the implication of this data to humans has not been firmly established.

The discussion of the neuroanatomical determinants of sexual functioning begins with an examination of the peripheral nervous system and moves through to an examination of the spinal chord and brain stem, the limbic structures, and, finally, the cortical structures and their compromise as a consequence of brain injury. The contributions of the various neural structures to sexual functioning are outlined in Table 9.1 below.

The peripheral nervous system

Both the male and female sexual organs receive sympathetic and parasympathetic innervation. In males, the sympathetic fibres originate from the mediolateral columns of the spinal chord, and form the hypogastric plexus, which provides both afferent and efferent innervation to the testes, prostate, seminal vesicles, and the *vas deferens*. The pelvic nerves, originating from the sacral spinal chord, provide parasympathetic innervation of the penis, prostate, seminal vesicles, and the *vas deferens* (Horn & Zasler, 1990).

Table 9.1 Correlations between the Neuroanatomical Structure and the Behavioural Correlates of Sexual Functioning

Neuroanatomical Structure	*Neuroanatomical Substructure*	*Behavioural Correlate*
Peripheral Nervous System	Autonomic Sympathetic Parasympathetic Somatic	Genital Sexual Functioning
Brain Stem	Reticular Activating System Afferent Input Efferent Output	Arousal and Alertness and Information Transfer
Subcortical	Hippocampus Amygdala Septal Complex Hypothalamus	Modulation of Sexual Behaviours and Genital Responses
Cortical	Pyriform Cortex Cingulate Cortex Frontal Lobes Temporal Lobes	Modulation of Drive, Initiation, and Sexual Activation

Adapted from Zasler, 1994.

As noted above, in the neurologically intact male, erections are mediated by both the reflexogenic and psychogenic pathways. The reflexogenic pathway is mediated primarily by the automatic sacral parasympathetic nerves and can be activated independently of conscious awareness. Psychogenic erection on the other hand involves supraspinal efferents and is thought to be mediated primarily by sympathetic innervation (Horn & Zasler, 1990). Psychogenic erection can be elicited by mental imagery and by nontactile sensory stimuli (Szasz, 1983). Reflex vasodilation of the genital vasculature in response to sexual stimuli is responsible for both male penile erection and female lubrication (Segraves, 1996). Neuroanatomical studies have demonstrated a dual innervation of the genitals in both sexes—sympathetic innervation from the T12-L4 segments of the spinal chord and parasympathetic sympathetic innervation from the S2-S4 chord segments. Stimulation of the sacral parasympathetic fibres elicits penile erection in many species, and ablation of these nerves interferes with reflexogenic erections. These fibres are also thought to mediate the lubrication response in the female (Segraves, 1996).

In the female, the sympathetic nerve supply is carried by the ovarian plexus. The parasympathetic nerve supply is mediated by the pelvic nerves via the uterine and hypogastric plexuses. The uterus and the ovaries receive sympathetic innervation only, whereas the vagina and the fallopian tubes receive mixed autonomic innervation (Goutier-Smith, 1986; Horn & Zasler, 1990). The autonomic nervous system does not appear to be as critical to fertility in females as it is in males. Furthermore, psychogenic stimulation does not appear to affect the vagina or vulva (Horn & Zasler, 1990).

Orgasm can be thought of as the cumulative sensory experience of a series of spinal chord reflexes. In the male, sensory impulses eliciting the ejaculatory reflex travel along the pudendal nerve to the sacral chord. Once a threshold value of simulation has been reached, contraction of the *vas deferens*, the seminal vesicles, and the prostatic smooth muscle occur resulting in the ejaculate being delivered into the pelvic urethra. Stimulation of the urethral bulb by the inflowing ejaculate elicits reflex closure of the bladder neck, preventing retrograde ejaculation, and rhythmic contractions of the perineal muscles and urethral bulb result in expulsion of the ejaculate (Kleerman, 1970; Segraves, 1996).

Female orgasm also appears to be a genital reflex. Sensory impulses travel to the sacral chord along the pudendal nerve, and efferent fibres innervate the ovary, fallopian tubes, vaginal musculature, and uterus. Rhythmic contractions of these structures appears to be mediated by α-adrenergic fibres, although the female sexual organs also have cholinergic innervation (Segraves, 1996).

High thoracic and cervical spinal chord injuries are extremely destructive to ejaculatory function (Yalla, 1994). Dependent upon the level of the lesion, both reflexogenic and psychogenic erections may remain intact. The former are maintained most frequently in patients with complete upper motor nerve lesions, especially in men with cervical lesions. Psychogenic erections are in tact most often with lower motor neurons lesions below T9 (Segraves, 1996).

There is, however, relatively little information concerning sexual behaviour in female patients with chord lesions, although Berard (1989) in his investigation of 15 chord-injured women noted that orgasm was impossible if the lesion was below T12 because of decreased sensation.

The brain stem

Several systems crucial to sexual functioning are located within the brain stem. The pontine and mesencephalic reticular activating systems, with attendant adrenergic and dopaminergic pathways, are required to initiate arousal and maintain mental alertness. These systems innervate limbic and frontal structures, and when dysfunctional may induce lethargy, decrease in attention, stupor, or even coma (Horn & Zasler, 1990). Specific activation within certain limbic and cortical structures may be required for libido and potency, initiated by externally (i.e., a partner or a movie) or internally generated stimuli (i.e., imagery or fantasy) (Coslett & Heilman, 1986; Miller, Cummings, McIntyre, Ebers, & Grodes, 1986).

Afferent sexual systems are closely associated with spinothalamic pathways in the anterolateral chord in the lateral medulla and pons, prior to their ascent to the thalamus (Boller & Frank, 1982; MacLean, 1975). In his extensive series of stimulation studies in the primate, MacLean noted that seminal discharge, sometimes preceding erection, was elicited only in those cases in which the electrodes impinged on the course of the spinothalamic pathway and its ancient medial ramifications into the caudal intralaminar region of the thalamus (MacLean, Dua, & Denniston, 1963). Stimulation at other sites could produce erection, but rarely ejaculation. Efferent systems to the spinal chord mainly pass from the hypothalamus with autonomic fibres in the dorsal longitudinal fasciculus and other descending pathways (Horn & Zasler, 1990).

Subcortical structures

The ascending sensory inputs from the genitalia appear to relay at the venterolateral and intralaminar nuclei of the thalamus prior to following their cortical pathway to the paracentral lobule (Horn & Zasler, 1990). Stimulation of thalamic areas may also result in erection (MacLean, 1975). The medial dorsal and anterior thalamus are sites that may be involved in the production of an erection. In these cases, input probably relays via the efferent tracts from the cingulum and frontal systems. Lesions in the thalamus have been associated with hypersexuality (Miller et al., 1986).

Limbic and paralimbic structures, particularly the hippocampus, septal complex, amygdala and several of the hypothalamic nuclei, play a crucial role in sexuality. MacLean (1975) postulated that the hippocampus exerts a modulating effect on penile tumescence. In primates, electrical stimulation of the fimbria of the hippocampus may lead to erection. After-discharges have also been seen in the hippocampus following erection-producing stimulation of septal and anterior thalamic sites (Horn & Zasler, 1990). Ablative and stimulation studies of the amygdala have been explored in relation to sexual behaviour. In primates, ablative studies have bilaterally removed large portions of the anterior temporal lobes, including the amygdala. The characteristic syndrome observed in the monkey following these ablations (i.e., the Klüver-Bucy syndrome) often induces sexual and oral activity with inappropriate objects (see the discussion of the clinical features and origins of Klüver-Bucy syndrome in chapter 8).

The form of "hypersexuality" noted in the Klüver-Bucy syndrome in man probably represents a failure to discriminate and effectively channel otherwise intact basic drives in the external world (Horn & Zasler, 1990; Mesulam, 1985, 2000a, 2000b). Throughout phylogeny eating, sexual, and aggressive behaviours have been consistently linked to limbic structures (Horn & Zasler, 1990), and direct stimulation of the amygdala often results in aggressive behaviours in primates and other animals (Horn & Zasler, 1990). In humans, complex partial seizures of temporal lobe origin (i.e., temporal lobe epilepsy: TLE) have been associated with disturbances in sexual functioning and demonstrates the clinical effects of recurrent amygdalar stimulation (Horn & Zasler, 1990). TLE may display itself as a "sexual seizure" with sexual genital sensations and autonomic changes associated with arousal (Boller & Frank, 1982; Freemon & Nevis, 1969). In certain cases, sexual activity may precipitate a seizure. Remmilard, Anderman, and Testa (1983) have reported 12 cases of women who observed epileptic sensations of sexual excitement or orgasm. In most cases, the EEG changes indicated temporal lobe epilepsy, the majority of which had a right-sided focus. The inter-ictal state for some patients with TLE may be characterised by hyposexuality, loss of libido, and unusual sexual practices (for example, transvestism or fetishism) (Boller & Frank, 1982; Freemon & Nevis, 1969; Miller et al., 1986).

Lesions of the limbic system or dysfunction at the hypothalamus and temporal lobe have also been associated with change in sexual preference (Miller et al., 1986). The left limbic region has been described as the area most likely affected in sex offenders who have brain injury, and dysfunction in this area has been reported to cause sexual sadism (Money, 1990).

The hypothalamus has been described as the major effector organ of the limbic system (Mesulam, 1985, 2000a, 2000b). Lesions of the hypothalamus often result in disturbances of sexual behaviour (Horn & Zasler, 1990). The anterior hypothalamus appears to be involved in endocrine activity and associated copulatory behaviours. Lesions here commonly produce hypogonadism and hyposexuality (Horn &

Zasler, 1990). The posterior hypothalamus and mammillary bodies may be part of an inhibitory system, as lesions in these structure may produce increased copulation and precocious puberty in some species (Boller & Frank, 1982).

The septal complex is located anteriorly in the wall of the third ventricle, behind the frontal lobe. Stimulation of the lower septum produces erection (MacLean, 1975), and in humans using self-stimulation procedures, it has been associated with pleasurable sexual sensations somewhat like the feeling of impending orgasm (Geschwind & Galaburda, 1985; Heath, 1964; Mesulam, 1985). Lesions of the septum are also associated with exaggerated emotional responses to threatening or unfamiliar stimuli. It has been postulated that the neurons of the septal complex help to link objects in the extrapersonal world with their motivational value (Mesulam, 1985, 2000a, 2000b), operating as part of the "pleasure circuit" originally described by Olds and Milner (1954).

In both the human male and female, direct stimulation of the septal region of the brain produces sexual orgasm and orgasm in the human is accompanied by electrical discharges in the septal area (Heath, 1963, 1972, 1975). Stimulation of the lower part of the septum and the adjoining medial preoptic area elicited full erection (MacLean & Ploog, 1962). Stimulation in some instances within the dorsal psalterium or fimbria of the hippocampus resulted in recruitment of hippocampal potentials and penile erection (MacLean, Denniston, Dua, & Ploog, 1962). Positive loci for erection were also found in mammillary bodies, along the course of the mammillothalamic tract, in the anterior thalamus, in the pregenual cingulate, and subcallosal cortex, all of which are known to receive projections from the anterior thalamic nuclei (MacLean, 1975). Stimulation at positive sites in the septum and the anterior thalamus commonly led to the development of self-sustained hippocampal after-discharges associated with throbbing of the penis and an increase in size of the erection (MacLean & Ploog, 1962), suggesting that the hippocampus exerts a modulatory influence on penile tumescence (MacLean, 1975). While many subcortical regions have been demonstrated to be responsive to electrical stimulation by producing erection, many points within the caudate, putamen, and globus pallidus elicit no genital response when stimulated (MacLean & Ploog, 1962), indicating that the circuitry is specific and not generalized.

Gorman and Cummings (1992) have reported two patients who developed markedly increased sexual behaviour following placement of ventriculoperitoneal shunts (VP) for the treatment of hydrocephalus. In both cases the catheter tip was located in the dorsal septal region as determined by subsequent CT imaging. Neither patient evidenced atypical sexual behaviour before the brain injury, although the second patient had disinhibited sexual behaviour while in a postencephalitic confusional state prior to shunt placement. There was, however, a dramatic exaggeration of sexual activity following the shunt insertion.

Gorman and Cummings (1992) also noted that no similar cases of hypersexuality with VP shunts in the absence of septal injury were noted in their series, or had been reported by other investigators. They reviewed extensive literature indicating that damage to the septum in animals and man had previously been associated with hypersexuality, including the case described by Heath and Fitzjarrell (1984) in which these investigators attempt to control seizures in a woman with epilepsy by placing a chemically stimulating cannula directly into the septum. When acetylcholine was introduced into the septal region, the patient became euphoric and experienced sexual orgasm on each of the 12 applications. An autopsy several years later confirmed the septal location of the cannula. Sem-Jacobsen (1968) made similar observations in relation to electrical stimulation of the septal area that consistently elicited sexual interest or orgasm. Gorman and Cummings (1992) concluded that the relationship between septal injury and hypersexuality in the two patients they described indicates that the septal nuclei play an important role in mediating sexual behaviour in humans.

Cortical structures

It is interesting to note that in the comprehensive series of stimulation studies conducted by Penfield (Penfield & Jasper, 1954) in his operations to treat epileptic disorders, despite stimulating the greater part of human neocortex as well as the limbic cortex of the insulo-temporal region, he rarely elicited signs or symptoms of a sexual nature (MacLean, 1975). Penfield and Rasmussen (1950) reported that stimulation of the posterior part of the post central gyrus produced genital sensations and patients with epilepsy who had lesions in the paracentral lobule reported genital sensations as a part of the aura (Smith & Khatri, 1979).

Stimulation of the cingulate gyrus and the transitional region between the medial frontal cortex and the limbic cortex of the anterior cingulate has been shown to produce genital hallucination and full penile erection in primates (Dua & MacLean, 1964; MacLean, 1975), although this reaction may be related to a general arousal and motivational system (Mesulam, 1985, 2000a, 2000b).

Lesions in the pyriform cortex, which is directly related to the olfactory circuit, have been related to sexual activity in many species and lesions in this area have been noted to produce hypersexuality (Mesulam, 1985).

The frontal lobes have been consistently implicated in the alteration in sexual function in numerous studies. Injury to the orbital region of the frontal lobes may produce disinhibited and sexually inappropriate behaviour. This behaviour may be only verbal in nature and lack any true sexual arousal or may be associated with true arousal associated with increased promiscuity (Horn & Zasler, 1990). This latter effect is much rarer and, in either case, there may be difficulties with erection and emission (Freemon & Nevis, 1969).

A case that illustrates this phenomenon was described by Miller, Cummings and colleagues (1991) in their description of a 33-year-old man who suffered traumatic brain injury in an automobile accident and had burr holes placed in the posttraumatic period. Contusions of the frontal and temporal lobes were noted at operation and in the years following surgery he became increasingly impulsive and had uncontrollable urges to expose himself in public and subsequently joined a nudist colony.

Injury to the dorsolateral convexity of the frontal lobe results in the apathetic constellation of behavioural changes (see chapter 3). Although the initiation of sexual behaviour is commonly impaired due to the adynamic state, erection and copulation are still possible (Walker, 1976). Frontal injury may also lead to problems of attentional functioning and inability to generate sexually arousing visual imagery. This in turn can compromise effective masturbation unless behavioural techniques are employed to maintain attention to the task (Horn & Zasler, 1990).

In an interesting study of normal subjects, Tiihonen et al. (1994) undertook HMPAO–SPECT (99mTc-hexamethyl propyleneamine oxime–single-photon emission computed tomography) scanning during orgasm in eight right-handed male volunteers. The scans indicated a decrease in cerebral blood flow in all areas of the brain with the single exception of the right prefrontal cortex where the flow was increased.

Aberrant sexual behaviours (ASB) following frontal lesions have also been noted. These include behaviours such as rape, child molestation, exhibitionism, and inappropriate touching, and it is estimated that 7.9% of men who sustain a TBI may display such behaviours postinjury (Simpson, Blaszczynski, & Hodgkinson, 1999). Similar to other disinhibited type behaviours following TBI this behaviour has been related to disinhibition of the usual social constraints associated with the ventromedial prefrontal cortex (VMPFC). The contribution of the preinjury personality, the sequelae of the injury, and the social environment (Simpson, Tate, Ferry, Hodgkinson, & Blaszczynski, 2001) are clearly not irrelevant. However, a number of case reports in the literature (Emory, Cole, & Myer, 1995; Goldberg & Buongiorno, 1982; Lehne, 1986; Miller et al., 1986; Regestein & Reich, 1978; Zencius et al., 1990) noted little evidence of prior sexual offending or the personality or social characteristics typical of offenders prior to the injury. As a result, the lion's share of the attribution of the behaviour change is ascribed to the brain changes.

Lishman (1968) noted that 6% of his sample of war veterans with severe brain injury demonstrated ASB and all of the lesions were frontal, mostly on the left side. Other reports note a frontotemporal focus (Graber, Hartman, Coffman, Huey, & Golden, 1982), a right frontal focus (Lehne, 1986), the basal forebrain, and the medial septal area (Miller et al., 1986) and the left limbic region (Money, 1990).

However, in a more comprehensive study Simpson et al. (2001) assessed 25 patients with ASB and 25 non-ASB brain-injured controls drawn from a pool of 477 patients with TBI who demonstrated 99 incidents of ASB (most commonly frotteurism, 45.5%; touching, 29.3%; exhibitionism, 17.2%; and sexual aggression, 8.1%), no differences were found with regard to premorbid psychosocial disturbance and there was not a higher proportion of frontal system injury, disorders of control, or impairments of executive function as demonstrated by neuropsychological measures in the ASB patients versus the non-ASB TBI controls.

These results lead the authors (Simpson et al., 2001) to conclude: "a simple attribution of SAB (sexually aberrant behaviours) to frontal system dysfunction is not tenable" (p. 569). Clearly the picture is more complex than the simple characterization that frontal lesion equals ASB as has been noted by a number of previous investigators (Levin & Grossman, 1978; Lishman, 1968; Sarapata, Herrmann, Johnson, & Aycock, 1998).

Neurohormonal influences

Clark et al. (1988) studied 33 patients who had loss of consciousness followed by a least a 24-hour posttraumatic amnesia. They demonstrated a fall in free testosterone, basal follicle stimulating hormone (FSH) and basal leutenizing hormone (LH) levels during the first three days following the head injury apparently due to dysfunction of the hypothalamus. The effect on testosterone, which correlated negatively with severity of the injury on admission, persisted at the 3- to 6-month follow-up in 5 out of the 21 patients who were re-tested. The stress of the injury itself can also alter sexual responses by increasing prolactin levels, thus leading to an automatic decrease in testosterone levels (Zasler, 1998).

It appears that androgen levels are closely linked to seminal emission and sex drive in the human male, and that there is a requirement for a certain minimal level of androgen to be available for sexual function to take place; however, excess amounts of androgen above these levels has minimum effect (Segraves, 1996). In the case of the female subject, current evidence suggests the oestrogen levels are essential to maintain vaginal epithelial integrity and lubrication whereas androgen levels may be related to libido (Segraves, 1996). Hyperprolactinaemia has been associated with decreased libido in both sexes (Segraves, 1988).

TBI can also have profound effects on pregnancy, including threats associated with mechanical trauma, unintended pharmacological injury, and the effect of brain injury on appropriate contraceptive regimes (Patel & Bontke, 1990). Crosby and Castilloe (1977), in their study of 441 pregnant women involved in motor vehicle accidents, noted that foetal loss is usually proportional to maternal injury. The leading cause of foetal death was maternal death and the second most frequent cause was placental separation.

Neuroendocrine disturbance following TBI continues to be a relatively poorly researched and understood aspect of these injuries and considerably more data is yet to emerge on the frequency, specificity, and implication of these changes.

Relationship changes

Brecher (1977) indicated that sexual activity in brain-injured males is associated with enhanced illness recovery rates, increased strength, increased immune responses, and produces a more global sense of well-being. However, diminished sexual frequency and physical dysfunction subsequent to closed head injury may also stem from emotional as well as physical problems and in the change in the relationship experienced by either or both partners (Miller, 1994). The sexual relationship is likely to be most satisfying when both partners are able to assume their respective adult roles. Many women report that subsequent to the closed head injury, their husbands became more egocentric, child-like, and animalistic and had a tendency to display dependency, impatience, decreased self-control, self-centredness, and inappropriate public behaviour. As a result of these changes, Miller (1994) noted that spouses often find themselves taking on a disciplinary parental role with the brain-injured spouse. One of Miller's (1994) spouses noted how hard it was to maintain a romantic frame of mind when her husband behaved "like a horny monkey in bed" (p. 15).

The personality changes noted in the injured partner inevitably have a powerful effect on the nature of the relationship within the couple. When we add to this the strain of caring for a "personality changed" partner in association with clinical levels of anxiety and depression in both the injured individual and the partner (Perlesz, Kinsella, & Crowe, 2000), the personality change of the patient, performance anxiety, self-consciousness, fear of rejection, and lack of recent experience (Miller, 1994) added to the environmental changes as a consequence of the injury including reduced income, pending medico-legal disputation, family strain associated with changed roles and responsibilities, and blame associated with the circumstances of the accident, these piled up stressors often contribute to deterioration in the marital relationship and as a result have a detrimental effect the sexual relationship (O'Carroll, Woodrow, & Maroun, 1991).

Allison (1993) notes that while sexual changes subsequent to the injury are common, they are not usually the reason that forces the couple to separate subsequent to the traumatic brain injury. Miller (1994) notes:

> Typically, the patient's wife will say that it is not her husband's erectile dysfunction that is the main problem, but that he just doesn't kiss, caress, cuddle, hold her or just talk to her the way he used to. Intimacy, in other words, is a multidimensional experience: there are many ways to lose it and many ways to get it back. (p. 16)

To summarise, numerous areas within the cerebral cortex, subcortex, brain stem, the peripheral nervous system, and the neuroendocrine system and the relationship of the individual are each important for the maintenance of appropriate sexual activity. Lesions studies have indicated that multiple sites and systems spanning the brain stem, limbic system, diencephalon, and cortex are each implicated in dysfunctional sexual behaviour following injury. Portions of the frontal and temporal lobes as well as the cingulate gyrus serve a regulating role in sexual behaviour, the ultimate expression of which is dependent upon the hypothalamus, pituitary, and basal forebrain nuclei (Ringman & Cummings, 2000). The anterior temporal and frontal structures are particularly susceptible to injury from TBI and the diffuse axonal injury effects of these injuries may compound specific lesion effects by further disconnecting the components of this complex distributed system. The discussion of the mechanics of the neuropathological and physiological alteration of sexual function associated with TBI begs the question: How frequently do sexual problems occur following TBI?

Methodological issues

As alluded to in the discussion of methodology in chapter 2, assessment of sexual changes consequent to closed head injury requires a differentiation between the source of the behavioural changes (Aloni & Katz, 1999). Primary sexual dysfunction refers to a dysfunction that is organic in origin and directly caused by the injury. This stands in contrast to secondary sexual dysfunction, which refers to the delayed aftereffect caused by the primary injury (Kaplan, 1983) that emerges as a consequence of the loss of function associated with the primary injury. Thus, an individual with TBI may not necessarily sustain damage to any of the complex matrix of neuroanatomical regions discussed above, but may develop a secondary depressive state associated with the loss of employment, quality of life, recreational pursuits, or intimate relationships with spouse, family, or friends and still have sexual dysfunction as a secondary effect of the injury mediated by the depression.

For example, in their study of self-reported sexual difficulties in a sample of 322 patients with TBI (193 men and 129 women), Hibbard Gordon, Flanagan, Haddad, and Labinsky (2000) noted that their TBIs reported more frequent physiological difficulties influencing sex drive (i.e., decreased energy, sex drive, ability to initiate sexual activities, or achieve orgasm); physical difficulties (i.e., problems with body positioning, movement, and sensation) and body-image difficulties (i.e., feeling attractive and comfortable having the partner view one's body during sexual activities). Yet in men with TBI and without disability the most sensitive predictor of sexual dysfunction was level of depression, whereas for women endocrine disorders were the best predictor. Due to the complex interacting forces of the organic, cognitive, and psychosocial consequences of brain injury, specific delineation of the nature of these effects can often be difficult to ascertain.

Prevalence and incidence of disturbances of sexual functioning

In this section I attempt to integrate the available literature on the frequency with which sexual functioning has been compromised as a consequence of traumatic brain injury. Unfortunately, the vast majority of data collected on this topic has centred around the examination of compromise in sexual function in male subjects due to their increased prevalence in head-injured samples and to their more obvious manifestation of sexually aberrant behaviours. Where possible, the available data on alteration in female subjects will also be presented.

Dimond (1980) reviewed the older and foreign language literature on the effects of brain injury on sexuality. Impotence has been associated with head injury for many years (Rojas, 1947; Stier, 1938), including boxers with cumulative traumatic encephalopathy (Maudsley & Ferguson, 1963). In examining sexual disturbances in a series of 100 patients with head injuries, Meyer (1955) found that 71% reported a decrease in sexual drive following injury (i.e., 30% mild and 41% severe) with the older patients more affected than the younger ones.

Walker and Jablon (1961) report that in a large sample of World War II veterans with head injury (739 men) the vast majority (87%) had no complaint about their sexual functioning subsequent to the injury. Eight percent complained of impotence or reduced libido, four reported an increase in sexual desire, and 14 reported other problems regarding their sexual appetites. The frontally injured subjects tended to have more sexual complaints than individuals injured in other brain regions. At the 25-year follow-up (Walker, 1972), an unspecified number of wives complained of diminution of sexual functioning in their spouses and wondered whether "anything might be done to enhance his sexual interest" (p. 8).

De Morsier and Gronek (1971) found that 47 of their 49 male patients reported impotence following TBI, and only two of their male patients reported increased sexual desire; there was no mention of decreased sexual desire.

In the more recent literature, the findings with regard to sexual functioning following from the brain injury have been mixed. Bond (1976) was one of the first investigators to address changes in sexuality of a social, physical, and cognitive nature subsequent to head trauma. Bond interviewed 47 males and 9 females at an unspecified time postinjury. The patients had a mean age of 30 years and 96% had suffered posttraumatic amnesia of at least seven days. Bond observed no association between the duration of posttraumatic amnesia, the level of physical disability or cognitive impairment, and the level of sexual activity. Oddy, Humphrey, and Utley (1978) studied 50 adults, six months subsequent to injury with a minimum period of 24 hours of posttraumatic amnesia. Of the 12 married patients, half reported an increase in sexual intercourse and half a decrease subsequent to the injury.

In a subsequent study one year after injury, Oddy and Humphrey (1980) noted that three of seven spouses reported feeling significantly less affectionate towards their injured partners. In one case, the patient suffered partial impotence, whereby he was physically capable of intercourse, but both partners reported curtailed functional ability and sexual satisfaction. Weddell and colleagues (1980) followed up TBI patients two years after injury. The participants were 31 males and 13 females with a mean age of 24.4 years (SD 6.2). Relatives of the participants also provided information in a structured interview. Information relating to alteration in sexual functioning was not specifically requested, and the questions focussed on personality changes. The highest personality change reported was irritability (as noted in the discussion of this matter in chapter 3) followed by alteration in the expression of affection. Eighteen percent of the sample was reported to be more affectionate than preinjury. Increased talkativeness, childishness, and disinhibition were also reported as common sequelae.

Rosenbaum and Najenson (1976) conducted a study investigating wives' reactions to traumatic injury in returned servicemen. Responses to a psychosocial outcome questionnaire were compared among wives of 10 severely brain injured, six spinal chord injured, and uninjured men who had fought in the Yom Kippur war in Israel. The majority of men in the brain-injured sample had suffered penetrating missile wounds, with only 2 out of the 10 sustaining closed head injuries. Analysis of the data revealed the largest reductions in sexual activity and the greatest distress regarding changes in sexual behaviour was in the spinal chord-injured group. Reduced sexual functioning and distress were also reported to be more common in the brain-injured group in comparison with the uninjured controls. The greatest level of mood disturbance was noted in the wives of the brain-injured patients in comparison to the spinal chord-injured patients and the control group, similar to our own observation of parallel levels of distress in the primary caregivers of traumatically brain-injured subjects and the subjects themselves (Perlesz et al., 2000).

Greater levels of mood disturbance were associated with diminished levels of sexual activity and, in addition, negative attitudes towards perceived sexual changes were associated with lower mood level. Overall, Rosenbaum and Najenson (1976) found an extreme reduction in postinjury sexual relations, but no clear-cut relationship between neuroanatomical locus of injury and the presence of sexual dysfunction. This may be because the locus of injury could not be clearly defined by self-report alone and required neurological evidence such as magnetic resonance imaging (MRI) or computed tomography (CT) scan to support information regarding site of injury.

Kosteljanetz, Jensen, Norgard et al. (1981) investigated sexual dysfunction in a sample of 19 males (mean age = 39 years) using both CT scan and questionnaire techniques. The participants had been unconscious for less than 15 minutes and noted postconcussive symptoms that endured for a minimum of six months postinjury. A 23-item questionnaire was administered soliciting information regarding sex drive and erectile dysfunction. Information regarding increased sex drive, frequency of sexual activities, and improved erectile capability was not requested. Ten patients (53%) reported reduced sex drive and 8 (42%) reported erectile dysfunction. The degree of dysfunction correlated highly with the extent of intellectual impairment and degree of cerebral atrophy noted on the CT scans.

Mauss-Clum and Ryan (1981) investigated the reactions of wives and mothers to male patients with brain injury. Half of the sample had received head injury while the other half had suffered brain dysfunction as a result of stroke or hypoxia due to cardiopulmonary disorder. Forty family members responded to the questionnaire in which several questions addressed sexual changes and marital relationships. Just under half the wives and mothers (47%) reported that the patients were either disinterested or preoccupied by sex (no delineation of level of reporting by relationship was outlined). Additionally, 42% of wives reported that they had no sexual outlet. A majority of respondents reported that the patients were dependent, impatient, irritable and had temper outbursts. Respondents also reported inflexibility (20%), self-centredness (43%), decrease of self-control (47%), and inappropriate public behaviour (40%). Emotional distress was frequently reported by wives including frustration (84%), irritability (74%), depression (79%) and anger (63%). Some wives (32%) indicated that they felt they were married to a stranger. Furthermore, nearly half of the wives reported that they were "married but did not have a husband," and felt ensnared. Approximately 25% of the wives reported that they had been verbally abused, threatened with physical violence, and had been accused of providing poor care by their spouses.

Sabhesan and Natarajan (1989) attempted to correlate evidence of persistent neurological damage with disturbances of sexual functioning in East Indian patients one year after head injury. A semi-structured interview was conducted by a psychiatrist and included an assessment of the patient's pretraumatic sexual behaviour, problems in marital life, present neurological status, changes in sexual behaviour, and associated psychological changes in both the patient and spouse. Thirty-four patients were used in the study ranging in age from 18 to 47. Participants were followed up daily from the time of admission to the time of discharge and were subsequently seen at three-month intervals. Four patients were unmarried at the time of the injury and five had either divorced or separated during the follow-up. One of the unmarried and two of the divorced patients were married during this period.

Over a period of one year, 13 of the 34 participants returned to their preinjury level of sexual functioning (Sabhesan & Natarajan, 1989). These 13 subjects then became controls for the remainder of the sample. The remainder demonstrated sexually inappropriate behaviour, total loss of sexual function, and sexual dysfunction. The deviant sexual behaviour included purposeful use of lewd language (9%), frotteurism (6%), exhibitionism (6%), sadism (6%), and rape (3%). Total loss of sexual behaviour was reported in 38% of patients. Approximately 57% of the patients reported decreased interest in sex while two reported increased interest in sex when compared with controls. Premature ejaculation was noted by 7 patients, and a similar number of patients noted postcoital symptoms. Patients with continuing sexual disturbance were distinguished from the controls by having an increased prevalence of delusional disorder, depression, and other neurotic features. The results of the frequency of sexual intercourse aspect of the study may well have been compromised by sociocultural effects. A voluntary restriction on intercourse to conserve health and strength mediated by the belief that spilling semen results in the dissipation of vital forces is apparently a commonly held view in this part of India.

Marital disharmony was reported by 57% of the "dysfunctional" patients compared to 15% of the control group (Sabhesan & Natarajan, 1989). Of the spouses, 62% developed clinically recognisable depression and 28% showed symptoms of anxiety. A random trial among these patients indicated that counselling, education and behavioural therapy were helpful.

Kreutzer and Zasler (1989) conducted a study aimed at assessing the psychosexual consequences of TBI. Their sample consisted of 21 males with a mean age of 39 years (SD 12.6). The mean number of months postinjury was 16.2 (SD 14.1). Five patients were single and the remaining 16 were married, all of whom had reported sexual contact in the past 3 months. They were administered an 11-item questionnaire, the Psychosexual Assessment Questionnaire, which was developed by the authors to assess changes in patients' sexual behaviour, affect, self-esteem, and heterosexual relationships. Each question was presented in a multiple-choice format and respondents were asked to rate changes in each area relative to their preinjury functioning. The results demonstrated that more than half (57%) reported a decrease in sex drive following injury. Fourteen percent indicated increase in sex drive subsequent to the injury and 28% reported no change in comparison to preinjury. The majority of respondents (57%) indicated that their ability to maintain an erection had diminished. An equal number of respondents reported either less time or more time spent in foreplay. Approximately half of the sample (52%) reported no change in ability to achieve orgasm in comparison to preinjury, while one-third reported greater difficulty and 14% reported improved ability to achieve orgasm. Nearly two-thirds (62%) reported diminished frequency of intercourse. Only one patient reported an increase in frequency of intercourse.

With regard to affect and self-esteem, the majority of respondents reported declines in self-confidence (67%), sex appeal (52%), and increased depression (71%: Kreutzer & Zasler, 1989). One-fifth of the sample reported no change in any of the three areas compared to preinjury. Of notable interest was that 14% of the sample reported increased self-confidence and 10% reported diminished depression subsequent to injury.

Data regarding quality of relationships was assessed only for the 16 married patients as none of the 5 single patients reported a steady heterosexual relationship (Kreutzer & Zasler, 1989). Overall, despite changes in sexual behaviour, there was evidence that the quality of marital relationships was preserved. Approximately 40% reported either a good or a very good relationship when compared to preinjury. One half of the sample indicated communication with their partner had remainder the same, 12% report improved communication, and 38% rated communication as worse. Affect and self-esteem were correlated with sexual behaviour, but none of the correlations was statistically reliable.

In our partial replication of the Kreutzer and Zasler (1989) study we (Crowe & Ponsford, 1999) noted 86% of our 14 TBI participants endorsed decrease in sex drive subsequent to the injury, a higher figure than Kreutzer and Zasler who noted this symptom in only 57% of their sample. While 86% of our sample indicated decrease in frequency of intercourse, Kreutzer and Zasler noted only 62%. The discrepancies between the figures were probably attributable to the recruitment method of our study as our sample participants were enrolled in the study because they had noted changes to sexual functioning subsequent to their injuries. This resulted in the participants endorsing a higher incidence of changes in sexual functioning overall. However, the similarity in the nature of the impairments noted is striking. Overall, our TBI participants seem to feature decrease in sex drive as well as decrease in frequency of intercourse in association with marked decrease in level of self-confidence, sex appeal, and affective state subsequent to the injury. The study also examined the possible cause of the diminution of sexual arousal as attributable to a decrease in the ability to generate, control, and manipulate arousing sexual imagery.

In a subsequent study undertaken by Jennie Ponsford (2003) on 208 participants with moderate to severe injury (two-thirds of the sample were male) followed up one to 5 years postinjury as compared to 150 controls, 36–54% of the TBI sample reported decrease in opportunity, importance, and frequency of sexual activity, reduced sex drive, decreased ability to engage in sexual activity, or to give their partner pleasure, and decreased enjoyment and ability to engage in sexual behaviours.

Kreuter, Dallhof, Gudjonsson, Sullivan, and Siosteen (1998) studied 92 individuals (65 men and 27 women) followed up 1 to 20 years postinjury and noted that 40% reported a decreased ability to be able to achieve orgasm, 47% reported decrease in the frequency of sexual intercourse, and 16% reported decreased sexual interest.

Garden, Bontke, and Hoffman (1990) conducted a further study evaluating sexual functioning and marital adjustment after TBI. Their participants (11 men and four women: mean age = 39.2 years) had experienced a single closed head injury at least two months before the study. The participants and their spouses were asked to respond to separate sexual history and functioning questionnaires. Intercourse frequency decreased for 75% of the female participants and their spouses, while 55% of male participants and spouses reported similar declines. Only one male patient and his spouse reported an increase in intercourse frequency after head injury. Forty-seven percent of all couples expressed dissatisfaction with their current sexual frequency, while 40% indicated no change in satisfaction. Five couples did not agree with each other about changes in the duration of foreplay. Of the 10 partners who did agree, foreplay duration increased for three couples (30%), remained the same for four couples (40%), and decreased for three couples (30%).

Erectile and ejaculatory problems were uncommon. One female participant's spouse and four male participants reported occasional erectile difficulties after as compared to before the injury (Garden et al., 1990). Seven (64%) of the female spouses experienced occasional or frequent anorgasmia after the spouse's injury as compared to three (27%) before the injury. Two of the injured female participants (50%) experienced problems with orgasm after the injury, while two had no change in orgasmic capability. Overall satisfaction with marital sexual adjustment since the TBI was recorded by eight (53%) spouses.

O'Carroll and colleagues (1991) conducted a postal questionnaire study and found a high incidence of sexual problems in a mixed sample of mild, moderate, and severely head-injured participants. The study failed to note any relationship between severity of injury and sexual dysfunction, and this was probably due to sampling error inherent within the design of the study. For the study as a whole there was only a 30% response rate, while in the group that was severely head injured, the response rate was 100%.

Sandel, Williams, Dellapietra, and Derogatis (1996) undertook a review of sexual functioning in 52 outpatients with a history of traumatic brain injury (39 men and 13 women; mean age = 34.6 [SD 11.25]; average length of posttraumatic amnesia (PTA) 53.82 days [55.22]; average length of time postinjury 3.71 year [SD 3.14]). The injured participants reported reduction in sexual functioning to below the levels noted in noninjured populations, but only at statistically significant levels on two scales of the Derogatis Interview of Sexual Functioning (DISF); orgasm and drive/desire. The authors noted that there was no relationship between sexual functioning and indices of severity of neuropsychological functioning, although the frontal lobe patients reported more sexual cognitions and fantasies and a higher overall satisfaction with their sexual functioning. Time since injury was inversely related to scores on the arousal scale, possibly suggesting some role of the injured frontal lobe/limbic system in hypersexual state in the early recovery after the injury. Patients with more recent injuries reported greater levels of arousal than those not recently injured. Right hemisphere injuries also correlated with higher scores on reports of sexual arousal and sexual experiences. The authors did note that one of the limitations of the study was the fact that only patients and not significant others were assessed regarding these changes, which may have lead to spurious effects due to the possibility of limitations in self-awareness.

Gosling and Oddy (1999) studied 18 heterosexual couples with regard to the quality of their marital and sexual relationships one to seven years after the male partner had suffered a severe closed head injury. The requirements for inclusion in the study were the necessity to be a heterosexual couple with a male partner who had sustained traumatic brain injury not less than one and not more than seven years prior to the assessment, the couple had to be in a stable relationship for at least three years prior to the injury, the couple were to still be together at the time of the study, and the period of PTA had to be of at least seven days. The mean age of the men was 42.1 years (SD 12.5), and of the women 39.2 years (SD 11.1). They had a mean duration of relationship of 16.2 years (SD 9.4). The mean number of years since the male partner's head injury was 4.1 years (SD 1.9), and the mean length of PTA for the men in the sample was 56.4 days (SD 33.3), indicating very severe injuries.

The females' partners rated their sexual satisfaction as significantly lower after the injury as compared to their evaluation of themselves before the injury (Gosling & Oddy, 1999). Two of the women did not complete the postinjury questionnaire since both reported a complete cessation of their sexual relationship. Another 12 rated their sexual relationship as worse since the injury, three as the same, and only one as improved. Seven women reported that their partner's level of sexual interest had decreased since his injury, seven reported no change, and three reported an increase in interest. Comparison of the female partners' ratings of marital satisfaction with

Table 9.2 Frequency of Alteration to Sexual Functioning Following TBI in a Mixed Group of Published Studies

Study	*Year*	*N*	*N (Male Patients)*	*% Not Changed**	*% Increased*	*% Decreased*
Meyer	1955	100	100	25	4	71
Walker & Jablon	1961	739	739	87	3	10
De Morsier & Gronek	1971	49	49	0	4	96
Oddy et al.	1978	54	NA	0	50	50
Kosteljanetz et al.	1981	19	19	32	10	58
Mauss-Clum & Ryan	1981	40	30	53	NA	NA
McKinlay, Brooks, Bond, Martinage, & Marshall	1981	55	46	52	NA	NA
Kreutzer & Zasler	1989	21	21	29	14	57
Sabhesan & Natarajan	1989	34	20	34	9	57
Davis & Schneider	1990	68	53	84	7	9
Garden et al.	1990	15	11	36	9	55
Kreuter et al.	1998	92	65	60	5	47
Crowe & Ponsford	1999	14	14	7	7	86
Gosling & Oddy	1999	18	17	41	18	41
Ponsford	2003	208	143	33	13	54
MEAN		101.7	94.8	38.2	11.8	53.2

* % not changed is determined by subtracting the number changed from the total number of subjects

those of the injured partner revealed a highly significant difference with the wives reporting much more dissatisfaction than their partners.

The qualitative aspect of the Gosling and Oddy's (1999) study observed a major role change experienced by the women, with many comparing the new role to that of a parent with total decision-making responsibility and the incompatibility of this role with that of sexual partner was noted by many. A tendency for the injured males to express gratitude but not to be able to communicate their feelings adequately was described by many women. Most of the women were resigned to the expectation that there would be little change in the future and, for most, the only positive aspect of the relationship was a sense of commitment and continuing companionship.

In an attempt to determine the level of hyper- or hyposexuality subsequent to TBI a compilation of some of the available data published in the literature is presented in Table 9.2. It should be stressed that the quality of this data is compromised by a number of issues including: (1) most of the data is self-reported; (2) there is no sense in which the samples could be considered to be representative of the TBI population overall as the patients were often selected on the basis of their report of sexual problems; (3) in some cases the data was interpolated from the published figures; (4) some of the older literature did not provide comprehensive enough data to be able to determine the variables of interest; (5) injury severity, period of PTA, and time since injury are various in the compared samples; and (6) data only for male patients was sufficiently plentiful to make any meaningful tabulation.

Despite these obvious shortcomings Table 9.2 does provide some insight into the frequency with which change to sexual function may occur in this selected sample of patients. About one third of male patients do not change as a consequence of the injury. More than half of the samples feature hyposexuality subsequent to the injury. Hypersexuality would appear to be rarer, occurring in less than 10% of cases. While, as noted above, hypersexual behaviour following brain injury is uncommon, when it does occur it is often associated with lesions to the base of forebrain, the diencephalon, and, most notably, the septum. Drugs that increase central monoamines may produce a similar syndrome.

Lesion location and mechanism of sexual dysfunction

Despite the issues raised concerning the site of lesions in TBI and their effect on sexual functioning, there has been surprisingly little support for specificity of localisation in the literature evaluating individuals subsequent to injury. This issue is necessarily confounded by the relatively diffuse nature of traumatic brain injury in its effect on the brain, and in the poor ability for older forms of imaging technology including CT, SPECT, and the earlier generation positron emission tomography (PET) scans to localise specific lesion sites.

Lishman (1973) noted that decreases in libido seem to be correlated with the severity of brain injury. Meyer (1971) made a similar observation. Bond (1976), on the contrary, found no association between the duration of posttraumatic amnesia, level of physical activity or cognitive impairment, and the level of sexual activity. Rosenbaum and Najenson (1976) found a drastic reduction in postinjury sexual relations, but no clear-cut relation between locus of injury and the presence of sexual dysfunction.

Kosteljanetz et al. (1981) noted the degree of sexual dysfunction observed in their sample was highly correlated with the extent of intellectual impairment and the degree of cerebral atrophy on CT, with sexual dysfunction more common in the impaired group. Sabhesan and Natarajan (1989) noted that in their sample of 34 patients, neurological parameters of severity such as duration of consciousness, PTA, early neurological deficit, presence of fracture, and the cause of injury were not significantly associated with the disability. However, they did note that sexually inappropriate behaviour was consistently noted in five of the eight patients that demonstrated evidence of frontal lobe damage. In the other three patients, there was a total loss of libido as a part of global amotivational state.

Zasler and Horn (1990) make a distinction between disinhibited sexual behaviour and hypersexual behaviour. In their view, true hypersexuality is more common in association with damage to the limbic system of the brain, whereas disinhibited sexual behaviour is a part of a general disinhibition phenomena thought to be related to involvement of the orbital (VMPFC) areas of the frontal lobes and associated structures. Hypersexuality of itself is thought to be related to a general loss of control in all aspects of behaviour rather than to greater sexual need per se (Aloni & Katz, 1999).

Griffith, Cole, and Cole (1990) propose that diffuse frontal injury with the involvement of the neural and endocrine systems is responsible for diminished sex drive. Garden (1991) proposes that medial temporal lesions account for hypersexuality whereas bilateral temporal lesions with lesions of the limbic system cause hyposexuality. Zasler (1998) contends that the frontal temporal areas, adjacent to the limbic structures of the right hemisphere, are responsible for arousal and sexual function. Lundberg (1992) concurs with Zasler and emphasises the contribution of the basal hypothalamus and the adjacent areas of the temporal lobe in regulating sexual desire. Rosenbaum and Hoggs (1989) note a drastic reduction in sexual relations, but no clear-cut relationship with locus of injury while Sandel et al. (1996) noted that most of their group were not experiencing major sexual dysfunction and not surprisingly observed that there was no relationship between sexual functioning and indices of the severity or neuropsychological functioning in their study. The frontal-lobe-injured patients reported more sexual cognitions and fantasies and a higher overall satisfaction with their sexual functioning, perhaps suggesting some role of injured frontal lobe/limbic system in hypersexual states in the early recovery period after injury.

Sexual disinhibition varies considerably in its nature and intensity and may include tactless attempts at intimacy, conversation loaded with sexual innuendo, inappropriate touching, lewd remarks, and, in more severe cases, indecent exposure and public masturbation (Miller, 1994).

Changes to sexual orientation have occasionally been noted in the wake of traumatic brain injury. These changes are more common with lesions of the limbic system, hypothalamus, and temporal lobe (Miller et al., 1986). For example, one patient with epilepsy who also engaged in fetishism and cross-dressing changed to a heterosexual pattern of sexual behaviour after temporal lobectomy (Mitchell, Falconer, & Hill, 1983). Horn and Zasler (1994) note that it is not uncommon for traumatic brain-injured patients who were heterosexual before their injury to turn to homosexual lifestyles or at least to engage in experimentation after injury. The authors consider this possibly occurs as a result of this being the only way that these individuals may be able to express their sexual feelings and meet their sexual needs due to the psychosocial concomitants of the injury. Brain injury may lead to paedophilia, and careful assessment of paedophilic patients may lead to discoveries of associated neurological abnormalities (Miller et al., 1986).

The evolution of sexual dysfunction following TBI

As with all aspects of behavioural change subsequent to traumatic brain injury, the nature of sexual function following the injury is subject to developmental effects that ensue in the period following the injury. Blackerby (1987) proposes that there are three phases of the development of sexual functioning following TBI. In the acute stage, the severely injured patient tends to be self-stimulating and exhibitionistic, which facilitates the patient's waking process (Blackerby, 1987; Ducharme & Gill, 1990). Sexual delusions may also be present. The second phase is characterised by inappropriate verbal allusions, confabulation, joking, and sexual approaches. These approaches may also be physical, accompanying the increase in sexual drive. The "reentry" phase is characterised by insensitivity to others, distractibility, poor judgement, memory disturbance, social isolation, medication effects, altered body image, and altered self-concept. The patient is faced with the changes in role as well as in reintegrating into the family and community. At this stage, the emotional reaction of the patient to the injury, including features of anxiety and depression, will often come into play (Blackerby, 1987; Ducharme & Gill, 1990). These deficits may effect a vicious circle of events triggering feelings of sexual inadequacy and incompetence that, in association with compromise in self-esteem and body image, may lead to social isolation and withdrawal.

Most TBI individuals sustain their injury during late adolescence and early adulthood. A number of developmental tasks must be undertaken during this time, the purpose of which is to facilitate the individuation process. The successful achievement of these tasks culminates in adult independence. The resolution of adolescence has been described as encompassing the achievement of six basic tasks: (1) attainment of separation and independence from the parents; (2) establishment of sexual identity; (3) commitment to work; (4) development of a personal value system; (5) development of a capacity for lasting relationships and sexual love; and (6) evolution of the relationship with parents into a state of relative parity (Committee on Adolescence, 1968). The period between ages 18 and 30 is the time in which the individual typically engages in activities that define and express his or her gender identity role through the formation of intimate relationships, the creation of family and the acquisition of the parenting role, a commitment to vocational activities, and involvement in social relationships and community roles (Gutman & Napier-Klemic, 1996).

In the ideal situation, substantial progress towards achievement of these aims would ordinarily transpire between the periods of 15 and 30 years. The impact of TBI, however, often results in regression to the dependency, irresponsibility, and immaturity more characteristic of earlier age levels (Blazyk, 1983). For many traumatically brain-injured individuals, normal development towards individuation and independence is disrupted or even reversed. This process is further disrupted as the individual brain injury means that these individuals may not have the same cognitive resources that were available prior to the injury or that other, non-brain-injured individuals would ordinarily possess (Blackerby, 1990). Consequently, while age-relevant issues regarding autonomy, sexuality, sexual orientation (Mapou, 1990), identity, self-image, relationships, and achievement remain, the capacity for positively resolving these issues is permanently diminished by the neuropsychological and psychosocial consequences of severe head trauma (Blazyk, 1983).

Conclusion

Alteration in sexual function following the injury comes about as a consequence of a combination of biopsychosocial factors. Clearly the contribution of each of these to compromise in sexual functioning added together produces a rich and complex cocktail of change as a consequence of the injury. TBI patients are usually in a regressive state subsequent to their injuries in which the need for care, attention, and love predominate. Mature sexual relations require the ability to interact, take initiative, and to adequately understand the needs of the other for their success (Benyakar et al., 1988). In the context of the injury then, it is thus not too surprising that things go awry.

10 Synthesis and conclusion

Putting it all together

The aim in this last chapter is to attempt to relate the nature of the initial injury to the final behavioural and emotional outcome for the postinjury individual. How sensible, then, is it for us to make an argument that the traumatic brain injury (TBI) has directly or indirectly caused the resulting outcome?

Kluckhohn and Murray (1953) note that "Everyman is in certain respects: (a) like all other men, (b) like some other men, and (c) like no other man" (p. 53). Clinical practice is based upon the nature of the individual case and, as a result, the interaction of forces that make each case simultaneously similar and distinct are at the heart of why two individuals respond in markedly different ways to the same brain injury.

Van Reekum, Cohen, and Wong (2000) noted the following criteria for determining the relationship between a particular cause and the ensuing disease state as originally adapted from the work of Sir Austin Bradford Hill (1965). The proposed criteria (van Reekum et al., 2000) for causation include:

> (1) consistently demonstrating an association between the causative agent and the purported outcome; (2) demonstrating a biologic gradient (i.e., that more of the causative agent causes more of the outcome); (3) demonstrating an appropriate temporal sequence (i.e., that the causative agent comes first in time); (4) providing a biologic rationale; (5) using analogous evidence (which is soft evidence in the sense that the pathophysiology of TBI is very different from that of any other neurological disorder); (6) finding experimental evidence for causation will not be available for TBI because clearly it is unethical to experimentally induce TBI in humans, and animal models of psychiatric illness are very limited); and (7) finding evidence of specificity of causation (this criterion has been deemphasized, because even in infectious diseases, it is clear that a single organism may produce a number of diseases and some disease may be produced by a number of infectious agents). (p. 317)

While these features may apply in more clearly biologically determined disease states such as an infection or metabolic disorder, the first four seem to be the most important areas of focus in the context of our discussion. Let's examine each of these in turn.

Consistently demonstrating an association between the causative agent and the purported outcome. There seems little doubt (as each of the areas we have surveyed so far have demonstrated) that there is an association between the TBI and various forms of behavioural and emotional sequelae. I believe that we can categorically endorse the view that the evidence does support this criterion.

Demonstrating a biologic gradient. It is difficult to contend that there is a direct and proportionate increase in the level of psychopathology and behavioural disturbance in those individuals who have more severe as compared to less severe injuries. For example, van Reekum et al. (2000), surveyed the incidence of major depression, bipolar affective disorder, generalized anxiety disorder, obsessive compulsive disorder, panic disorder, posttraumatic stress disorder, schizophrenia, substance abuse, and personality disorder subsequent to TBI and noted that the support for the association was mixed at best and, in the case of PTSD, there was "compelling evidence for a reverse gradient (i.e., increased risk of PTSD with milder TBI)" (p. 324). This is a similar conclusion to the one noted in chapter 4.

This seems to weaken the case for a direct association between the trauma and the presentation. It may perhaps provide some support for the notion that in individuals affected by TBI there is some specifically vulnerable area or areas of the brain that are always affected irrespective of severity of the blow. The neuropathological literature surveyed in chapter 1 consistently indicates that the effect of the TBI is diffuse rather than specific and the mechanism of a "specific" area of vulnerability, such as the ascending neuromodulatory tracts for dopamine, noradrenaline, acetylcholine, and serotonin that supply the cortex, might be an important possibility, but the mechanisms for such a process would require considerable further exposition.

A second issue here is the degree to which a lack of insight associated with a more severe injury (see chapter 6) may result in a behavioural syndrome in which the level of the stressor was not to be apprehended or accommodated due to the inability on the part of the individual to grasp the meaning and implication of any postinjury changes, thereby acting as a protective mechanism against the development of the more severe forms of psychopathology.

Certainly it is the case that length of coma, duration of posttraumatic amnesia, the presence of seizure, and the type of brain injury (i.e., complicated versus uncomplicated mild traumatic brain injury [MTBI]) (William, Levin, & Eisenberg, 1990) are associated with the outcome of TBI (Alexander, 1995; Johnston & Hall, 1994; Ruff, Crouch et al., 1994), but at best, the association between the severity of the injury and the behavioural and emotional outcome is not a direct one. Van Reekum et al. (2000), keen not to throw the baby out with the bath water on this point, note that the absence of a biologic gradient in and of itself is a fascinating finding and does not definitively lessen the support for causation, and instead they note that the presence of the injury, irrespective of severity, may convey an increased risk for the development of the behavioural and emotional disorders.

Van Reekum et al. (2000) note, for example, that the relative risk (i.e., the risk of developing the diagnosis after a TBI as compared to the risk for those who do not have a TBI) of developing major depression after TBI was 7.5. A relatively high level of risk was also noted for developing bipolar affective disorder with an increased risk of 5.5. The level of risk (2.0) for developing anxiety disorders was less powerful with the exception of panic disorder that increased the risk by 5.8. The risk for schizophrenia and substance abuse were quite low with the risks less than or equal to 1, indicating little or no increased risk of the disorder following the injury (van Reekum et al., 2000).

Demonstrating an appropriate temporal sequence. While there does tend to be support for the idea that the TBI comes first and then the behavioural changes ensue, I could certainly not argue that this was consistently and always the case. In the emergence of postinjury psychosis discussed in chapter 6, the lead times can be very long indeed, and at any stage through this process it is impossible to disentangle the injury-related effects from those that occur as a consequence of changes in circumstance, ability, and interpersonal responding, which of themselves have been proven to contribute to the emergence of these presentations in non-brain-injured individuals.

Providing a biologic rationale. Once again the support for this association has been less than powerful. Premorbid characteristics of the patient have been consistently demonstrated to influence the likely outcome for an individual subjected to a TBI. For example, an individual with a prior history of alcohol or drug abuse or psychopathology is more vulnerable to the physiological and long-term behavioural and emotional sequelae of the injury (e.g., Corrigan, 1995; Dikmen, et al., 1995; Solomon & Malloy, 1992), than an individual without this history (see chapter 8). Preexisting differences in personality, social role, adjustment, education, and intellect have also been associated with the level of persisting disability (e.g., Gans, 1983; MacMillan, Hart, Martelli, & Zasler, 2002; Thomsen, 1992), and individuals who have a history of psychological adversity prior to their injury have poorer recovery and more marked "late" symptoms than those who do not (MacMillan et al., 2002). Once again, it would be hard to definitively say that the injury itself is at fault if the substrate to which the injury has been added of itself conveys a vulnerability to the injury.

It is clear through our analysis of the various behavioural and emotional complications that can ensue in the wake of TBI that the relationship between these entities and the physical nature of the original injury in a sizeable percentage of cases is not a direct one. Each individual case will result in a different structural and behavioural pathology dependent upon the nature and severity of the injury and the physical forces of the impact, as well as the age, sex, genetic endowment, and experience of the individual at the time of injury. These effects will be further mediated by the individual's response to the injury as well as how the circumstances affecting the individual physically, cognitively, emotionally, socially, or economically have changed. Thus, while TBI can be treated as if it were a common diagnostic entity, the nature of the individual component in terms of the blow, the neural substrate, and the individual who sustains the injury each contribute unique variance to the explanation of the postinjury outcome. Nonetheless, I doubt that any of us would concede that there is no association between the injury and the final outcome. How, then, are we to conceptualise this relationship?

A biopsychosocial model of response to TBI

There is now almost universal agreement in the area of psychiatry that the biopsychosocial model of psychopathology is one of the most effective ways to characterise the diverse features of these disorders (Dilts, 2001). This model was originally proposed by George Engel in the early 1980s (Engel, 1980), and its principal theoretical position is that all illnesses have biological, psychological, and social causes.

The biological model of mental illness proposes that mental illness is caused by dysfunction of tissues and cells. The psychological model proposes that mental disorders are the result of previous patterns of thinking, feeling, perceiving, cognating, and behaving. The social model proposes that mental disorders are caused by dysfunctional interpersonal interactions including, importantly, developmental and childhood experiences. The model contends that each of these domains interacts with and influences the others in producing the final outcome (Dilts, 2001).

Most psychiatric syndromes described in the *DSM-IV-TR* (APA, 2000) can be characterized as either primary (i.e., arising directly from a particular biological state related to the given disorder) or secondary (i.e., resulting from the effects of general medical disorders of neurologic, cardiologic, oncologic, or endocrinologic functioning). Clearly, in the context of TBI, both sources of psychopathology may be at work and each needs to be explored in turn.

One useful way of looking at the evolution of the behavioral and emotional disorders following TBI is to consider them in the context of the "diathesis stress" model. This model proposes that individuals vary in terms of their sensitivity to stress-induced biological responses, due to their genetic endowment and their exposure to stressful life events (SLE), both in the presence of the injury and during their pre-injury lives. As discussed in chapter 4, stressful experiences may alter endocrine processes to the extent that normal homeostatic processes become compromised and thus psychopathology ensues. A stressful experience may thus exhaust psychological coping by compromising underlying biological and motivational processes.

The contribution of prior SLEs to the emergence of psychopathology has been clearly demonstrated in a number of psychopathological entities including depression and a variety of the anxiety-related conditions (Abramson, Alloy, & Metalsky, 1988; Angst & Vollrath, 1991; Brown & Bifulco, 1985; Ingram & Luxton, 2005; Overholser, Norman, & Miller, 1990; Paykel & Dowlatshahi, 1988; Scher, Ingram, & Segal, 2005; Traill & Gotlib, 2006). The effects of SLEs on other forms of psychopathology including schizophrenia have also been numerously reported in the literature (Mason & Beavan-Pearson, 2005; O'Flynn, Gruzelier, Bergman, & Siever, 2003), and a number of theorists (e.g., Warren & Zgourides, 1991; Rasmussen & Eisen, 1991) have also proposed that SLEs might be implicated in the onset of obsessive-compulsive disorder (OCD).

One study that attempted to differentiate between the types of events involved in particular patterns of symptomatology found that events involving loss were more likely to lead to depressive symptoms, whereas events involving threat and danger were more likely to lead to anxiety symptoms (Finlay-Jones & Brown, 1981). On the other hand, other studies have found that recent SLEs often play an important role in mixed forms of depression/anxiety whereas they appear to only play a minor role in "pure" forms of depression and anxiety where childhood and genetic factors are thought to be of greater importance (Alnaes & Torgersen, 1988; Torgersen, 1985a, 1985b).

It thus seems that there is little doubt that SLEs of themselves can contribute to the emergence of significant psychopathology. The other side of the coin, however, (i.e., what is the nature of the diathesis?) has proven more elusive (Ingram & Luxton,

2005). A good example of this is the cognitive vulnerability model (Beck, Rush, Shaw, & Emery, 1979; Clark & Beck, 1999).

The cognitive vulnerability model proposes that schemas in the form of poorly adaptive attitudes, beliefs and assumptions about the world, the self, and the future contribute to the onset of depression when they occur in the context of other predisposing factors. Thus individuals with the cognitive vulnerability are at greater risk of developing depression because of their greater tendency to appraise life events as negative (Alloy, Abramson, Hogan et al. 2000; Alloy, Abramson, Whitehouse et al., 2006). The three aetiological hypotheses concerning cognitive vulnerability are stability, onset, and relapse (Clark & Beck, 1999). The stability hypothesis proposes that the cognitive structures contributing to the vulnerability for depression are relatively stable, although inaccessible until unmasked by an internal or external stimulus (Clark & Beck, 1999). The onset hypothesis contends that negative events that match the maladaptive content of the schema will lead to a greater risk of depression in individuals who have not previously proven to be depressed. The depression recurrence hypothesis indicates that "a negative event that matches the content of the self-referent schemas ...will lead to a heightened risk of recurrence of depression" in individuals who have previously had a history of depression (Clark & Beck, 1999, p. 268).

While there is support for these models, contrary findings have also emerged. For example, the remitted depression studies (i.e., the maladaptive cognitive patterns are concomitants rather than vulnerabilities for depression) (Haeffel, Abramson et al., 2005; Teasdale & Barnard, 1993), indicate that the effects of antidepressants that reduce depressive thinking support the conclusion that the negative thinking is mood dependent rather than an enduring characteristic of vulnerable individuals (Teasdale, 1993). In response to this sort of evidence, a third possibility is that a third intervening variable that correlates with measures of cognitive responsivity to therapy has been proposed (Ingram, Miranda, & Segal, 1998).

Another example of the predisposing factors that may relate to this issue is the notion of psychosis-proneness. Researchers studying the causes of schizophrenia have long recognised the need to isolate indicators of the disorder that appear before its clinical manifestation (Overby, 1992). Accurate and early assessment of individuals at risk for schizophrenia is important, as the timely application of effective behavioural interventions (e.g., social skills training, cognitive behavioural therapy, and occupational therapy: Liberman, Musser, & Wallace, 1986) have been shown to lessen relapse rates of the condition and make the study of early and prophylactic use of medication a more sensible enterprise.

Traditionally, "at risk" research has targeted the families of affected individuals, yet the majority of those affected has no detected expression of schizophrenia among their first-degree relatives (Gottesman & Shields, 1972). The development of psychometric measures of risk has allowed sampling of the population on a much broader scale. Chapman and Chapman (1985) among others (e.g., Mason, Claridge, & Jackson, 1995) have developed a set of scales based on Meehl's (1962, 1990) constructs of schizotypy and schizoidy. Isolation of psychosis-prone individuals using this technique relies on accurate self-assessment on several scales reflecting schizophrenia-related symptomatology. Psychosis-prone individuals exhibit a multitude of abnormalities reflective of schizophrenia including information-processing deficits and neuropsychological deficits (Asarnow, Neuchterlein, & Marner, 1983; Avons et al., 2003; Gruzelier et al., 2003; Kimble et al., 2000) and thought and language disorders (Allen & Schuldberg, 1989; Liddle et al., 2002; Niznikiewicz et al., 2002).

In one of our studies (McLaren & Crowe, 2003) we took this notion of susceptibility and invoked a similar argument regarding the emergence of OCD, which is one of the most debilitating and prevalent anxiety disorders, with a cross-cultural lifetime prevalence of about 2.5% (Karno, Golding, Sorenson, & Burnam, 1988; Nelson & Rice, 1997; Stein, Forde, Anderson, & Walker, 1997; Trivedi, 1996; Weissman, Bland, Canino, Greenwald, Hwu, Lee, Newman, Oakley-Browne, Rubio-Stipec, Wickramarathe, Wittchen, & Yeh, 1994). Sufferers typically spend excessive time obsessing about intrusive phenomena and feel compelled to carry out extensive rituals that are distressing and time-consuming (Abramowitz, 1997).

A number of laboratory studies have demonstrated that subjects who display a strong tendency to suppress their thoughts experience an increased frequency of the suppressed thoughts in what has become known as the "rebound effect" (Clark, Ball, & Pape, 1991; Lavy & van den Hout, 1990; Wenzlaff, Wegner, & Klein, 1991). In addition, some researchers have found that people with OCD tend to suppress their thoughts more than non-OCD subjects (Muris, Merckelbach, & Horselenberg, 1996; Salkovskis, 1985). In line with this, the "rebound" phenomenon has been postulated as an important factor in the maintenance of OCD symptomatology, particularly the obsessive component of the disorder (Salkovskis & Campbell, 1994). However, the relationship between thought suppression and psychopathology remains unclear since researchers have failed to identify thought suppression as a predictor variable for increased intrusive phenomena (Kelly & Kahn, 1994; Roemer & Borkovec, 1994; Salkovskis & Campbell, 1994).

While considerable evidence is now available indicating that there is a major genetic contribution to the emergence of the disorder (e.g., Pauls & Alsobrook, 1999; Pollock & Carter, 1999) and to its comorbidity with Tourette's syndrome (Pauls, Towbin, Leckman, Zahner, & Cohen, 1986), fewer studies have focused upon the environmental factors that might govern the initial onset of OCD.

It can be argued that SLEs involve different degrees of controllability, some where life changes, although stressful, are controllable (i.e., deciding to move, taking a new job, terminating a relationship) while others can affect the individual when there is little or no perceived capacity to control the events (i.e., being evicted, being fired, or having a relationship terminated). Some research has linked OCD with the notion of control, and, in particular with a lack of perceived mental control of the stressful events (Clark & Purdon, 1995; Edwards & Dickinson, 1987; Freeston, Ladouceur, Rheaume, Letarte, Gagnon, & Thibodeau, 1994). Studies employing human subjects have found that uncontrollable stress leads to higher levels of anxiety than controllable stress (Netter, Croes, Merz, & Müller, 1991; Sanderson, Rapee, & Barlow, 1989). Huether's extensive review of this literature (1998) observed that long-lasting uncontrollable stress that activated sustained levels of glucocorticoid release was associated with the destabilisation and reorganisation of neuronal networks in the cortical and limbic brain structures of young children.

Taken together, these studies suggest a relationship between SLE and the psychological states observed in anxiety and depression. A number of researchers (Freeston, Ladouceur, Rheaume, Letarte, Gagnon, & Thibodeau, 1994) have identified lack of perceived mental control as a possible determining factor in OCD. Some controlled studies indicate that the extent of perceived control over stressful events could be an important factor in determining responses to stress and, hence, psychopathological outcome.

It seems likely that uncontrollable SLE could lead to heightened levels of fear and anxiety, and a heightened sense of subjective threat relative to controllable life events. If such an uncontrollable life event was combined with a tendency towards thought suppression, then OCD could be a predictable outcome. This contention is supported by previous studies with posttraumatic stress disorder (PTSD) indicating that trauma reactions are, at least in part, maintained by thought suppression (Ehlers & Clark, 2000). This suggestion has also been noted in the context of the discussion of blame surrounding the injury. If one assumes one has responsibility for the event, this may then provide a buffer against the long-term distress associated with it because it suggests that, at least at some level, one had control over the outcome (Brewin, 1984; Bulman & Wortman, 1977; Delahanty, Herberman, Craig, Hayward, Fullerton, Ursano, & Baum, 1997; Williams, Williams, & Ghadiali, 1998).

We tested these conjectures in our study (McLaren & Crowe, 2003) to determine if the suggested relationships did apply. The overall results of the study with both clinical and nonclinical samples of participants supported the notion that strong efforts to suppress thoughts (i.e., the diathesis) coupled with a low perceived capacity to control a recent SLE (i.e., the stress) are associated with increased OCD symptoms and diagnosis.

The strength of this correlation suggested that while low perceived control over stressful life events is a clear factor in OCD symptomatology, the effect of high levels of thought suppression was even more profound. These findings reinforce other research that indicates that thought suppression exerts a strong main effect upon the manifestations of psychopathology. The findings from the study extended this suggestion by specifically associating high thought suppression in combination with a lack of perceived control over SLE in the occurrence of OCD symptoms.

At this stage it is unclear exactly how these variables are exerting their influence. It may be that people who are high thought suppressors are inclined to "attract" SLEs and then perceive themselves as lacking control over those events. However, according to Wegner and Zanakos (1994) it is more probable that the tendency towards thought suppression *follows* unwanted experiences rather than acting as a cause of sensitivity to those unwanted experiences. It is conceivable that people might differ in their proclivity to adopt more vigilant mental control strategies than others due to either an experiential or genetically derived predisposition to these behaviours or both. The ready adoption of such avoidance strategies where thoughts and feelings are deliberately suppressed, might inadvertently lead the person into an OCD-type cycle as he or she fails to habituate to the relevant fear stimuli.

It is worth noting an unexpected finding of the study: Respondents who reported that they had *not* undergone a stressful life event in the preceding 18 months but who showed a high tendency towards thought suppression also produced high scores on the anxiety, OCD, and depression self-report measures. There are several possible explanations for this finding. First, it might be that respondents have experienced earlier high-magnitude stressful life events that are impinging on present psychopathological symptoms, but that these earlier events were not reported. Alternatively, it could indicate the overarching effect of thought suppression on many psychopathological symptoms. Whether the notion of thought suppression suggests an innate tendency or whether the thought suppression has come about as a means of attempting to maintain control during a past high-magnitude stressful life event remains a question for future research.

The conclusion to be drawn from our study is that the psychological nature of the individual who goes on to have the uncontrolled stressful life event such as sustaining a TBI significantly contributes to the subsequent pathology that emerges for that individual. It is difficult to be definitive about what the diathesis for each individual might be and how this might culminate in the final pathological outcome for those individuals who sustain a TBI. Certainly in the case of the individual who goes on to develop OCD subsequent to the TBI the diathesis in my view would be high levels of thought suppression. For the emergence of psychosis, possibly psychosis-proneness, and for the emergence of depression, the previous pattern of loss, or the perception of the loss of how life could have been without the TBI, culminates in the behavioural and emotional complications of the condition.

These thoughts are echoed by MacMillan and colleagues (2002) who note:

> Brain injury results in multiple cognitive, emotional, social and physical demands that constitute, singularly and in combination, severe stressors that not only challenge the coping capabilities of the individual, but also directly diminish available resources through the loss of pre-morbid skills coupled with reductions in social and financial supports. (p. 47)

While the cumulative multistressor account of the behavioural and emotional complication following a TBI is compelling (e.g., Evered, Ruff, Baldo, & Isomura, 2003; Ruff et al., 1996; Ruff & Richardson, 1999) it should be emphasised that support for the model continues to be theoretical and definitive studies in support of this contention are yet to be completed (Iverson, 2005).

Is it possible for us then to make a more succinct account of how these complex susceptibilities in association with the injury act together to produce the final outcome for the individual? A good place to complete this process is by examining the model proposed by Thomas Kay (1993, 1999).

Kay's model of the interaction of preinjury status, injury variables, psychological and sociological variables to the evolution of behavioural and emotional dysfunction following TBI

A particularly attractive model of some of these phenomena in the context of TBI was developed by Thomas Kay (Kay, 1993; 1999; Kay, Newman, Cavallo, Ezrachi, & Resnick, 1992). Kay contends that after a traumatic event potentially causes

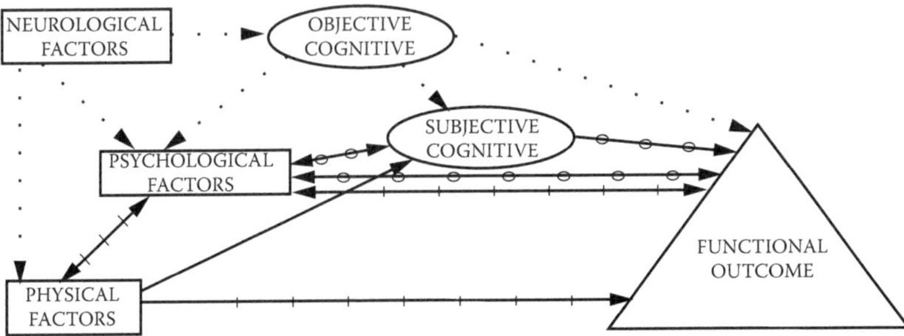

Figure 10.1 A neuropsychological model of functional outcome after MTBI.

brain damage, neurological, physical, cognitive, and psychological factors may each interact to determine the person's resultant level of functioning (Kay, 1999). Kay's model is a dynamic one in which forces move from one influence to another and the resultant level of functional outcome for the individual arises as a consequence of the interaction of each of these variables. Kay's model is presented in Figure 10.1.

A central concept to the model is the notion of relative "vulnerability," a similar concept to the one we have just been considering in the context of our discussion of the diasthesis. Along each of the dimensions of the model, neurological, physical, cognitive, and psychological, the person is considered to have relative strengths or vulnerabilities that help determine the impact of the trauma on his or her ability to function in the wake of the injury sustained. The principal areas of vulnerability include all of the previous psychological factors in the individual's life history prior to the injury contributing to the substrate on which the injury reacts. As Kay (1999) notes:

> The predisposing psychological factors include prior psychological history, personality style and coping mechanisms, the emotional response to the injury, and the psychological realities of the person's work and home environments including their interpersonal relationships and family situations. Individuals with preexisting psychiatric or personality disorders have poorer outcomes after central nervous insult. However, certain individuals who appeared to be functioning within the normal range pre-morbidly may nevertheless carry the psychological ingredients for vulnerability to the effects of trauma, physical injury and pain or loss of cognitive function. (p. 154)

A person who has experienced significant sexual, physical, or emotional trauma in the past, may achieve the appearance of emotional stability in the present by dissociating those experiences. The integrity of the personality is thus sustained by denying, suppressing, or repressing the previous trauma (Kay, 1999): In the wake of the additional stress associated with the TBI, in which the original mechanisms of coping with the preinjury trauma become overtaxed, that the decompensation occurs and culminates in the emergence of psychiatric morbidity.

Kay (1999) draws a distinction between brain dysfunction (a term implying abnormal brain function not necessarily associated with structural change) and brain damage or impairment (a term referring to the permanent structural changes within the brain). Kay maintains that psychological factors such as anxiety, depression, and emotional disruption independent of or due to reactivated prior emotional trauma, as well as physical factors such as fatigue, pain, and medication effects, can each affect cognitive function above and beyond damage to the brain. Kay's point is well taken and it is clear that the constellation of deficits occurring for the individual is the crucial determinant of the final outcome, irrespective of whether these are due to objective neurologically based deficits or to more subjective psychological and social phenomena.

Kay (1999) also makes a distinction between objective and subjective cognitive components. He contends that the objective cognitive component is the true cognitive potential of the individual as defined by neurological factors only. However, the final cognitive outcome for the individual occurs as a consequence of these objective deficits combined with the subjective cognitive components that represents the person's experience of his or her own cognitive capacities at any given point in time.

Under the conditions of the decompensation associated with preexisting trauma coupled with the compromise of function arising from the contemporary injury—especially when depression, anxiety or dissociation are present—the cognitive capacity for attention, new learning, and organisation may break down in a way that may mimic brain injury (Kay, 1999). The hallmarks of these situations include: the presence of extreme subjective complaints that are not borne out or appear inconsistent on neuropsychological testing, a history consistent with emotional destabilisation, and a strongly emotional (and often regressive) representation on the part of the patient especially when recounting the details of the injury.

As previously noted, Kay's model proposes a powerful theoretical account of the variety of internally and externally mediated factors that may contribute to the emergence of the behavioural and emotional complications of TBI. The one aspect that is not clearly characterised, however, is why one patient featuring a TBI might go on to develop a PTSD while another may develop depression and a third develop some form of neurovegetative disturbance. I contend that the notion of the different forms of diatheses discussed above may, at least in part, account for these differences.

Following a TBI the variety of individual differences—environment, history, and injury-related factors—interact to create a unique constellation of effects for each individual. The factors and influences that arise as direct effects of the injury interact with the change in circumstances and life situation to produce the variety of emotional and behavioural disturbances that occur subsequent to TBI.

Conclusion

As noted in the introduction, it is hard to imagine what it must be like for an individual following the personal crisis and catastrophe that ensues as a result of a serious traumatic brain injury. The individual is confronted with a huge range of alterations in his or her normal functioning at the biological, psychological, and social levels. From the neurological perspective, a range of primary and secondary neurological events occur culminating in pain, seizures, compromise in movement, sensation, perception, orthopaedic and other injuries, neuropsychological compromise including disorientation, confusion, retrograde and anterograde memory deficits, decrease in attention and concentration, slowed speed of information processing, executive deficits including concreteness in idea generation, disinhibition and impulsivity, psychological deficits including diminished self-esteem, loneliness, a renewed dependency on parents or spouse, infantilization by the wider community, diminution of sexual functioning and interest, depression, anxiety and social isolation, economic deficits including loss of income, loss of one's employment as a defining feature of one's social persona, medical costs, loss of treasured interests or hobbies, and the unenviable role of the plaintiff in any medico-legal proceedings surrounding the claim. All of these changes are occurring to an individual who has just had a near-death experience, culminating in the not too surprising reflection upon "Who am I?" and "Why am I here?"

As a result, some of these individuals develop a wide range of behavioral, emotional, and psychiatric conditions following the injury including depression, bipolar disorder, secondary mania, psychotic states, posttraumatic stress disorder, obsessive compulsive disorder, phobic disorders, and generalised anxiety disorders to name only a few. These individuals can also be subject to a number of neuropsychiatric syndromes including disorders of drive and impulse control, and disturbance of neurovegetative functioning including disruptions of sleep, eating, and sexual function, and may try to cope with these changes by adopting or resorting to a previous behavioural pattern of substance abuse.

The relationship between the injury and the final outcome for the individual is by no means a direct one and there are many levels of interaction at the biochemical, cellular, organic, systemic, individual, psychological, and social levels that can significantly alter the final result. Nonetheless, there is a predictability about many of these effects and I hope that in reading this book that some of these relationships and rules for prediction have emerged for you.

References

Abramowitz, J.S. (1997). Effectiveness of psychological and pharmacological treatments for obsessive-compulsive disorder: A quantitative review. *Journal of Consulting and Clinical Psychology, 65*(1), 44–52.

Abramson, L.Y., Alloy, L.B., & Metalsky, G.I. (1988). The cognitive diathesis-stress theories of depression: Toward an adequate evaluation of the theories' validities. In L.B. Alloy (Ed.), *Cognitive processes in depression.* New York: Guilford.

Achte, K.A., Hillbom, E., & Aalberg, V. (1969). Psychoses following war brain injuries. *Acta Psychiatrica Scandinavica, 45*(1), 1–18.

Adams, J.H., Graham, D.I., Scott, G., Parker, L.S., & Doyle, D. (1980). Brain damage in fatal non-missile head injury. *Journal of Clinical Pathology, 33*(12), 1132–1145.

Adair, R.K. (1990). *The physics of baseball.* New York: Harper and Row.

Adler, A. (1945). Mental symptoms following head injury: A statistical analysis of two hundred cases. *Archives of Neurology and Psychiatry, 53*, 34–43.

Adolphs, R., Damasio, H., Tranel, D., Cooper, G., & Damasio, A.R. (2000). A role for somatosensory cortices in the visual recognition of emotion as revealed by three-dimensional lesion mapping. *Journal of Neuroscience, 20*(7), 2683–2690.

Adolphs, R., Damasio, H., Tranel, D., & Damasio, A.R. (1996). Cortical systems for the recognition of emotion in facial expressions. *Journal of Neuroscience, 16*(23), 7678–7687.

Adolphs, R., Tranel, D., Damasio, H., & Damasio, A. (1994). Impaired recognition of emotion in facial expressions following bilateral damage to the human amygdala. *Nature, 372*(6507), 669–672.

Ahmed, S., Bierley, R., Sheikh, J.I., & Date, E.S. (2000). Post-traumatic amnesia after closed head injury: A review of the literature and some suggestions for further research. *Brain Injury, 14*, 765–780.

Alderman, N. (2003). Contemporary approaches to the management of irritability and aggression following traumatic brain injury. *Neuropsychological Rehabilitation, 13*(1), 211–240.

Alexander, M.P. (1995). Mild traumatic brain injury: Pathophysiology, natural history, and clinical management. *Neurology, 45*, 1253–1260.

Alfano, D.P., Paniak, C.E., & Finlayson, M.A.J. (1993). The MMPI and closed head injury: A neurocorrective approach. *Neuropsychiatry, Neuropsychology, and Behavioral Neurology, 6*, 111–116.

Allen, C.C., & Ruff, R.M. (1990). Self-rating versus neuropsychological performance of moderate versus severe head–injured patients. *Brain Injury, 4*(1), 7–17.

Allen, J., & Schuldberg, D. (1989). Positive thought disorder in an hypothetically psychosis-prone population. *Journal of Abnormal Psychology, 98*, 491–494.

Allen, L.M., Conder, R.L., Green, P., & Cox, D.R. (1997) *CARB'97 Manual for the computerized assessment of response bias.* Durham, NC: CogniSyst.

Allgulander, C., & Nilsson, B. (2000). Victims of criminal homicide in Sweden: A matched case-control study of health and social risk factors among all 1,739 cases during 1978–1994. *American Journal of Psychiatry, 157*(2), 244–247.

Allison, M. (1993). The effect of brain injury on marriage: Identifying relationships at risk. *Headlines, May/June*, 2–6.

Alloy, L., Abramson, L., Whitehouse, W., Hogan, M., Panzella, C., & Rose, D. (2006). Prospective incidence of first onsets and recurrences of depression in high and low cognitive risk for depression. *Journal of Abnormal psychology, 115(1)*, 145–156.

Alloy, L.B., Abramson, L.Y., Hogan, M.E., Whitehouse, W.G., Rose, D.T., Robinson, M.S., Kim, R.S., & Lapkin, J.B. (2000). The Temple–Wisconsin Cognitive Vulnerability to Depression (CVD) Project: Lifetime history of Axis I psychopathology in individuals at high and low cognitive risk for depression. *Journal of Abnormal Psychology, 109*, 403–418.

Alnaes, R., & Torgersen, S. (1988). Major depression, anxiety disorders and mixed conditions. Childhood and precipitating events. *Acta Psychiatrica Scandinavica, 78*(5), 632–638.

Aloni, R., & Katz, S. (1999). A review of the effect of traumatic brain injury on the human sexual response. *Brain Injury, 13*, 269–280.

Alves, E.M., Colohan, A.R.T., O'Leary, T.J., Rimel, R.W., & Jane, J.A. (1986). Understanding post-traumatic symptoms after minor head injury. *Journal of Head Injury Rehabilitation, 1*, 1–121.

Alves, W.M., Macciocchi, S.N., & Barth, J.T. (1993). Postconcussive symptoms after uncomplicated mild head injury. *The Journal of Head Trauma and Rehabilitation, 8*, 48–59.

American Congress of Rehabilitation Medicine (ACRM). (1993). Definition of mild traumatic brain injury. *Journal of Head Trauma Rehabilitation, 8*, 86–87.

American Congress of Rehabilitation Medicine (ACRM). (1995). Recommendations for use of uniform nomenclature pertinent to patients with sever alterations in consciousness. *Archives of Physical Medicine and Rehabilitation, 76*, 205–209.

American Psychiatric Association. (1987). *Diagnostic and statistical manual of mental disorders–Revised* (3rd ed.) (DSM–III–R). Washington, DC: American Psychiatric Association.

American Psychiatric Association. (1994). *Diagnostic and statistical manual of mental disorders* (4th ed.). Washington DC: American Psychiatric Association.

American Psychiatric Association. (2000). *Diagnostic and statistical manual of mental disorders–Text revision* (4th ed.). Washington DC: American Psychiatric Association.

Andary, M.T., Crewe, N., Ganzel, S.K., Haines-Pepi, P.C., Kulkarni, M.R., Stainton, D.F., Thompson, A., & Yosef, M. (1997). Traumatic brain injury/chronic pain syndrome: A case comparison study. *The Clinical Journal of Pain, 13*, 244–250.

Andersen, G., Vestergaard, K., & Ingeman-Nielsen, M., & Jensen, T.S. (1995). Incidence of central poststroke pain. *Pain, 61*(2), 187–193.

Anderson, C. (1942). Chronic head cases. *Lancet, 2*, 1–4.

Anderson, C.V., Bigler, E.D., & Blatter, D.D. (1995). Frontal lobe lesions, diffuse damage, and neuropsychological functioning in traumatic brain-injured patients. *Journal of Clinical and Experimental Neuropsychology, 17*(6), 900–908.

Anderson, S.D. (1995). Postconcussional disorder: Common result of head injury. *Canadian Journal of Diagnostics, 12(4)*, 77–86.

Anderson, S.D. (1996). Postconcussional disorder and loss of consciousness. *Bulletin of the American Academy of Psychiatry and Law, 24(4)*, 493–504.

Andersson, S., & Bergedalen, A.M. (2002). Cognitive correlates of apathy in traumatic brain injury. *Neuropsychiatry, Neuropsychology and Behavioral Neurology, 15*(3), 184–191.

Andersson, S., Gundersen, P.M., & Finset, A. (1999). Emotional activation during therapeutic interaction in traumatic brain injury: effect of apathy, self-awareness and implications for rehabilitation. *Brain Injury, 13*(6), 393–404.

Andersson, S., Krogstad, J.M., & Finset, A. (1999). Apathy and depressed mood in acquired brain damage: relationship to lesion localization and psychophysiological reactivity. *Psychological Medicine, 29*(2), 447–456.

Andreasen, N.C. (1983). *Scale for the assessment of negative symptoms.* Iowa City: University of Iowa.

Andreasen, N.C. (1984). *Scale for the assessment of positive symptoms.* Iowa City: University of Iowa.

Andreasen, N.C., & Carpenter, W.T., Jr. (1993). Diagnosis and classification of schizophrenia. *Schizophrenia Bulletin, 19*(2), 199–214.

Andreasen, N.C., & Olsen, S. (1982). Negative versus positive schizophrenia: Definition and reliability. *Archives of General Psychiatry, 39,* 789–794.

Angst, J., Gamma, A., Benazzi, F., Ajdacic, V., Eich, D., & Rossler, W. (2003). Toward a redefinition of sub-threshold bipolarity: Epidemiology and proposed criteria for bipolar-II, minor bipolar disorders and hypomania. *Journal of Affective Disorders, 73,* 133–146.

Angst, J., & Volrath, M. (1991). The natural history of anxiety disorders. *Acta Psychiatric Scandinavica, 84,* 446–452.

Annegers, J.F., Grabow, J.D., Groover, R.V., Laws, E.R., Elveback, L.R., & Kurland, L.T. (1998). Seizures after head trauma: A population study. *Neurology, 30,* 683–689.

Anstey, K.J., Butterworth, P., Jorm, A.F., Christensen, H., Rodgers, B., & Windsor, T.D. (2004). A population survey found an association between self-reports of traumatic brain injury and increased psychiatric symptoms. *Journal of Clinical Epidemiology, 57,* 1202–1209.

Arbisi, P.A., & Ben-Porath, Y.S. (1995). An MMPI-2 infrequent response scale for use with psychopathological populations: The F(p) Scale. *Psychological Assessment, 7,* 424–431.

Arciniegas, D.B., & Silver, J.M. (2001). Regarding the search for a unified definition of mild traumatic brain injury. *Brain Injury, 15(7),* 649–52.

Arenth, P.M., Bogner, J.A., Corrigan, J.D., & Schmidt, L. (2001). The utility of the Substance Abuse Subtle Screening Inventory–3 for use with individuals with brain injury. *Brain Injury, 15*(6), 499–510.

Asarnow, R.F., Neuchterlein, K.H., & Marner, S.R. (1983). Span of apprehension performance, neuropsychological functioning, and indices of psychosis–proneness. *Journal of Nervous and Mental Disease, 171,* 662–669.

Ashman, T.A., Schwartz, M.E., Cantor, J.B., Hibbard, M.R., & Gordon, W.A. (2004). Screening for substance abuse in individuals with traumatic brain injury. *Brain Injury, 18*(2), 191–202.

Austin, M.P., Ross, M., Murray, C., O'Carroll, R.E., Ebmeier, K.P., & Goodwin, G.M. (1992). Cognitive function in major depression. *Journal of Affective Disorders, 25,* 21–30.

Avons, S.E., Nunn, J.A., Chan, L., & Armstrong, H. (2003). Executive function assessed by memory updating and random generation in schizotypal individuals. *Psychiatry Research, 120,* 145–154.

Baddeley, A. (1990). *Human memory: theory and practice.* London: Erlbaum.

Bagley, S.I. (1979). Funny bones: A review of the problem of heterotopic bone formation. *Orthopaedic Review, 8*, 113–120.

Barker, L.H., Bigler, E.D., Johnson, S.C., Anderson, C.V., Russo, A.A., Boineau, B., & Blatter, D.D. (1999). Polysubstance abuse and traumatic brain injury: Quantitative magnetic resonance imaging and neuropsychological outcome in older adolescents and young adults. Journal of the International Neuropsychological Society, *5*(7), 593–608.

Barnhill, L.J., & Gaultieri, C.T. (1989). Two cases of late-onset psychosis after closed head injury. *Neuropsychiatry, Neuropsychology, and Behavioral Neurology, 2,* 211– 217.

Bar-On, R., Tranel, D., Denburg, N.L., & Bechara, A. (2003). Exploring the neurological substrate of emotional intelligence. *Brain, 126*, 1790–2000.

Barrett, D.H., Green, M.L., Morris, R., Giles, W.H., & Croft, J.B. (1996). Cognitive functioning and posttraumatic stress disorder. *American Journal of Psychiatry, 153(11)*, 1492–1494.

Barth, J.T., Macciocchi, S.N., Giordani, B., Rimel, R., Jane, J.A., & Boll, T.J. (1983). Neuropsychological sequelae of minor head injury. *Neurosurgery, 13(5),* 529–533.

Baxter, L.R. Jr, Schwartz, J.M., Bergman, K.S., Szuba, M.P., Guze, B.H., Mazziotta, J.C., Alazraki, A., Selin, C.E., Ferng, H.K., & Munford, P. (1992). Caudate glucose metabolic rate changes with both drug and behavior therapy for obsessive-compulsive disorder. *Archives of General Psychiatry, 49(9)*, 681–689.

Bazarian, J.J., Wong, T.M., Harris, M., Leahey, N., Mookerjee, S., & Dombovy, M.L. (1999). Epidemiology and predictors of postconcussive syndrome after minor head injury in an emergency population. *Brain Injury, 13*, 173–189.

Bechara, A. (2003). Risky business: emotion, decision-making, and addiction. *Journal of Gambling Studies, 19*(1), 23–51.

Bechara, A., Damasio, H., & Damasio, A.R. (2000). Emotion, decision making and the orbitofrontal cortex. *Cerebral Cortex, 10*(3), 295–307.

Bechara, A., Damasio, A.R., Damasio, H., & Anderson, S.W. (1994). Insensitivity to future consequences following damage to human prefrontal cortex. *Cognition, 50*(1–3), 7–15.

Bechara, A., Damasio, H., Damasio, A.R., & Lee, G.P. (1999). Different contributions of the human amygdala and ventromedial prefrontal cortex to decision-making. *Journal of Neuroscience, 19*(13), 5473–5481.

Bechara, A., Damasio, H., Tranel, D., & Anderson, S.W. (1998). Dissociation of working memory from decision making within the human prefrontal cortex. *Journal of Neuroscience, 18*(1), 428–437.

Bechara, A., Damasio, H., Tranel, D., & Damasio, A.R. (1997). Deciding advantageously before knowing the advantageous strategy. *Science, 275*(5304), 1293–1295.

Bechara, A., Dolan, S., Denburg, N., Hindes, A., Anderson, S.W., & Nathan, P.E. (2001). Decision-making deficits, linked to a dysfunctional ventromedial prefrontal cortex, revealed in alcohol and stimulant abusers. *Neuropsychologia, 39*(4), 376–389.

Bechara, A., Tranel, D., & Damasio, H. (2000). Characterization of the decision-making deficit of patients with ventromedial prefrontal cortex lesions. *Brain, 123 (Pt 11)*, 2189–2202.

Bechara, A., Tranel, D., & Damasio, H. (2002). The somatic marker hypothesis and decision-making. In J. Grafman (Ed.), *Handbook of neuropsychology* (2nd ed.) (Vol. 7, pp. 117–143).

Bechara, A., Tranel, D., Damasio, H., & Damasio, A.R. (1996). Failure to respond autonomically to anticipated future outcomes following damage to prefrontal cortex. *Cerebral Cortex, 6*(2), 215–225.

Beck, A. (2005). The current state of cognitive therapy: A 40-year retrospective. *Archives of General Psychiatry, 62*, 953–959.

Beck, A., Brown, G., Steer, R., Eidelson, J., & Riskind, J. (1987). Differentiating anxiety and depression: A test of the cognitive content–specificity hypothesis. *Journal of Abnormal Psychology, 96(3),* 179–183.

Beck, A., Rush, A., Shaw, B., & Emery, G. (1979). *Cognitive therapy for depression.* New York: Guilford Press.

Beck, A., & Steer, R. (1987). *Beck Depression Inventory Manual.* New York: The Psychological Corporation.

Beetar, J.T., Guilmette, T.J., & Sapradeo, F.R. (1996). Sleep and pain complaints in symptomatic traumatic brain injury and neurologic populations. *Archives of Physical Medicine and Rehabilitation, 77,* 1298–1302.

Bennazi, F. (2003). Lifetime prevalence of manic/hypomanic syndromes in young adults. *European Neuropsychopharmacology, 13*(Suppl. 14), 5178.

Bennett, D.R., Fuenning, S.I., Sullivan, G., & Weber, J. (1980). Migraine precipitated by head trauma in athletes. *The American Journal of Sports Medicine, 8*(3), 202–205.

Benyakar, M., Tadir, M., Groswasser, Z., & Stern, M.J. (1988). Dreams in head-injured patients. *Brain Injury, 2,* 351–356.

Berard, E.J.J. (1989). The sexuality of spinal cord injured women: Physiology and pathophysiology: A review. *Paraplegia, 27,* 99–112.

Berent, S., & Schwartz, C. (1999). Essential psychometrics. In J. Sweet (Ed.), *Forensic neuropsychology: Fundamentals and practice* (pp. 3–26). Exton, P.A: Swets & Zeitlinger.

Bergamasco, B., Bergamini, L., Doriguzzi, T., & Fabiani, D. (1968). EEG sleep patterns as a prognostic criterion in post-traumatic coma. *Electroencephalography and Clinical Neurophysiology, 24*(4), 374–377.

Beric, A. (1998). Central pain and dysesthesia syndrome. *Neurologic Clinics, 16*(4), 899–918.

Berlin, R.M. (1983). Psychiatric problems in neurologic patients. *American Journal of Psychiatry, 140*(9), 1270–1271.

Bernard, L.C., McGrath, M.J., & Houston, W. (1996). The differential effects of simulating malingering, closed head injury, and other CNS pathology on the Wisconsin Card Sorting Test: support for the "pattern of performance" hypothesis. *Archives of Clinical Neuropsychology, 11*(3), 231–245.

Bernstein, D.M. (1999). Recovery from mild head injury. *Brain Injury, 13(3),* 151–172.

Berry, D. (1998). *Methodological issues in evaluation of validity scales from child self–report inventories.* Presented at 106th Annual Meeting of the American Psychological Association, San Francisco, CA: August 18.

Berry, D.T., Baer, R.A., & Harris, M.J. (1991). Detection of malingering on the MMPI: A meta-analysis. *Clinical Psychology Review, 11,* 585–598.

Berry, D.T., & Butcher, J.N. (1998). Detection of feigning of head injury symptoms on the MMPI-2. In C. Reynolds (Ed.), *Detection of malingering in head injury litigation*. New York: Plenum.

Berry, D., Wetter, M., Baer, R., Youngjohn, J., Gass, C., Lamb, D., Franzen, M., MacInnes, W., & Bucholz, D. (1995). Overreporting of closed head injury symptoms on the MMPI-2. *Psychological Assessment, 7,* 517–523.

Berthier, M.L., Kulisevsky, J., Gironell, A., & Heras, J.A. (1996). Obsessive–compulsive disorder associated with brain lesions: clinical phenomenology, cognitive function, and anatomic correlates. *Neurology, 47*(2), 353–361.

Berthier, M.L., Kulisevsky, J.J., Gironell, A., & Lopez, O.L. (2001). Obsessive compulsive disorder and traumatic brain injury: behavioral, cognitive, and neuroimaging findings. *Neuropsychiatry Neuropsychology and Behavioral Neurology, 14*(1), 23–31.

Bieliauskas, L.A. (1993). Depressed or not depressed? That is the question. *Journal of Clinical and Experimental Neuropsychology, 15(1),* 119–134.

Bienenfeld, D., & Brott, T. (1989). Capgras syndrome following minor head trauma. *Journal of Clinical Psychiatry, 50*(2), 68–69.

Bigler, E.D. (2001). The lesion(s) in traumatic brain injury: Implications for clinical neuropsychology. *Archives of Clinical Neuropsychology, 16(2),* 95–131.

Bigler, E.D., Blatter, D.D., Johnson, S.C., Anderson, S.V., Russo, A.A., Gale, S.D., Ruser, D.K., McNamara, S., & Bailey, B. (1996). Traumatic brain injury, alcohol and quantitative neuroimaging: Preliminary findings. *Brain Injury, 10,* 197–206.

Bigler, E.D., & Clement, P. (1997). *Diagnostic clinical neuropsychology* (3rd ed.). Austin, TX: University of Texas Press.

Bigler, E.D., Johnson, S.C., & Blatter, D.D. (1999). Head trauma and intellectual status: relation to quantitative magnetic resonance imaging findings. *Applied Neuropsychology, 6,* 217–225.

Bigler, E.D., & Snyder, J.L. (1995). Neuropsychological outcome and quantitative neuroimaging in mild head injury. *Archives of Clinical Neuropsychology, 10,* 159 –174.

Binder, L.M. (1993). Assessment of malingering after mild head trauma with the Portland Digit Recognition Test. *Journal of Clinical and Experimental Neuropsychology, 15*(2), 170–182.

Binder, L.M., & Kelly, M.P. (1996). Portland Digit Recognition Test performance by brain dysfunction patients without financial incentives. *Assessment, 3,* 403–409.

Binder, L.M., & Willis, S.C. (1991). Assessment of motivation after financially compensable minor head trauma. *Psychological Assessment, 3,* 175–181.

Binder, L.M., Villanueva, M.R., Howieson, D., & Moore, R.T. (1993). The Rey AVLT recognition memory task measures motivational impairment after mild head trauma. *Archives of Clinical Neuropsychology, 8*(2), 137–147.

Bishara, S.N., Partridge, F.M., Godfrey, H.P.D., & Knight, R.G. (1992). Post-traumatic amnesia and Glasgow Coma Scale related to outcome in survivors in a consecutive series of patients with severe closed-head injury. *Brain Injury, 6,* 373–380.

Bittner, R.M., & Crowe, S.F. (2006). The relationship between naming difficulty and FAS performance following traumatic brain injury. Brain Injury, 20(9), 971–980.

Blackerby, W. (1987). Disruption of sexuality following a head injury. *National Head Injury Foundation News, 7,* 8.

Blackerby, W.F. (1990). A treatment model for sexuality disturbance following brain injury. *Journal of Head Trauma Rehabilitation, 5,* 73–82.

Blair, R.J. (1995). A cognitive developmental approach to mortality: investigating the psychopath. *Cognition, 57,* 1–29.

Blair, R.J. (2001). Neurocognitive models of aggression, the antisocial personality disorders, and psychopathy. *Journal of Neurology Neurosurgery and Psychiatry, 71*(6), 727–731.

Blair, R.J. (2004). The roles of orbital frontal cortex in the modulation of antisocial behavior. *Brain and Cognition, 55*(1), 198–208.

Blair, R.J., & Cipolotti, L. (2000). Impaired social response reversal. A case of "acquired sociopathy." *Brain, 123 (Pt 6),* 1122–1141.

Blair, R.J., Jones, L., Clark, F., & Smith, M. (1997). The psychopathic individual: A lack of responsiveness to distress cues? *Psychophysiology, 34,* 192–198.

Blair, R.J., Mitchell, D., & Blair, K. (2005). *The psychopath: Emotion and the brain.* Oxford, UK: Blackwell Publishing.

Blake, D.D., Weathers, F.W., Nagy, L.M., Kaloupek, D.G., Klauminzer, G., Charney, D.S., & Keane, T.M. (1990) A clinician rating scale for assessing current and lifetime PTSD: the CAPS–1. *The Behavior Therapist, 13*, 187–188.

Blanchard, E.B., & Hickling, E.J. (1997). *After the crash*. Washington, DC: American Psychological Association.

Blanchard, E.B., & Hickling, E.J. (2004). *After the crash* (2nd ed.). Washington, DC: American Psychological Association.

Blanchard, R.J., Blanchard, DC., & Takahashi, L.K. (1977). Reflexive fighting in the albino rat: Aggressive or defensive behavior? *Aggressive Behavior, 3*, 145–155.

Blanchard, E.B., Hickling, E.J., Taylor, A.E., Loos, W.R., Forneris, C.A., & Jaccard, J. (1996). Who develops PTSD from motor vehicle accidents? *Behavior Research Therapy, 34(1)*, 1–10.

Blanchard, E.B., Hickling, E.J., Taylor, A.E., Loos, W.R., & Gerardi, R.J. (1994). Psychological morbidity associated with motor vehicle accidents. *Behavior Research Therapy, 32(3)*, 283–90.

Blazyk, S. (1983). Developmental crisis in adolescents following severe head injury. *Social Work in Health Care, 8*, 55–67.

Bleiberg, J., Garmoe, W.S., Halpern, E.L., Reeves, D.L., & Nadler, J.D. (1997). Consistency of within-day and across-day performance after mild brain injury. *Neuropsychiatry, Neuropsychology and Behavioral Neurology, 10*(4), 247–253.

Bleuler, E. (1911). *Dementia praecox or the group of schizophrenias* (German ed.). New York: International Universities Press.

Blumbergs, P.C., Scott, G., Manavis, J., Wainwright, H., Simpson, D.A., & McLean, A.J. (1995). Topography of axonal injury as defined by amyloid precursor protein and the sector scoring method in mild and severe closed head injury. *Journal of Neurotrauma, 12*, 565–572.

Blumer, D., & Benson, D.F. (1975). Personality changes with frontal and temporal lobe lesions. In D.F. Benson, & D. Blumer (Eds.), *Psychiatric aspects of neurologic disease*. New York: Grune & Stratton.

Boake, C., Millis, S.R., High, Jr.W.M., Delmonico, R.L., Kreutzer, J.S., Rosenthal, M., Sherer, M., & Ivanhoe, C.B. (2001) Using early neuropsychological testing to predict long term productivity outcome from traumatic brain injury. *Archives of Physical Medicine & Rehabilitation, 82*, 761–8.

Boffeli, T.J., & Guze, S.B. (1992). The simulation of neurological disease. *Psychiatric Clinics of North America, 15*, 301–310.

Bohnen, N., & Jolles, J. (1992). Neurobehavioral aspects of postconcussive symptoms after mild head injury. *The Journal of Nervous and Mental Disease, 180*(11), 683–692.

Bohnen, N., Jolles, J., & Twijnstra A. (1992). Neuropsychological deficits in patients with persistent symptoms six months after mild head injury. *Neurosurgery, 30(5)*, 692–5.

Bohnen, N.I., Jolles, J., Trinjstra, A., Melink, R., & Winjen, G. (1995). Late neurobehavioural symptoms after mild head injury. *Brain Injury, 9*, 27–33.

Boller, F., & Frank, E. (1982). *Sexual dysfunction in neurological disorders: Diagnosis, management and rehabilitation*. New York: Raven Press.

Bombadier, C.H., & Rimmele, C.T. (1998). Alcohol use and readiness to change after spinal cord injury. *Archives of Physical Medicine and Rehabilitation, 79*, 1110–1115.

Bombadier, C.H., Rimmele, C.T., & Zintel, H. (2002). The magnitude and correlates of alcohol and drug use before traumatic brain injury. *Archives of Physical Medicine Rehabilitation, 83*, 1765–1773.

Bond, M.R. (1976). Assessment of psychosocial outcome of severe head injury. *Acta Neurochirurgica, 34*, 57–70.

Bond, M.R. (1984). The psychiatry of closed head injury. In N. Brooks (Ed.), *Closed head injury. Psychological, social and family consequences* (pp. 148–178). Oxford: Oxford University Press.

Bonica, J.J., & Loeser, J.D. (2001). Applied anatomy relevant to pain. In J.D. Loeser, S.H. Butler, C.R. Chapman, & D.C. Turk (Eds.), *Bonica's management of pain* (3rd ed). Philadelphia: Lippincott Williams & Wilkins.

Bonne, O., Brandes, D., Gilboa, A., Gomori, J.M., Shenton, M.E., Pitman, R.K., & Shalev, A.Y. (2001). Longitudinal MRI study of hippocampal volume in trauma survivors with PTSD. *American Journal of Psychiatry, 158*(8), 1248–1251.

Bontke, C. (Ed.). (1996). Do patients with mild brain injuries have posttraumatic stress disorder too? *Journal of Head Trauma Rehabilitation, 11,* 95–102.

Bontke, C.F., Lehmkuhl, D.L., Englander, J.S., Mann, N., Ragnarsson, K.T., Zasler, N.D., Graves, D.E., Thoi, L.L., & Jung, C. (1993). Medical complications and associated injuries of persons treated in Traumatic Brain Injury Model Systems Programs. *Journal of Head Trauma Rehabilitation, 8*, 34.

Bornstein, R.A., Miller, H.B., & van Schoor, J.T. (1989). Neuropsychological deficit and emotional disturbance in head-injured patients. *Journal of Neurosurgery, 70*(4), 509–513.

Borod, J.C. (1996). Emotional disorders (emotion). In J.G. Beaumont, P.M. Kenealy, & M.J.C. Rogers (Eds.), *The Blackwell dictionary of neuropsychology* (pp. 312–320). Oxford, England: Blackwell.

Bowen, A., Chamberlain, M.A., Tennant, A., Neumann, V., & Conner, M. (1999). The persistence of mood disorders following traumatic brain injury: A 1 year follow-up. *Brain Injury, 13*(7), 547–553.

Bowers, D., Blonder, L.X., & Heilman, K.M. (1992). *The Florida affect battery.* Center for Neuropsychological Studies, University of Florida, Gainesville, FL.

Bowsher, D. (1996). Central pain: clinical and physiological characteristics. *Journal of Neurology, Neurosurgery and Psychiatry, 61*(1), 62–69.

Branca, B., & Lake, A. (2004). Psychological and neuropsychological integration in multidisciplinary pain management after TBI. *Journal of Head Trauma Rehabilitation, 19*, 40–57.

Brecher, J. (1977). Sex, stress and health. *International Journal of Health Services, 7,* 89–101.

Bremner, J.D., Randall, T., Scott, T.M., Brunen, R.A., Seibyl, J.P., Southwick, S.M., Delaney, R.C., McCarthy, G., Charney, D.S., & Innis, R.B. (1995). MRI–based measurement of hippocampal volume in patients with combat-related posttraumatic stress disorder. *American Journal of Psychiatry, 152*, 973–981.

Bremner, J.D., Innis, R.B., Ng, C.K., Staib, L.H., Salomon, R.M., Bronen, R.A., Duncan, J., Southwick, S.M., Krystal, J.H., Rich, D., Zubal, G., Dey, H., Soufer, R., & Charney, D.S. (1997). Positron emission tomography measurement of cerebral metabolic correlates of yohimbine administration in combat-related posttraumatic stress disorder. *Archives of General Psychiatry, 54*(3), 246–254.

Breslau, N., Davis, G.C., Andreski, P., & Peterson, E. (1991). Traumatic events and posttraumatic stress disorder in an urban population of young adults. *Archives of General Psychiatry, 48(3),* 216–22.

Brewin, C.R. (1984). Attributions for industrial accidents: Their relationship to rehabilitation outcome. *Journal of Social and Clincial Psychology, 2*, 156–164.

Brewin, C.R., Andrews, B., Rose, S., & Kirk, M. (1999). Acute stress disorder and posttraumatic stress disorder in victims of violent crime. *American Journal of Psychiatry, 156(3),* 360–6.

Brewin, C.R., Dalgleish, T., & Joseph, S. (1996). A dual representation theory of posttraumatic stress disorder. *Psychology Review, 103(4),* 670–86.

Brickley, M.R., & Shepherd, J.P. (1995). The relationship between alcohol intoxication, injury severity and Glasgow Coma score in assault patients. *Injury, 26*, 311–314.

Britton, K.R. (1998). Medroxyprogesterone in the treatment of aggressive hypersexual behaviour in traumatic brain injury. *Brain Injury, 12,* 703–707.

Brom, D., Kleber, R.J., & Hofman, M.C. (1993). Victims of traffic accidents: incidence and prevention of post-traumatic stress disorder. *Journal of Clinical Psychology, 49*(2), 131–40.

Brooks, D.N., Aughton, M.E., Bond, M.R., Jones, P., & Rizvi, S. (1980). Cognitive sequelae in relationship to early indices of severity of brain damage after severe blunt head injury. *Journal of Neurology, Neurosurgery and Psychiatry, 43*, 529–534.

Brooks, N. (1984). *Closed head injury: psychological, social and family consequences.* Oxford: Oxford University Press.

Brooks, N. (1988). Personality change after severe head injury. *Acta Neurochirurigica (Supplementary), 44*, 59–64.

Brooks, N., Campsie, L., Symington, C., Beattie, A., & McKinlay, W. (1986). The five year outcome of severe blunt head injury: A relatives' view. *Journal of Neurology, Neurosurgery and Psychiatry, 49*, 764–770.

Brooks, S.C. (1990). Management of patients with head injuries. *British Medical Journal, 300*(6728), 876.

Brown, G.W., & Bifulco, A. (1985). In I. Sarason, & B. Sarason (Eds.), *Social support: theory, research and applications.* Boston: Martins Nijhoff.

Brown, G., Chadwick, O., Shaffer, D., Rutter, M., & Traub, M. (1981). A prospective study of children with head injuries: III. Psychiatric sequelae. *Psychological Medicine, 11,* 63–78.

Brown, G.W., Harris, T.O., & Hepworth, C. (1995). Loss, humiliation and entrapment among women developing depression: A patient and non–patient comparison. *Psychological Medicine, 25*, 7–21.

Bruck, D., & Broughton, R.J. (2004). Diagnostic ambiguities in a case of post-traumatic narcolepsy with cataplexy. *Brain Injury, 18*(3), 321–326.

Brunas-Wagstaff, J., Bergquist, A., & Wagstaff, G.F. (1994). Cognitive correlates of functional and dysfunctional impulsivity. *Personality and Individual Differences, 17*, 289–292.

Brussel, J.A., & Hitch, K.S. (1943). The military malingerer. *The Military Surgeon, 93,* 33–44.

Bryant, R.A. (1996). Posttraumatic stress disorder, flashbacks, and pseudomemories in closed head injury. *Journal of Traumatic Stress, 9(3),* 621–629.

Bryant, R.A. (2001). Posttraumatic stress disorder and mild brain injury: controversies, causes and consequences. *Journal of Clinical and Experimental Neuropsychology, 23(6),* 718–28.

Bryant, R.A., & Harvey, A.G. (1995). Acute stress response: A comparison of head injured and non-head injured patients. *Psychological Medicine, 25*(4), 869–873.

Bryant, R.A., & Harvey, A.G. (1996). Initial posttraumatic stress responses following motor vehicle accidents. *Journal of Traumatic Stress, 9(2),* 223–34.

Bryant, R.A., & Harvey, A.G. (1998). Relationship between acute stress disorder and posttraumatic stress disorder following mild traumatic brain injury. *American Journal of Psychiatry, 155*(5), 625–629.

Bryant, R.A., & Harvey, A.G. (1999). The influence of traumatic brain injury on acute stress disorder and post-traumatic stress disorder following motor vehicle accidents. *Brain Injury, 13*(1), 15–22.

Bryant, R.A., & Harvey, A.G. (2000). New DSM-IV diagnosis of acute stress disorder. *American Journal of Psychiatry, 157(11)*, 1889–91.

Bryant, R.A., Marosszeky, J.E., Crooks, J., Baguley, I., & Gurka, J. (2000). Coping style and post-traumatic stress disorder following severe traumatic brain injury. *Brain Injury, 14(2)*, 175–80.

Buchanan, R.W., & Carpenter, W.T. (1994). Domains of psychopathology: An approach to the reduction of heterogeneity in schizophrenia. *Journal of Nervous and Mental Diseases, 182,* 193–204.

Buchsbaum, M.S. (1995). Positron emission tomography studies of abnormal glucose metabolism in schizophrenic illness. *Clinical Neuroscience, 3*(2), 122–130.

Buchsbaum, M.S., Potkin, S.G., Siegel, B.V., Jr., Lohr, J., Katz, M., Gottschalk, L.A., Gulasekaram, B., Marshall, J.F., Lottenberg, S., Teng, C.Y., Abel, L., Plon, L., & Bunney, W.E.Jr. (1992). Striatal metabolic rate and clinical response to neuroleptics in schizophrenia. *Archives of General Psychiatry, 49*(12), 966–974.

Buckley, P., Stack, J.P., Madigan, C., O'Callaghan, E., Larkin, C., & Redmond, O. (1993). Magnetic resonance imaging of schizophrenia-like psychoses associated with cerebral trauma: clinicopathological correlates. *American Journal Psychiatry, 150*, 146–148.

Bullock, R. (1997). Head Injury Committee report. *AANS/CNS Joint Section on Neurotrauma and Critical Care Newsletter, Winter/Spring*, 4–5.

Bulman, R.J., & Wortman, C.B. (1977). Attributions on blame and coping in the "real world": Severe accidents survivors react to their lot. *Journal of Personality and Social Psychology, 35*, 351–363.

Burges, C., & McMillan, T.M. (2001). The ability of naive participants to report symptoms of post-traumatic stress disorder. *British Journal of Clinical Psychology, 40(2)*, 209–14.

Burgess, P.W., & Shallice, T. (1996). Bizarre responses, rule detection and frontal lobe lesions. *Cortex, 32*(2), 241–259.

Busch, C.R., & Alpern, H.P. (1998). Depression after mild traumatic brain injury: A review of current research. *Neuropsychology Review, 8*(2), 95–108.

Butler, R.J. (1994). Neuropsychological investigation of amateur boxers. *British Journal of Sport Medicine, 28*, 187–190.

Caine, E.D. (1986). The neuropsychology of depression: the pseudodementia syndrome. In I. Grant, & K.M. Adams (Eds.), *The assessment of neuropsychiatric disorders*. Oxford: Oxford University Press.

Calder, A.J., Young, A.W., Rowland, D., Perrett, D.I., Hodges, J.R. and Etcoff, N.L. (1996) Face perception after bilateral amygdala damage: Differentially severe impairment of fear. *Cognitive Neuropsychology, 13,* 699–745.

Calev, A., Pollina, D.A., Fennig, S., & Banerjee, S. (1999). Neuropsychology of mood disorders. In A. Calev (Ed.), *Assessment of neuropsychological functions in psychiatric disorders*. Washington, DC: American Psychiatric Press.

Carson, A.J., MacHale, S., Allen, K., Lawrie, S.M., Dennis, M., House, A., Sharpe, M., & Warlow, C. (2000). Depression after stroke and lesion location: A systematic review. *Lancet, 356*(9224), 122–126.

Carter, J.E., & McCormick, A.Q. (1983). Whiplash shaking syndrome: retinal hemorrhages and computerized axial tomography of the brain. *Child Abuse and Negligence, 7(3)*, 279–286.

Cartlidge, N.E.F. (1977). Post-concussional syndrome. *Scottish Medical Journal, 23*, 103.

Castriotta, R.J., & Lai, J.M. (2001). Sleep disorders associated with traumatic brain injury. *Archives of Physical Medicine and Rehabilitation, 82*, 1403–1406.

Centers for Disease Control and Preventions Mild Traumatic Brain Injury Working Group. (2003). *Report to Congress on mild traumatic brain injury in the United States: Steps to prevent a serious public health problem.* National Center for Injury Prevention and Control. Atlanta, GA: Centers for Disease Control and Prevention.

Chapman, L.J., & Chapman, J.P. (1985). Psychosis proneness. In M. Alpert (Ed.), *Controversies in schizophrenia* (pp. 157–174). New York: Guilford.

Chen, S.H., Kareken, D.A., Fastenau, P.S., Trexler, L.E., & Hutchins, G.D. (2003). A study of persistent post-concussion symptoms in mild head trauma using positron emission tomography. *Journal of Neurology, Neurosurgery and Psychiatry, 74*, 326–332.

Cherner, M., Temkin, N., Machamer, J., & Dikmen, S.S. (2001). Utility of a composite measure to detect problematic alcohol use in persons with traumatic brain injury. *Archives of Physical Medicine and Rehabilitation, 82*, 780–786.

Childers, M.K., Holland, D., Ryan, M.G., & Rupright, J. (1998). Obsessional disorders during recovery from severe head injury: report of four cases. *Brain Injury, 12(7),* 613–616.

Cicerone, K., & Kalmar, K. (1997). Does premorbid depression influence post-concussive symptoms and neuropsychological functioning? *Brain Injury, 11*, 643–648.

Clark, D., & Beck, A. (1999). *Scientific foundations of cognitive theory and therapy of depression.* New York: John Wiley and Sons.

Clark, D.A., & Purdon, C.L. (1995). The assessment of unwanted intrusive thoughts: A review and critique of the literature. *Behaviour Research and Therapy, 33*(8), 967–976.

Clark, D.M., Ball, S., & Pape, D. (1991). An experimental investigation of thought suppression. *Behaviour Research and Therapy, 29*(3), 253–257.

Clark J.D.A., Raggatt, P.R., & Edwards, O.M. (1988). Hypothalamic hypogonadism following major head injury. *Clinical Endocrinology, 29,* 153–16.

Clifton, G.L., Ziegler, M.G., & Grossman, R.G. (1981). Circulating catecholamines and sympathetic activity after head injury. *Neurosurgery, 8*, 10–14.

Clinchot, D.M., Bogner, J., Mysiw, J., Corrigan, J., & Fugate, L. (1996). Defining sleep disturbance after brain injury. *Archives of Physical Medicine and Rehabilitation, 77,* 947.

Cohen, M., Oksenberg, A., Snir, D., Stern, M.J., & Grosswasser, Z. (1992). Temporally related changes of sleep complaints in traumatic brain injured patients. *Journal of Neurology, Neurosurgery and Psychiatry, 55,* 313–5.

Cohn, C.K., Wright, J.R., & DeVaul, R.A. (1977). Post head trauma syndrome in an adolescent treated with lithium carbonate-case report. *Diseases of the Nervous System, 38*(8), 630–631.

Committee on Adolescence, Group for the Advancement of Psychiatry (1968). *Normal adolescence.* New York: Charles Scribner's Sons.

Conder, R., Allen, L., & Cox, D. (1992). *Manual for the computerized assessment of response bias.* Durham, NC: CogniSyst, Inc.

Contole, J., & PACS Team. (1996). *Dealing with challenging behaviours after acquired brain injury.* Victoria: Bouverie Publications.

Corcoran, C., McAllister, T.W., & Malaspina, D. (2005). Psychotic disorders. In J.M. Silver, T.W. McAllister, & S.C. Yudofsky (Eds.), *Textbook of traumatic brain injury* (pp. 213–229). Washington, DC: American Psychiatric Publishing.

Corrigan, J.D. (1989). Development of a scale for assessment of agitation following traumatic brain injury. *Journal of Clinical and Experimental Neuropsychology, 11*, 261–277.

Corrigan, J.D. (1995). Substance abuse as a mediating factor in outcome from traumatic brain injury. *Archives of Physical Medicine and Rehabilitation, 76*(4), 302–309.

Corrigan, J.D., Lamb-Hart, G.L., & Rust, E. (1995). A programme of intervention for substance abuse following traumatic brain injury. *Brain Injury, 9*(3), 221–236.

Corrigan, P.W. (1997). The social perceptual deficits of schizophrenia. *Psychiatry, 60*(4), 309–326.

Coslett, H., & Heilman, K. (1986). Male sexual function: impairment after right hemisphere stroke. *Archives of Neurology, 43,* 1036–1039.

Costanzo, R.M., & Becker, D.P. (1986). Smell and taste disorders in head injury and neurosurgery patients. In H.L. Meiselman, & R.S. Rivlin (Eds.), *Clinical measurement of taste and smell* (pp. 565–578). New York: Macmillan.

Costanzo, R.M., & Zasler, N.D. (1991). Head trauma. In V. Getchell, L.M. Bartoshuk, R.L. Doty, & J.B. Snow (Eds.), *Smell and taste in health and disease* (pp. 711–730). New York: Raven Press.

Costanzo, R.M., & Zasler, N.D. (1992). Epidemiology and pathophysiology of olfactory and gustatory dysfunction in head trauma. *Journal of Head Trauma Rehabilitation, 7,* 15–24.

Courville, C.B. (1937). *Pathology of the central nervous system.* Mountain View, CA: Pacific Press Publishing Association.

Courville, C.B. (1942). Coup-contrecoup mechanism of cranio-cerebral injuries. *Archives of Surgery, 45,* 19–43.

Courville, C.B. (1952). Traumatic alterations in the neurons of the human brain incident to cranio-cerebral injury: A comparison with Cajal's observations on experimental animals. *Bulletin of Los Angeles Neurological Society, 17,* 71–93.

Crewe, N.M. (1984). Sexually inappropriate behavior. In D.S. Bishop (Ed.), *Behavioural problems and the disabled: Assessment and management* . Malabar, FL: Robert E. Krieger.

Crompton, M.R. (1971). Hypothalamic lesions following closed head injury. *Brain, 94,* 165–172.

Crosby, W.M., & Costilloe, J.P. (1977). Safety of lap belt restraint for pregnant victims of automobile collisions. *New England Journal of Medicine, 284,* 632.

Crow, T.J. (1980). Molecular pathology of schizophrenia: more than one disease process. *British Medical Journal, 280,* 66–68.

Crowe, H. (1964a). A new diagnostic sign in neck injuries. *California Medicine, 100*(1), 12–13.

Crowe, H. (1964b). The conservative management of neck injuries. *California Medicine, 101*(4), 257–259.

Crowe, S.F. (1992). Dissociation of two frontal lobe syndromes by a test of verbal fluency. *Journal of Clinical and Experimental Neuropsychology, 14*(2), 327–39.

Crowe, S.F. (1996). The performance of schizophrenic and depressed subjects on tests of fluency: Support for a compromise in dorso-lateral pre-frontal functioning. *Australian Psychologist, 31,* 204–209.

Crowe, S.F. (1998). *The neuropsychological effects of the psychiatric disorders.* Amsterdam, Netherlands: Harwood Academic Publishers.

Crowe, S.F. (2000). Traumatic brain injury without loss of consciousness: A case study. *Brain Impairment, 1*(2), 105–110.

Crowe, S.F., & Hoogenraad, K. (2000). Differentiation of dementia of the Alzheimer's type from depression with cognitive impairment on the basis of a cortical versus subcortical pattern of cognitive deficit. *Archives of Clinical Neuropsychology, 15*(1), 9–19.

Crowe, S.F., & Kuttner, M. (1991). Differences between schizophrenia and the schizophrenia-like psychosis of the temporal lobe epilepsy: Support for the two process view of schizophrenia. *Neuropsychiatry, Neuropsychology and Behavioural Neurology, 4,* 127–135.

Crowe, S.F., Ng, K.T., & Gibbs, M.E. (1989a). Effect of retraining trials on memory consolidation in weakly reinforced learning. *Pharmacology, Biochemistry and Behaviour, 33*(4), 889–894.

Crowe, S.F., Ng, K.T., & Gibbs, M.E. (1989b). Memory formation processes in weakly reinforced learning. *Pharmacology, Biochemistry and Behaviour, 33*(4), 881–887.

Crowe, S.F., Ng, K.T., & Gibbs, M.E. (1990). Memory consolidation of weak training experiences by hormonal treatments. *Pharmacology, Biochemistry and Behaviour, 37*(4), 729–734.

Crowe, S.F., & Ponsford, J. (1999). The role of imagery in sexual arousal disturbances in the male traumatically brain injured individual. *Brain Injury, 13,* 347–354.

Culebras, A. (1992a). Neuroanatomic and neurologic correlates of sleep disturbances. *Neurology, 42*(7) (Suppl. 6), 19–27.

Culebras, A. (1992b). The neurology of sleep. Introduction. *Neurology, 42*(7 Suppl. 6), 6–8.

Cullum, C.M., Heaton, R.K., & Grant, I. (1991). Psychogenic factors influencing neuropsychological performance: Somatoform disorders, factitious disorders and malingering. In H.O. Doerr, & A.S. Carlin (Eds.), *Forensic neuropsychology: Legal and scientific basis.* New York: Guilford Press.

Cummings, J.L. (1985). Organic delusions: phenomenology, anatomical correlations, and review. *The British Journal of Psychiatry, 146,* 184–197.

Cummings, J.L. (1986). Subcortical dementia. *British Journal of Psychiatry, 149,* 682–697.

Cunnien, A. (1997). Psychiatric and medical syndromes associated with deception. In R. Rogers (Ed.), *Clinical assessment of malingering and deception* (2nd ed.). New York: Guilford Press.

Curran, C.A., Ponsford, J.L., & Crowe, S.F. (2000). Coping strategies and emotional outcome following traumatic brain injury: A comparison with orthopaedic patients. *Journal of Head Trauma Rehabilitation, 15,* 1256–1274.

Damasio, A.R. (1994). *Descartes' error: Emotion, reason and the human brain.* New York: GP Putnam.

Damasio, A.R. (1996). The somatic marker hypothesis and the possible functions of the prefrontal cortex. *Philosophical Transactions of the Royal Society of London. Series B, Biological sciences, 351*(1346), 1413–1420.

Damasio, A.R. (1995). Consciousness. Knowing how, knowing where. *Nature, 375*(6527), 106–107.

Damasio, A.R. (1998). Emotion in the perspective of an integrated nervous system. *Brain Research: Brain Research Reviews, 26*(2–3), 83–86.

Damasio, A.R., & Anderson, S.W. (1993). The frontal lobes. In K.M. Heilman, & E. Valenstein (Eds.), *Clinical neuropsychology* (pp. 409–460). New York: Oxford University Press.

Damasio, A.R., Grabowski, T.J., Bechara, A., Damasio, H., Ponto, L.L., Parvizi, J., & Hichwa, R.D. (2000). Subcortical and cortical brain activity during the feeling of self–generated emotions. *Nature Neuroscience, 3*(10), 1049–1056.

Damasio, A.R., Tranel, D., & Damasio, H. (1990). Individuals with sociopathic behavior caused by frontal damage fail to respond autonomically to social stimuli. *Behavioural Brain Research, 41*(2), 81–94.

David, A.S. (1992). Frontal lobology—Psychiatry's new pseudoscience. *British Journal of Psychiatry, 161,* 244–248.

David, A.S., & Prince, M. (2005). Psychosis following head injury: A critical review. *Journal of Neurology, Neurosurgery, and Psychiatry, 76*(Suppl. 1), 53–60.

Davis, D.L., & Schneider, L.K. (1990). Ramifications of traumatic brain injury for sexuality. *Journal of Head Trauma Rehabilitation, 5,* 31–37.

Davison, G.C., & Neale, J.M. (2004). *Abnormal psychology* (9th ed.) New York: John Wiley and Sons.

Davison, K., & Bagley, C.K. (1969). Schizophrenia-like psychosis associated with organic disorder of the CNS. *British Journal of Clinical Psychology, 4*(Suppl.), 13–184.

Deans, G.T., McGalliard, J.N., & Rutherford, W.H. (1986). Incidence and duration of neck pain among patients injured in car accidents. *British Medical Journal, 292,* 94–5.

Deb, S., Lyons, I., & Koutzoukis, C. (1998). Neuropsychiatric sequelae one year after a minor head injury. *Journal of Neurology Neurosurgery and Psychiatry, 65*(6), 899–902.

Deb, S., Lyons, I., & Koutzoukis, C. (1999). Neurobehavioural symptoms one year after a head injury. *British Journal of Psychiatry, 174*, 360–365.

Deb, S., Lyons, I., Koutzoukis, C., Ali, I., & McCarthy, G. (1999). Rate of psychiatric illness 1 year after traumatic brain injury. *American Journal of Psychiatry, 156*(3), 374–378.

De Benedittis, G., & De Santis, A. (1983). Chronic post-traumatic headache: clinical, psychopathological features and outcome determinants. *Journal of Neurosurgical Science, 27*(3), 177–186.

de Kruijk, J.R., Twinstra, A., & Leffers, P. (2001). Diagnostic criteria and differential diagnosis of mild traumatic brain injury. *Brain Injury, 15,* 99–106.

Delahunty, A., Morice, R., Frost, B., & Lambert, F. (1991). Neurocognitive rehabilitation in schizophrenia eight years post head injury: A case study. *Cognitive Rehabilitation, 9*(5), 24–28.

Delahanty, D.L., Herberman, H.B., Craig, K.J., Hayward, M.C., Fullerton, C.S., Ursano, R.J., & Baum, A. (1997). Acute and chronic distress and posttraumatic stress disorder as a function of responsibility for serious motor vehicle accidents. *Journal of Consulting and Clinical Psychology, 65*(4), 560–567.

Delay, J., & Deniker, P. (1956). Chlorpromazine and neuroleptic treatments in psychiatry. *Journal of Clinical and Experimental Psychopathology, 17,* 19–24.

DelBello, M.P., Soutullo, C.A., Zimmerman, M.E., Sax, K.W., Williams, J.R., McElroy, S.L., & Stratowski, S.M. (1999). Traumatic brain injury in individuals convicted of sexual offences with and without bipolar disorder. *Psychiatry Research, 89*, 281–286.

Delmonico, R.L., Hanley-Peterson, P., & Englander, J. (1998). Group psychotherapy for persons with traumatic brain injury: Management of frustration and substance abuse. *Journal of Head Trauma Rehabilitation, 13*(6), 10–22.

De Mol, J., Violon, A., & Brihaye, J. (1982). [Post traumatic schizophrenic bouts: with regard to 6 cases of traumatic schizophrenia (author's transl)]. *Encephale, 8*(1), 17–24.

De Morsier, G., & Gronek, B. (1971). [Post-traumatic headache and neck pain, and pain from pressure on the nerve of Arnold]. *Schweizer Archiv für Neurologie, Neurochirurgie und Psychiatri, 109*(2), 245–271.

Dencker, P.G. (1944). The postconcussion syndrome: prognosis and evaluation of the organic factors. *New York State Journal of Medicine, 44*, 379–84.

Derogatis, L.R., Lipman, R.S., & Covi, L. (1973). SCL-90: An outpatient psychiatric rating scale– preliminary report. *Psychopharmacology Bulletin, 9,* 13–28.

Devinsky, O., Morrell, M.J., & Vogt, B.A. (1995). Contributions of anterior cingulate cortex to behaviour. *Brain, 118* (Pt 1), 279–306.

Diamond, R., Barth, J.T., & Zillmer, E.A. (1988). Emotional correlates of mild closed head trauma: the role of the MMPI. *International Journal of Clinical Neuropsychology, 10,* 35–40.

Diamond, D.M., Fleshner, M., & Rose, G.M. (1994). Psychological stress repeatedly blocks hippocampal primed burst potentiation in behaving rats. *Behavioural Brain Research, 62*(1), 1–9.

DiCarlo, M.A., Gfeller, J.D., & Oliveri, M.V. (2000). Effects of coaching on detecting feigned cognitive impairment with the Category test. *Archives of Clinical Neuropsychology, 15*(5), 399–413.

Dieckmenn, G., Schneider-Jonietz, B., & Schneider, H. (1988). Psychiatric and neuropsychological findings after stereotactic hypothalamotomy in cases of extreme sexual aggressivity. *Acta Neurochirurgica* (Suppl.), *44,* 163–166.

Dikmen, S., Bombadier, C.H., Machamer, J.E., Fann, J.E., & Temkin, N.R. (2004). Natural history of depression in traumatic brain injury. *Archives of Physical Medicine and Rehabilitation, 85,* 1457–1464.

Dikmen, S., Machamer, J., Donovan, D., Winn, R., & Temkin, N.R. (1995). Alcohol use before and after traumatic brain injury. *Annals of Emergency Medicine, 26,* 167–176.

Dikmen, S., McLean, A., Jr., Temkin, N.R., & Wyler, A.R. (1986). Neuropsychologic outcome at one-month post-injury. *Archives of Physical Medicine and Rehabilitation, 67*(8), 507–513.

Dikmen, S., & Reitan, R.M. (1977). Emotional sequelae of head injury. *Annals of Neurology, 2,* 492–494.

Dikmen, S., Reitan, R.M., & Temkin, N.R. (1983). Neuropsychological recovery in head injury. *Archives of Neurology, 40*(6), 333–338.

Dikmen, S.S., Temkin, N., & Armsden, G. (1989). Neuropsychological recovery: Relationship to psychosocial functioning and post-concussional complaints. In H.S. Levin, H.M. Eisenberg, & A.L. Benton (Eds.), *Mild head injury* (pp. 229–241). New York, NY: Oxford University Press.

Dikmen, S.A., Temkin, N., Machamer, J., Hulubkov, A.L., Fraser, R.T., & Winn, R. (1994). Employment following traumatic head injuries. *Archives of Neurology, 51,* 177–186.

Dikmen, S.A., Temkin, N., McLean, A., Wyler, A., & Machamer, J. (1987) Memory and head injury severity. *Journal of Neurology, Neurosurgery and Psychiatry, 50,* 1613–1618.

Dilley, M., & Fleminger, S. (2006). Advances in neuropsychiatry: clinical implications. *Advances in Psychiatric Treatment, 12,* 23–34.

Dilts, S.L. (2001). *Models of the mind.* Philadelphia, PA: Brunner-Routledge.

Dimond, S.J. (1980). *Neuropsychology: A textbook of systems and psychological functions of the human brain.* London: Butterworth's.

Dolan, R.J., Bench, C.J., Brown, R.G., Scott, L.C., & Frackowiak, R.S. (1994). Neuropsychological dysfunction in depression: the relationship to regional cerebral blood flow. *Psychological Medicine, 24*(4), 849–857.

Dolberg, O.T., Barkai, G., Gross, Y., & Schreiber, S. (2005). Differential effects of topiramate in patients with traumatic brain injury and obesity—A case series. *Psychopharmacology, 179*(4), 838–845.

Donovan, N.J., & Barry, J.J. (1994). Compulsive symptoms associated with frontal lobe injury. *American Journal of Psychiatry, 151*(4), 618.

Drevets, W.C. (1999). Prefrontal cortical-amygdalar metabolism in major depression. *Annals of the New York Academy of Science*, 877, 614–637.

Drubach, D.A., Kelly, M.P., Winslow, M.M., & Flynn, J.P. (1993). Substance abuse as a factor in the causality, severity, and recurrence rate of traumatic brain injury. *Maryland Medical Journal, 42*(10), 989–993.

Drummond, L.M., & Gravestock, S. (1988). Delayed emergence of obsessive-compulsive neurosis following head injury. Case report and review of its theoretical implications. *British Journal of Psychiatry, 153*, 839–842.

Dua, S., & MacLean, P.D. (1964). Localization for penile erection in medical frontal lobe. *American Journal of Physiology, 207,* 1425–1434.

Ducharme, S., & Gill, K.M. (1990). Sexual values, training and professional roles. *Journal of Head Trauma Rehabilitation, 5,* 38–45.

Duman, R.S., Heninger, G.R., & Nestler, E.J. (1997). *Archives of General Psychiatry, 54*(7), 597–606.

Duong, T.T., Englander, J., Wright, J., Cifu, D.X., Greenwald, B.D., & Brown, A.W. (2004). Relationship between strength, balance, and swallowing deficits and outcome after traumatic brain injury: A multicenter analysis. *Archives of Physical Medicine and Rehabilitation, 85*(8), 1291–1297.

Eames, P. (1988). Behavior disorders after severe head injury: their nature and causes and strategies for management. *Journal of Head Trauma Rehabilitation, 3,* 1–6.

Eames, P. (1990). Organic bases of behaviour disorder after traumatic brain injury. In R.L. Wood (Ed.), *Neurobehavioural sequelae of traumatic brain injury.* London: Taylor & Francis.

Edna, T.H. (1987). Disability 3–5 years after minor head injury. *Journal of Oslo City Hospital, 37,* 41–48.

Edna, T.H., & Cappelen, J. (1987). Late post-concussional symptoms in traumatic head injury. An analysis of frequency and risk factors. *Acta Neurochirurgica (Wien), 86,* 12–17.

Edwards, S., & Dickinson, M. (1987). Intrusive unwanted thoughts: A two-stage model of control. *British Journal of Medical Psychology, 60,* 317–328.

Ehlers, A., & Clark, D. (2000). A cognitive model of posttraumatic stress disorder. *Behavior Research and Therapy, 38,* 319–345.

Ehrlich, J., & Sipesk, A. (1985). Group treatment of communication skills for head trauma patients. *Cognitive Rehabilitation, 13,* 32–37.

Ekman, P., & Friesen, W.V. (1976). Measuring facial movement. *Environmental Psychology and Nonverbal Behavior, 1*(1), 56–75.

Ellenberg, J.H., Levin, H.S., & Saydjari, C. (1996). Posttraumatic amnesia as a predictor of outcome after severe closed head injury: prospective assessment. *Archives of Neurology, 53,* 782–791.

Elliott, M.L., & Biever, L.S. (1996). Head injury and sexual dysfunction. *Brain Injury, 10,* 703–717.

Elliott, R., Baker, S.C., Rogers, R.D., O'Leary, D.A., Paykel, E.S., Frith, C.D., Dolan, R.J., & Sahakian, B.J. (1997). Prefrontal dysfunction in depressed patients performing a complex planning task: A study using positron emission tomography. *Psychological Medicine, 27*(4), 931–942.

Elsass, L., & Kinsella, G. (1989). Development of a scale for measuring behaviour change following closed head injury. In V. Anderson & M. Bailey (Eds.), *Proceedings of the fourteenth Annual Brain Impairment Conference.* Melbourne: Australian Society for the Study of Brain Impairment.

Emory, L.E., Cole, C.M., & Myer, W.J. (1995). Use of Depo-Provera to control sexual aggression in persons with traumatic brain injury. *Journal of Head Trauma Rehabilitation, 10,* 47–58.

Engel, G.L. (1980). The clinical application of the biopsychosocial model. *American Journal of Psychiatry, 137*(5), 535–544.

Endicott, J., & Spitzer, R.L. (1978). A diagnostic interview: the schedule for affective disorders and schizophrenia. *Archives of General Psychiatry, 35*(7), 837–844.

Enoch, M.D., & Trethowan, W.H. (1979). *Uncommon psychiatric syndromes* (2nd ed.). Bristol: John Wright & Sons.

Enticott, P.G., & Ogloff, J.R.P. (2006). Elucidation of impulsivity. *Australian Psychologist, 41*(1), 3–14.

Epstein, R.S., & Ursano, R.J. (1994). Anxiety disorders. In J.M. Silver, S.C. Yudofsky, & R.E. Hales (Eds.), *Neuropsychiatry of traumatic brain injury* (pp. 285–311). Washington, DC: American Psychiatric Press.

Eslinger, P.J., & Damasio, A.R. (1985). Severe disturbance of higher cognition after bilateral frontal lobe ablation: patient EVR. *Neurology, 35*(12), 1731–1741.

Eslinger, P.J., Grattan, L.M., & Geder, L. (1995). Impact of frontal lobe lesions on rehabilitation and recovery from acute brain injury. *Neuropsychological Rehabilitation, 5*, 161–182.

Essleman, P.C., & Uomoto, J.M. (1995). Classification of the spectrum of mild traumatic brain injury. *Brain Injury, 9(4)*, 417–24.

Etcharry-Bouyx, F., & Dubas, F. (2000). Obsessive–compulsive disorders in association with focal brain lesions. In J. Bogousslavsky, & J.L. Cummings (Eds.), *Behavior and mood disorders in focal brain lesions* (pp. 304–326). Cambridge, U.K: Cambridge University Press.

Etcoff, L.M., & Kampfer, K.M. (1996). Practical guidelines in the use of symptom validity and other psychological tests to measure malingering and symptom exaggeration in traumatic brain injury cases. *Neuropsychology Review, 6*(4), 171–201.

Evans, R.W. (1992). The postconcussion syndrome and the sequelae of mild head injury. *Neurology Clinics, 10*(4), 815–847.

Evans, R.W. (2004). Post-traumatic headaches. *Neurology Clinics of North America, 22*, 237–249.

Evans, R.W., Evans, R.I., & Sharp, M.J. (1994). The physician survey on the postconcussion and whiplash syndromes. *Headache, 34*(5), 268–274.

Evered, L., Ruff, R., Baldo, J., & Isomura, A. (2003). Emotional risk factors and postconcussional disorder. *Assessment, 10*, 420–427.

Ewing, R., McCarthy, D., Gronwall, D., & Wrightson, P. (1980). Persisting effects of minor head injury observable during hypoxic stress. *Journal of Clinical Neuropsychology, 2*, 147–155.

Ezrachi, O., Ben-Yishay, Y., Kay, T., Diller, L., & Rattock, J. (1991). Predicting employment in traumatic brain injury following neuropsychological rehabilitation. *Journal of Head Trauma Rehabilitation, 6*(3), 71–84.

Fann, J. (1997). Traumatic brain injury and psychiatry. *Journal of Psychosomatic Research, 43*, 335–343.

Fann, J.R., Burington, B., Leonetti, A., Jaffe, K., Katon, W.J., & Thompson, R.S. (2004). Psychiatric illness following traumatic brain injury in an adult health maintenance organization population. *Archives of General Psychiatry*, 61, 53–61.

Fann, J., Katon, W., Uomoto, J., & Esselman, P. (1995). Psychiatric disorders and functional disability in outpatients with traumatic brain injuries. *The American Journal of Psychiatry, 152*(10), 1493–1500.

Fann, J., Uomoto, J., & Katon, W. (2000). Sertraline in the treatment of major depression following mild traumatic brain injury. *Brain Injury, 12*, 226–232.

Farrow, T.F., Zheng, Y., Wilkinson, I.D., Spence, S.A., Deakin, J.F., Tarrier, N., Griffiths, P.D., Woodruff, P.W. (2001). Investigating the functional anatomy of empathy and forgiveness. *Neuroreport, 12*, 2433–2438.

Fedoroff, J.P., Starkstein, S.E., Forrester, A.W., Geisler, F.H., Jorge, R.E., Arndt, S.V., & Robinson, R.G. (1992). Depression in patients with acute traumatic brain injury. *American Journal of Psychiatry, 149(7)*, 918–923.

Feighner, J.P., Robins, E., Guze, S.B., Woodruff, R.A., Jr., Winokur, G., & Munoz, R. (1972). Diagnostic criteria for use in psychiatric research. *Archives of General Psychiatry, 26*(1), 57–63.

Feinstein, A., Hershkop, S., Ouchterlony, D., Jardine, A., & McCullagh, S. (2002). Posttraumatic amnesia and recall of a traumatic event following traumatic brain injury. *Journal of Neuropsychiatry and Clinical Neuroscience, 14*(1), 25–30.

Fenton, G., McClelland, R., Montgomery, A., MacFlynn, G., & Rutherford, W. (1993). The postconcussional syndrome: social antecedents and psychological sequelae. *The British Journal of Psychiatry, 162*, 493–497.

Ferguson, S.M., & Rayport, M. (1984). Psychosis in epilepsy. In D.P. Blumer (Ed.), *Psychiatric aspects of epilepsy* (pp. 229–270). Washington, DC: American Psychiatric Press.

Feutchwanger, E. (1923). *Die Funktionen des stirnhirns:Ihre pathologie und psychologie.* Berlin: Springer.

Fichtenberg, N.L., Millis, S.R., Mann, R.N., Zafonte, R.D., & Millard, A.E. (2000). Factors associated with insomnia among post-acute traumatic brain injury survivors. *Brain Injury, 14*(7), 659–667.

Fichtenberg, N.L., Zafonte, R.D., Putnam, S., Mann, N.R., & Millard, A.E. (2002). Insomnia in a post–acute brain injury sample. *Brain Injury, 16*, 197–206.

Filley, C.M., & Jarvis, P.E. (1987). Delayed reduplicative paramnesia. *Neurology, 37*(4), 701–703.

Finlay-Jones, R., & Brown, G.W. (1981). types of stressful life event and the onset of anxiety and depressive disorders. *Psychological Medicine, 11*(4), 803–815.

Fisher, C.M. (1983). Honoured guest presentation: Abulia minor versus agitated behavior. *Clincial Neurosurgery, 31*, 9–31.

Fisher, J. (1985). Cognitive and behavioral consequences of closed head injury. *Seminars in Neurology, 5*(3).

Flashman, L.A., Amador, X., & McAllister, T.W. (2005). Awareness of deficits. In J.M. Silver, T.W. McAllister, & S.C. Yudofsky (Eds.), *Textbook of traumatic brain injury* (pp. 353–367). Washington, DC: American Psychiatric Publishing Inc.

Fleming, J., Tooth, L., Hassell, M., & Chan, W. (1999). Prediction of community integration and vocational outcome 2–5 years after traumatic brain injury rehabilitation in Australia. *Brain Injury, 13*, 417–431.

Fleminger, S., Oliver, D.L., Williams, W.H., & Evans, J. (2003). The neuropsychiatry of depression after brain injury. *Neuropsychological Rehabilitation, 13(1/2)*, 65–87.

Flor-Henry, P. (1974). Psychosis, neurosis and epilepsy. *British Journal of Psychiatry, 124*, 144–150.

Flor-Henry, P. (1976). Lateralized Temporal-Limbic Dysfunction and. Psychopathology. *Annals of the New York Academy of Science, 380*, 777–797.

Foa, E.B., Keane, T.M., & Friedman, M.J. (2000). *Effective treatments for PTSD: Practice guidelines from the International Society for Traumatic Stress Studies.* New York: Guilford Press.

Foa, E.B., Riggs, D.S., Dancu, C.V., & Rothbaum, B.O. (1993). Reliability and validity of a brief instrument for assessing post-traumatic stress disorder. *Journal of Traumatic Stress, 6*, 459–473.

Fodor, J.A. (1983). The modularity of mind: An essay on faculty psychology. Cambridge, MA: Bradford/MIT Books.

Fodor, J.A. (1985). Précis of The Modularity of Mind. *Behavioral and Brain Sciences, 8*, 1–42.

Fodor, J.A. (2000). *The mind doesn't work that way: the scope and limits of computational psychology.* Cambridge, Mass: MIT Press.

Foreman, M.M., & Hall, J.L. (1987). Effects of D2–dopaminergic receptor stimulation on male rat sexual behavior. *Journal of Neural Transmission, 68*(3–4), 153–170.

Formisano, R., Voogt, R.D., Buzzi, M.G., Vinicola, V., Penta, F., Peppe, A., & Stanzione, P. (2004). Time interval of oral feeding recovery as a prognostic factor in severe traumatic brain injury. *Brain Injury, 18*(1), 103–109.

Forrester, G., Encel, J., & Geffen, G. (1994). Measuring post-traumatic amnesia (PTA): An historical review. *Brain Injury, 8*(2), 175–184.

Fortune, N., & Wren, X. (1999). *The definition, incidence and prevalence of acquired brain injury in Australia.* Australian Institute of Health and Welfare, cat no. DIS 15, Canberra: Australian Institute of Health and Welfare.

Fortuny, A.Y.L., Briggs, M., Newcombe, F., Ratcliffe, G., & Thomas, C. (1980). Measuring the duration of post-traumatic amnesia. *Journal of Neurology, Neurosurgery and Psychiatry, 43*, 377–379.

Fox, D.D., Lees-Haley, P.R., Earnest, K., & Dolezal-Wood, S. (1995). Base rates of postconcussive symptoms in health maintenance organization patients and controls. *Neuropsychology, 9*, 606–611.

Frankowski, R.F. (1986). Descriptive epidemiological studies of head injury in the United States: 1974–1984. *Advances in Psychosomatic Medicine, 16*,153–172.

Franulic, A., Horta, E., Maturana, R., Scherpenisse, J., & Carbonell, C. (2000). Organic personality disorder after traumatic brain injury: Cognitive, anatomic, and psychosocial factors. A 6 month follow-up. *Brain Injury, 14*(5), 431–439.

Freeland, J. (1996). Awareness of deficits: A complex interplay of neurological, social and rehabilitation factors. *i.e. Magazine, 4*, 32–34.

Freeston, M. H., Ladouceur, R., Rheaume, J., Letarte, H., Gagnon, F., & Thibodeau, N. (1994). Self-report of obsessions and worry. *Behaviour Research and Therapy, 32*(1), 29–36.

Freemon, F., & Nevis, A. (1969). Temporal lobe sexual seizures. *Neurology, 19*, 87–90.

Frieboes, R.M., Müller, U., Murck, H., Yves von Cramon, D., Holsboer, F., & Steiger, A. (1999). Nocturnal hormone secretion and the sleep EEG in patients several months after traumatic brain injury. *Journal of Neuropsychiatry and Clinical Neurosciences, 11*(3), 354–360.

Friedman, M. (1983). *Head injury.* New York, NY: CIBA Geigy Corporation.

Fujii, D., & Ahmed, I. (1996). Psychosis secondary to traumatic brain injury. *Neuropsychiatry, Neuropsychology and Behavioral Neurology, 9*, 133–138.

Fujii, D., & Ahmed, I. (2002). Characteristics of psychotic disorder due to traumatic brain injury: An analysis of case studies in the literature. *Journal of Neuropsychiatry and Clinical Neuroscience, 14*(2), 130–140.

Fujii, M., Fujita, K., Hiramatsu, H., & Miyamoto, T. (1998). Cases of two patients whose food aversions disappeared following severe traumatic brain injury. *Brain Injury, 12*(8), 709–713.

Fuller, M.G., Fishman, E., Taylor, C.A., & Wood, R.B. (1994). Screening patients with traumatic brain injuries for substance abuse. *Journal of Neuropsychiatry and Clinical Neurosciences, 6*(2), 143–146.

Fuster, J.M. (1989). *The prefrontal cortex: Anatomy, physiology, and neuropsychology of the frontal lobe.* New York: Raven.

Fuster, J.M. (2003). *Cortex and mind.* Oxford, UK: Oxford University Press.

Gabbard, G.O., Twemlow, S.W., & Jones, F.C. (1981). Do "near death experiences" occur only near death? *Journal of Nervous and Mental Disease, 169*(6), 374–377.

Gaetz, M., & Weinberg, H. (2000). Electrophysiological indices of persistent post–concussion symptoms. *Brain Injury, 14*(9), 815–832.

Galbraith, S., Murray, W., Patel, A., & Knill-Jones, R. (1976). The relationship between alcohol and head injury and its effects on the conscious level. *British Journal of Surgery, 63*, 128–130.

Gandolfo, R. (1995). MMPI–2 profiles of worker's compensation claimants who present with complaints of harassment. *Journal of Clinical Psychology, 51*(5), 711–715.

Gans, J.S. (1983). Psychological adaptation. *Seminars in Nuerology, 3*, 201–211.

Ganser, S.J.M. (1898). Über einen eigenartigen hysterischen dämmerzustand. *Archiv für Psychiatrie und Nervenkrankheiten, Berlin, 30*, 633–640.

Garden, F. (1991). Incidence of sexual dysfunction in neurological disabilities. *Sexuality and Disability, 9,* 1–6.

Garden, F., Bontke, C., & Hoffman, M. (1990). Sexual functioning and marital adjustment after traumatic brain injury. *Journal of Head Trauma Rehabilitation, 5,* 53–59.

Garland, D.E., & Bailey, S. (1981). Undetected injuries in head-injured adults. *Clinical Orthopaedics and Related Research, 155*, 162–165.

Gasquoine, P.G. (2000). Postconcussional symptoms in chronic back pain. *Applied Neuropsychology, 7(2)*, 83–89.

Gass, C.S. (1991). MMPI-2 interpretation and closed head injury: A correction factor. *Psychological Assessment, 3*, 27–31.

Gazzaniga, M.S., Ivry, R., & Mangun, G.R. (2002). *Cognitive neuroscience: The biology of the mind* (2nd ed.). New York: W.W. Norton.

Geerts, W.H., Code, K.I., Jay, R.M., Chen, E., & Szalai, J.P. (1994). A prospective study of venous thromboembolism after major trauma. *New England Journal of Medicine, 331*(24), 1601–1606.

Geffen, G.M., Encel, J.S., & Forrester, G.M. (1991). Stages of recovery during post traumatic amnesia and subsequent everyday memory deficits. *Neuroreport, 2*, 105–108.

Gellman, I., Keenan, M.A., & Botte, M.J. (1996). Recognition and pain management of upper extremity pain syndromes in the patient with brain injury. *Journal of Head Trauma Rehabilitation, 11*(4), 23–30.

Gennarelli, T.A., & Graham, D.I. (2005). Neuropathology. In J.M. Silver, T.W. McAllister, & S.C. Yudofsky (Eds.), *Textbook of traumatic brain injury* (pp. 27–50). Washington, DC: American Psychiatric Publishing Inc.

Gennarelli, T.A., Thibault, L.E., Adams, J.H., Graham, D.I., Thompson, C.J., & Marcinin, R.P. (1982). Diffuse axonal injury and traumatic coma in the primate. *Annals of Neurology, 12*, 564–574.

Gennarelli, T.A., Thibault, L.E., & Graham, D.I. (1998). Diffuse axonal injury: An important form of traumatic brain damage. *Neuroscientist, 4*, 202–215.

Gerberding, J.L., & Binder, S. (2003). *Report to Congress on mild traumatic brain injury in the United States: Steps to prevent a serious public health problem*. National Center for Injury Prevention and Control. Atlanta, GA: Centers for Disease Control and Prevention.

Gerner, R.H. (1993). Treatment of acute mania. *Psychiatry Clinics of North America, 16*(3), 443–460.

Gervais, R.O., Rohling, M.L., Green, P., & Ford, W. (2004). A comparison of WMT, CARB, and TOMM failure rates in non–head injury disability claimants. *Archives of Clinical Neuropsychology, 19*(4), 475–487.

Geschwind, N., & Galaburda, A. (1985). Cerebral lateralization: Biological mechanisms, associations and pathology: I. A hypothesis and a program for research. *Archives of Neurology, 42*, 428–459.

Gilbert, P. (1989). *Human nature and suffering.* Hove, U.K.: Erlbaum.

Gilbertson, M.W., Shenton, M.E., Ciszewski, A., Kasai, K., Lasko, N.B., Orr, S.P., & Pitman, R.K. (2002). Smaller hippocampal volume predicts pathologic vulnerability to psychological trauma. *Nature Neuroscience, 5,* 1242–1247.

Glaesser, J., Neuner, F., Lutgehetmann, R., Schmidt, R., & Elbert, T. (2004). Posttraumatic stress disorder in patients with traumatic brain injury. *BMC Psychiatry, 4*, 5.

Gold, P.W., Goodwin, F.K., & Chrousos, J.P. (1988). Clinical and biochemical manifestations of depression. *New England Journal of Medicine, 319*, 348–353.

Goldberg, E. (1995). The rise and fall of modular orthodoxy. *Journal of Clinical and Experimental Neuropsychology, 17*, 193–208.

Goldberg, R.L., & Buongiorno, P.A. (1982). The use of Carbamazepine for the treatment of paraphilias in a brain damaged patient. *International Journal of Psychiatry Medicine, 12*, 275–279.

Golden, Z., & Golden, C.J. (2003). The differential impacts of Alzheimer's dementia, head injury, and stroke on personality dysfunction. *International Journal of Neuroscience, 113*(6), 869–878.

Goldney, R.D. (2004). A note on the association of bipolar disorders after head injury: Causal or coincidental? *Psychiatry, Psychology and Law, 11*, 50–52.

Goldney, R.D. (2005). A note on the association of schizophrenia after head injury: causal or coincidental? *Psychiatry, Psychology and the Law, 12*(1), 103–106.

Goldstein, F.C., Levin, H.S., Goldman, W.P., Clark, A.N., & Altonen, T.K. (2001). Cognitive and neurobehavioral functioning after mild versus moderate traumatic brain injury in older adults. *Journal of the International Neuropsychological Society, 7*(3), 373–383.

Goldstein, F.C., Levin, H.S., Goldman, W.P., Kalechstein, A.D., Clark, A.N., & Kenehan–Altonen, T. (1999). Cognitive and behavioral sequelae of closed head injury in older adults according to their significant others. *The Journal of Neuropsychiatry and Clinical Neurosciences, 11*, 38–44.

Gómez, P.A., Lobato, R.D., Ortega, J.M., & De La Cruz, J. (1996). Mild head injury: Differences in prognosis among patients with a Glasgow Coma Scale score of 13 to 15 and analysis of factors associated with abnormal CT findings. *British Journal of Neurosurgery, 10(5)*, 453–460.

Gordon, W.A., Haddad, L., Brown, M., Hibbard, M.R., & Sliwinski, M. (2000). The sensitivity and specificity of self–reported symptoms in individuals with traumatic brain injury. *Brain Injury, 14*, 21–33.

Gorman, D.G., & Cummings, J.L. (1992). Hypersexuality following septal injury. *Archives of Neurology, 49*, 308–310.

Gosling, J., & Oddy, M. (1999). Rearranged marriages: marital relationships after head injury. *Brain Injury, 13*, 785–796.

Gotsch, K., Annest, J.L., Holmgreen, P., & Gilchrist, J. (2002). Nonfatal sports- and recreation-related injuries treated in emergency departments–United States, July 2000–June 2001. *Morbidity and Mortality Weekly Report, 51*, 736–740.

Gottesman, I.I., & Shields, J. (1972). *Schizophrenia and genetics: A twin study vantage point.* New York: Academic Press.

Goutier-Smith, P.C. (1986). Sexual function and dysfunction. *Clinical Neurobiology, 1*, 634–642.

Gouvier, W.D., Uddo-Crane, M., & Brown, L.M. (1988). Base rates of post–concussional symptoms. *Archives of Clinical Neuropsychology, 3(3)*, 273–278.

Graber, B., Hartman, K., Coffman, J.A., Huey, C.J., & Golden, C.J. (1982). Brain damage among mentally disordered sex offenders. *Journal of Forensic Science, 27*, 125–134.

Grafman, J., Vance, S.C., Weingartner, H., Salazar, A.M., & Amin, D. (1986). The effects of lateralized frontal lesions on mood regulation. *Brain, 109*, 1127–1148.

Graham, D.I. (1996). Blunt head injury: Prospects for improved outcome. *Neuropathology and Applied Neuropsychology, 22*(6), 505–509.

Graham, D.I., & Gennarelli, T.A. (1997). Chapter 5: Trauma. In D.I. Graham, & P.L. Lantos (Eds), *Greenfield's neuropathology* (6th ed.) (p. 197–262). United Kingdom: Arnold.

Graham, D.I., & McIntosh, T.K. (1996). *Neuropathology of brain injury.* Philadelphia, PA: WB Saunders.

Grant, I., & Alves, W. (1987). Psychiatric and psychosocial disturbances in head injury. In H.S. Levin, J. Grafman, & H.M. Eisenberg (Eds.), *Neurobehavioral recovery from head injury* (pp. 232–261). New York: Oxford University Press.

Grant, S., Contoreggi, C., & London, E.D. (2000). Drug abusers show impaired performance in a laboratory test of decision making. *Neuropsychologia, 38*(8), 1180–1187.

Grattan, L.M., & Eslinger, P.J. (1989). Empirical study of empathy. *American Journal of Psychiatry, 146*(11), 1521–1522.

Gray, J.A. (1987). *The psychology of fear and stress.* Cambridge, England: Cambridge University Press.

Gray, J.A., & McNaughton, N. (1996). The neuropsychology of anxiety: reprise. *Nebraska Symposium on Motivation, 43*, 61–134.

Green, R.E., Turner, G.R., & Thompson, W.F. (2004). Deficits in facial emotion perception in adults with recent traumatic brain injury. *Neuropsychologia, 42*(2), 133–141.

Green, P., Allen, L.M., & Astner, K. (1996). *Manual for the Computerized Word Memory Test.* Durham, NC: Cognisyst.

Green, P., Rohling, M.L., Lees-Haley, P.R., & Allen, L.M., 3rd. (2001). Effort has a greater effect on test scores than severe brain injury in compensation claimants. *Brain Injury, 15*(12), 1045–1060.

Greiffenstein, M.F., Baker, W.J., & Gola, T. (1994). Validation of malingered amnesia measures with a large clinical sample. *Psychological Assessment, 6,* 218–224.

Greiffenstein, M.F., Baker, W.J., & Gola, T. (1996). Motor dysfunction profiles in traumatic brain injury and postconcussion syndrome. *Journal of the International Neuropsychological Society, 2*(6), 477–485.

Greiffenstein, M.F., Baker, W.J., & Gola, T. (2002). Brief report: Anosmia and remote outcome in closed head injury. *Journal of Clinical and Experimental Neuropsychology, 24*(5), 705–709.

Greiffenstein, M.F., Baker, W.J., & Gola, T. (2003). Straw man walking: Reply to Varney (2002). *Journal of Clinical and Experimental Neuropsychology, 25*(1), 152–154.

Greve, K.W., Bianchini, K.J., Mathias, C.W., Houston, R.J., & Crouch, J.A. (2003). Detecting malingered performance on the Wechsler Adult Intelligence Scale. Validation of Mittenberg's approach in traumatic brain injury. *Archives of Clinical Neuropsychology, 18*(3), 245–260.

Greve, K.W., Sherwin, E., Stanford, M.S., Mathias, C., Love, J., & Ramzinski, P. (2001). Personality and neurocognitive correlates of impulsive aggression in long-term survivors of severe traumatic brain injury. *Brain Injury, 15*(3), 255–262.

Greyson, B. (1983). The near-death experience scale: construction, reliability, and validity. *Journal of Nervous and Mental Disease, 171*, 369–375.

Greyson, B. (1998). Biological aspects of near-death experiences. *Perspectives in Biology and Medicine, 42*(1), 14–32.

Greyson, B. (2001). Posttraumatic stress symptoms following near-death experiences. *American Journal of Orthopsychiatry, 71*(3), 368–373.

Greyson, B., & Stevenson, I. (1980). The phenomenology of near-death experiences. *American Journal of Psychiatry, 137*(10), 1193–1196.

Griffith, E., Cole, S. & Cole, T. (1990). Sexuality and sexual dysfunction. In M. Rosenthal, E. Griffith, M. Bond, & D. Miller (Eds.), *Rehabilitation of the adult and child with traumatic brain injury* (pp. 206–224). Philadelphia, PA: F. A. Davis.

Grigsby, J., & Kaye, K. (1993). Incidence and correlates of depersonalization following head trauma. *Brain Injury, 7*(6), 507–513.

Groher, M. (1977). Language and memory disorders following closed head trauma. *Journal of Speech and Hearing Research, 20*, 212–223.

Groleau, G.A., Tso, E.L., Olshaker, J.S., Barish, R.A., & Lyston, D.J. (1993). Baseball bat assault injuries. *Journal of Trauma, 34(3),* 366–372.

Gronwall, D., & Wrightson, P. (1974). Delayed recovery of intellectual function after minor head injury. *Lancet, 2*, 605–609.

Gronwall, D., & Wrightson, P. (1975). Cumulative effect of concussion. *Lancet, 2*, 995–997.

Gronwall, D., & Wrightson, P. (1980). Duration of post-traumatic amnesia after mild head injury. *Journal of Clinical Neuropsychology, 2*, 51–60.

Gronwall, D., Wrightson, P., & Waddell, P. (1990). *Head injury: The facts. A guide for families and caregivers.* Oxford: Oxford University Press.

Gruzelier, J.H. (2003). Theory, methods and new directions in the psychophysiology of the schizophrenic process and schizotypy. *International Journal of Psychophysiology, 48*, 221–245.

Gualtieri, C.T. (1991). *Neuropsychiatry and behavioral pharmacology.* New York: Springer-Verlag.

Gualtieri, C.T., & Cox, D.R. (1991). The delayed neurobehavioural sequelae of traumatic brain injury. *Brain Injury, 5(32),* 219–232.

Guerrero, J.L., Thurman, D.J., & Sniezek, J.E. (2000). Emergency department visits associated with traumatic brain injury: United States, 1995–1996. *Brain Injury, 14(2),* 181–186.

Guilleminault, C., Faull, K.F., Miles, L., & van de Hoed, J. (1983). Posttraumatic excessive daytime sleepiness. A review of 20 patients. *Neurology (Cleveland), 33,* 1584–1589.

Guilleminault, C., Yuen, K.M., Gulerick, M.G., Karadeniz, D. (2000). Hypersomnia after head–neck trauma: A medicolegal dilemma. *Neurology, 54*, 653–659.

Gujral, I., Stallones, L., Gabella, B., Keefe, T.J., & Chen, P. (2006). Sex differences in mortality after traumatic brain injury, Colorado 1994–1998. *Brain Injury, 20*(3), 283–291.

Gurgo, R. D., Bedi, K. S., & Nurcombe, V. (2002). Current concepts in central nervous system regeneration. *Journal of Clinical Neuroscience, 9*(6), 613–617.

Gurney, J.G., Rivara, F.P., Mueller, B.A., Newell, D.W., Copass, M.K., & Jurkovich, G.J. (1992). The effects of alcohol intoxication on the initial treatment and hospital course of patients with acute brain injury. *Journal of Trauma–Injury Infection and Critical Care, 33*(5), 709–713.

Gurvits, T.V., Shenton, M.E., Hokama, H., Ohta, H., Lasko, N.B., Gilbertson, M.W., Orr, S.P., Kikinis, R., Jolesz, F.A., McCarley, R.W., & Pitman, R.K. (1996). Magnetic resonance imaging study of hippocampal volume in chronic, combat–related posttraumatic stress disorder. *Biol Psychiatry, 40*(11), 1091–1099.

Guth, P.E. (2000). The effects of depression in head injured adults as related to educational level, gender, and activity level. *Dissertation Abstracts International: Section B: the Sciences & Engineering, 61*, 1803, U.S.: Univ. Microfilms International.

Gutman, S.A. & Napier-Klemic, J. (1996). The experience of head injury on the impairment of gender identity and gender role. *The American Journal of Occupational Therapy, 50,* 535–544.

Guze, B.H., & Gitlin, M. (1994). The neuropathologic basis of major affective disorders: nauroanatomic insights. *The Journal of Neuropsychiatry and Clinical Neurosciences, 6*, 114–121.

Haboubi, N.H., Long, J., Koshy, M., & Ward, A.B. (2001). Short-term sequelae of minor head injury (6 years experience of minor head injury clinic). *Disability Rehabilitation, 23*(14), 635–638.

Haeffel, G.J., Abramson, L.Y., Metalsky, G.I., Dykman, B.M., Donovan, P., Hogan, M.E., Voelz, Z.R., Halberstadt, L., & Hankin, B.L. (2005). Negative cognitive styles, dysfunctional attitudes, and the remitted depression paradigm: A search for the elusive cognitive vulnerability to depression factor among remitted depressives. *Emotion, 5(3)*, 343–348.

Hagen, C. (1984). Language disorders in head trauma. In A. Holland (Ed.), *Language disorders in adults* (pp. 245–281). San Diego, CA: College-Hill.

Haglund, Y., & Bergstrand, G. (1990). Does Swedish amateur boxing lead to chronic brain damage? 2. A retrospective study with CT and MRI. *Acta Neurologica Scandinavica, 82*, 297–302.

Haglund, Y., & Eriksson, E. (1993). Does amateur boxing lead to chronic brain damage? A review of some recent investigations. *American Journal of Sports Medicine, 21*, 97–109.

Haglund, Y., & Persson, H.E. (1990). Does Swedish amateur boxing lead to chronic brain damage? A retrospective clinical neurophysiological study. *Acta Neurologica Scandinavica, 82*, 353–360.

Hamner, M.B., Lorberbaum, J.P., & George, M.S. (1999). Potential role of the anterior cingulate cortex in PTSD: review and hypothesis. *Depress Anxiety, 9*(1), 1–14.

Harper, C.G., Doyle, D., Adams, J.H., & Graham, D.I. (1986). Analysis of abnormalities in pituitary gland in nonmissile head injury: Study of 100 consecutive cases. *Journal of Clinical Pathology, 39*, 769–773.

Harris, E.C., & Barraclough, B. (1997). Suicide as an outcome for mental disorders. A meta–analysis. *British Journal of Psychiatry, 170*, 205–228.

Harris, P., Nagy, S., & Vardaxis, N. (Eds.). (2006). *Mosby's dictionary of medicine, nursing & health professions* (Australian and New Zealand Edition). Sydney: Mosby.

Hart, R.P., Martelli, M.F., & Zasler, N.D. (2000). Chronic pain neuropsychological functioning. *Neuropsychological Review, 10*(3), 131–149.

Hart T., Giovannetti T., Montgomery M.W., & Schwartz M.F. (1998). Awareness of errors in naturalistic action following traumatic brain injury. *Journal of Head Trauma and Rehabilitation, 13*, 16–28.

Harvey, A.G., Brewin, C.R., Jones, C., & Kopelman, M.D. (2003). Coexistence of posttraumatic stress disorder and traumatic brain injury: Towards a resolution of the paradox. *Journal of the International Neuropsychological Society, 9*(4), 663–676.

Harvey, A.G., & Bryant, R.A. (1998). Acute stress disorder after mild traumatic brain injury. *Journal of Nervous and Mental Disease, 186*(6), 333–337.

Hasen, S. (1982). Spiral control of sexual behavior: effects of intrathecal administration of lisuride. *Neuroscience Letters, 33*, 329–332.

Haslam, C., Batchelor, J., Fearnside, M.R., Haslam, S.A., Hawkins, S., & Kenway, E. (1994). Post-coma disturbance and post-traumatic amnesia as nonlinear predictors of cognitive outcome following severe closed head injury: Findings from the Westmead Head Injury Project. *Brain Injury, 6*, 519–528.

Hayman, M.A., & Abrams, R. (1977). Capgras' syndrome and cerebral dysfunction. *British Journal of Psychiatry, 130*, 68–71.

Heath, R.G. (1964). Pleasure response of human subjects to direct stimulation of the brain: physiologic and psychodynamic considerations. In R.G. Heath (Ed.), *The role of pleasure in behaviour* (pp. 219–243). New York: Harper and Row.

Heath, R.G. (1963). Electrical self–stimulation of the brain in man. *American Journal of Psychiatry, 120*, 571–577.

Heath, R.G. (1972). Pleasure and brain activity in man: deep and surface electroencephalograms during orgasm. *Journal of Nervous and Mental Disease, 154*, 3–18.

Heath, R.G. (1975). Brain function and behavior. *Journal of Nervous and Mental Disease, 160,* 159–175.

Heath, R.G. & Fitzjarrell, A.T. (1984). Chemical stimulation to deep forebrain nuclei in parkinsonism and epilepsy. *International Journal of Neurology, 18,* 163–178.

Heaton, R.K., Smith, H.H., Jr., Lehman, R.A., & Vogt, A.T. (1978). Prospects for faking believable deficits on neuropsychological testing. *Journal of Consulting and Clinical Psychology, 46*(5), 892–900.

Heilbronner, R.L., Henry, G.K., & Carson-Brewer, M. (1991). Neuropsychologic test performance in amateur boxers. *American Journal of Sports Medicine, 19*, 376–380.

Heinemann, A., Goranson Ginsburg, K., & Schnoll, S. (1989). Alcohol use and activity patterns following spinal cord injury. *Rehabilitation Psychology, 34*, 191–205.

Heinemann, A., Keen, M., Donohue, R., & Schnoll, S. (1988). Alcohol use by persons with recent spinal cord injury. *Archives of Physical Medicine and Rehabilitation, 69*, 619–624.

Heinemann, A.W., Mamott, B.D., & Schnoll, S. (1990). Substance use by persons with recent spinal cord injuries. *Rehabilitation Psychology, 35*, 217–228.

Hibbard, M.R., Bogdany, J., Uysal, S., Kepler, K., Silver, J.M., Gordon, W.A., & Haddad, L. (2000). Axis II psychopathology in individuals with traumatic brain injury. *Brain Injury, 14*, 45–61.

Hibbard, M.R., Gordon, W.A., Flanagan, S., Haddad, L., & Labinsky, E. (2000). Sexual dysfunction after traumatic brain injury. *NeuroRehabilitation, 15*, 107–120.

Hibbard, M.R., Uysal, S., Kepler, K., Bogdany, J., & Silver, J. (1998). Axis I psychopathology in individuals with traumatic brain injury. *Journal of Head Trauma Rehabilitation, 13*(4), 24–39.

Hickling, E.J., Gillen, R., Blanchard, E.B., Buckley, T., & Taylor, A. (1998). Traumatic brain injury and posttraumatic stress disorder: A preliminary investigation of neuropsychological test results in PTSD secondary to motor vehicle accidents. *Brain Injury, 12*(4), 265–274.

High, W.M., Levin, H.S., & Gary, H.E. (1990). Recovery of orientation following closed-head injury. *Journal of Clinical and Experimental Neuropsychology, 12*, 703–714.

Hilbom, E. (1960). After–effects of brain injuries. *Acta Psychiatrica et Neurologica Scandinavica 142*(Suppl.), 1–195.

Hill, A.B. (1965). The environment and disease: Association or causation? *Proceedings of the Royal Society of Medicine, 58*, 293–300.

Hiott, D.W., & Labbate, L. (2002). Anxiety disorders associated with traumatic brain injuries. *Neurorehabilitation, 17*(4), 345–55.

Hirschfeld, R.M., Calabrese, J.R., Weissman, M.M., Reed, M., Davies, M.A., Frye, M.A., Keck, P.E., Jr., Lewis, L., McElroy, S.L., McNulty, J.P., & Wagner, K.D. (2003). Screening for bipolar disorder in the community. *Journal of Clinical Psychiatry, 64*, 53–59.

Hof, P.R., Bouras, C., Buee, L., Delacourte, A., Perl, D.P., & Morrison, J.H. (1992). Differential distribution of neurofibrillary tangles in the cerebral cortex of dementia pugilistica and Alzheimer's disease cases. *Acta Neuropathologica, 85*, 23–30.

Hoffman, R.M. (1995). Disclosure habits after near-death experiences: influences, obstacles, and listeners selection. *Journal of Near-Death Studies, 14,* 29–48.

Holtzheimer, P.E., & Nemeroff, C.B. (2006). Advances in the treatment of depression. *NeuroRx, 3*, 42–56.

Horn, L. & Zasler, N. (1990). Neuroanatomy and neurophysiology of sexual function. *Journal of Head Trauma Rehabilitation, 5,* 1–13.

Hornak, J., Rolls, E.T., & Wade, D. (1996). Face and voice expression identification in patients with emotional and behavioural changes following ventral frontal damage. *Neuropsychologia, 34*, 247–261.

Horner, M.D., & Hamner, M.B. (2002). Neurocognitive functioning in posttraumatic stress disorder. *Neuropsychology Review, 12*(1), 15–30.

Hough, S. (1989). Sexuality within the head-injury rehabilitation setting: A staff's perspective. *Psychological Reports, 65,* 745–746.

Hsiang, J.N., Yeung, T., Ashley, L.M., & Poon, W.S. (1997). High risk head injury. *Journal of Neurosurgery*, 87, 234–238.

Huether, G. (1998). Stress and the adaptive self-organization of neuronal connectivity during early childhood. *International Journal of Developmental Neuroscience, 16*(3–4), 297–306.

Hunt, C.J., Andrew, G., & Sumich, H.J. (1995). The management of mental disorders. *Handbook for the affective disorders* (Vol. 3). Sydney, NSW: World Health Organization.

Ingram, R.E, Miranda, J., & Segal, Z. (1998). *Cognitive vulnerability to depression.* New York: Guilford Press.

Ingram, R.E., & Luxton, D.D. (2005).Vulnerability–stress models. In B.L. Hankin, & J.R.Z. Abela (Eds.), *Development of psychopathology: A vulnerability–stress perspective.* (pp. 32–46). Thousand Oaks, CA: Sage Publications.

Inman, T.H., & Berry, D.T. (2002). Cross-validation of indicators of malingering: A comparison of nine neuropsychological tests, four tests of malingering, and behavioral observations. *Archives of Clinical Neuropsychology, 17*(1), 1–23.

Insel, T.R. (1992a). Neurobiology of obsessive compulsive disorder: A review. *International Clinical Psychopharmacology, 7*(Suppl. 1), 31–33.

Insel, T.R. (1992b). Toward a neuroanatomy of obsessive–compulsive disorder. *Archives of General Psychiatry, 49*(9), 739–744.

Insel, T.R., & Akiskal, H.S. (1986). Obsessive–compulsive disorder with psychotic features: A phenomenologic analysis. *American Journal of Psychiatry, 143*(12), 1527–1533.

International Headache Society, Headache Classification Committee. (1988). Proposed classification and diagnostic criteria for headache disorders, cranial neuralgias and facial pain. *Cephalagia, 8*(Suppl. 7), 9–96.

Ivanhoe, C.B., & Hartman, E.T. (2004). Clinical caveats on medical assessment and treatment of pain after TBI. *Journal of Head Trauma Rehabilitation, 19*(1), 29–39.

Iverson, G.L. (2005). Outcome from mild traumatic brain injury. *Current Opinion in Psychiatry, 18*, 301–317.

Iverson, G.L., & Lange, R.T. (2003). Examination of "postconcussion-like" symptoms in a healthy sample. *Applied Neuropsychology, 10*(3), 137–44.

Iverson, G.L., & McCracken, L.M. (1997). 'Postconcussive' symptoms in persons with chronic pain. *Brain Injury, 11*(11), 783–90.

Iverson, G.L., & Tulsky, D.S. (2003). Detecting malingering on the WAIS-III. Unusual Digit Span performance patterns in the normal population and in clinical groups. *Archives of Clinical Neuropsychology, 18*(1), 1–9.

Jablensky, A. (1995). Schizophrenia: Recent epidemiological issues. *Epidemiological Review, 17,* 10–20.

Jackson, H.F., & Moffat, N.J. (1987). Impaired emotional recognition following severe head injury. *Cortex, 23*(2), 293–300.

Jackson, J.H. (1875). On temporary mental disorders after Epileptic Paroxysms. *West Riding Lunatic Asylum Medical Reports, 5*, 240–262.

Jackson, R.D., & Mysiw, W.J. (1989). Abnormal cortisol dynamics after traumatic brain injury: lack of utility in predicting agitation or therapeutic response to tricyclic antidepressants. *American Journal of Physical Medicine and Rehabilitation, 68*, 18–23.

Jacobson, L., & Mariano, A.J. (2001). General considerations of chronic pain. In J.D. Loeser, S.H. Butler, C.R. Chapman, & D.C. Turk (Eds.), *Bonica's management of pain* (3rd ed.). Philadelphia: Lippincott Williams & Wilkins.

Jenike, M.A., & Brandon, A.D. Obsessive–compulsive disorder and head trauma: A rare association. *Journal of Anxiety Disorders, 2,* 353–359.

Jennett, B. (1996). Epidemiology of head injury. *Journal of Neurology, Neurosurgery and Psychiatry, 60*, 362–369.

Jennett, B. (1990). Scale and scope of the problem. In M. Rosenthal, M.R. Bond, E.R. Griffiths & J.D. Miller (Eds.). *Rehabilitation of the adult and child with traumatic brain injury* (2nd ed.). Philadelphia, PA: F.A. Davis.

Jennett, B., & Bond, M. (1975). Assessment of outcome after severe brain damage. *The Lancet, March 1*, 480–484.

Jennett, B., & Teasdale, G. (1981). *Management of head injuries.* Philadelphia, PA: F.A. Davis.

Jeret, J.S., Mandell, M., Anziska, B., Lipitz, M., Vilceus, A.P., Ware, J.A., & Zesiewicz, T.A. (1993). Clinical predictors of abnormality disclosed by computed tomography after mild head trauma. *Neurosurgery, 32(1),* 9–16.

Johnston, M.V., & Hall, K.M. (1994). Outcomes evaluation in TBI Rehabilitation. Part I: overview and system principles. *Archives of Physical Medicine and Rehabilitation, 75*(12), SC1–9.

Jones, D.K., Dardis, R., Ervine, M., Horsfield, M.A., Jeffree, M., Simmons, A., Jarosz, J., & Strong, A. (2000). Cluster analysis of diffusion tensor magnetic resonance images in human head injury. *Neurosurgery, 47(2)*, 306–314.

Jorge, R.E. (2005). Neuropsychiatric consequences of traumatic brain injury: A review of recent findings. *Current Opinion in Psychiatry, 18*(3), 289–299.

Jorge, R.E., & Robinson, R.G. (2002). Mood disorder following traumatic brain injury. *Neurorehabilitation, 17*(4), 311–324.

Jorge, R.E., Robinson, R.G., Arndt, S.V., Starkstein, S.E., Forrester, A.W., & Geisler, F. (1993). Depression following traumatic brain injury: A 1 year longitudinal study. *Journal of Affective Disorders, 27*(4), 233–243.

Jorge, R.E., Robinson, R.G., Moser, D., Tateno, A., Crespo-Facorro, B., & Arndt, S. (2004). Major depression following traumatic brain injury. *Archives of General Psychiatry, 61*, 42–50.

Jorge, R.E., Robinson, R.G., Starkstein, M.D., & Arndt, S.V. (1994). Influence of major depression on 1-year outcome in patients with traumatic brain injury. *Journal of Neurosurgery, 81*, 726–733.

Jorge, R.E., Robinson, R.G., Starkstein, S.E., Arndt, S.V., Forrester, A.W., & Geisler, F.H. (1993). Secondary mania following traumatic brain injury. *American Journal of Psychiatry, 150,* 916–921.

Joseph, R. (1998). Traumatic amnesia, repression, and hippocampus injury due to emotional stress, corticosteroids and enkephalins. *Child Psychiatry and Human Development, 29(2)*, 169–185.

Kahlbaum, K.L. (1863). *Die gruppierung der psychishen kranke.* Danzing: AW Kafemann.

Kalsbeek, W.D., McLaurin, R.L., Harris, B.S.H., & Miller, J.D. (1980). The national head and spinal cord injury survey: major findings. *Journal of Neurosurgery, 53*, S19–S31.

Kant, R., Duffy, J.D., & Pivovarnik, A. (1998). Prevalence of apathy following head injury. *Brain Injury, 12*(1), 87–92.

Kaplan, H.S. (1983). *The evaluation of sexual disorders.* New York: Brunner/Mazel.

Kaplan, C.A., & Corrigan, J.D. (1992). Effect of blood alcohol level on recovery from severe closed head injury. *Brain Injury, 6*, 337–349.

Karno, M., Golding, J.M., Sorenson, S.B., & Burnam, M.A. (1988). The epidemiology of obsessive-compulsive disorder in five US communities. *Archives of General Psychiatry, 45*(12), 1094–1099.

Karzmark, P. (1992). Prediction of long-term cognitive outcome of brain injury with neuropsychological, severity of injury, and demographic data. *Brain Injury, 6*(3), 213–217.

Karzmark, P., Hall, K., & Englander, J. (1995). Late-onset post-concussion symptoms after mild brain injury: The role of premorbid, injury-related, environmental, and personality factors. *Brain Injury, 9*, 21–26.

Katz, D.I., & Alexander, M.P. (1994). Predicting outcome and course of recovery in patients admitted to rehabilitation. *Archives of Neurology, 51*, 661–670.

Kaufmann, D.M. (1981). Neurological aspects of sexual dysfunction. *Clinical neurology for psychiatrists*. San Francisco, CA: Grune & Stratton.

Kawasaki, H., Adolphs, R., Kaufman, O., Damasio, H., Damasio, A.R., Granner, M., Bakken, H., Hori, T., & Howard, M.A. (2001). Single-unit responses to emotional visual stimuli recorded in human ventral prefrontal cortex. *Nature Neuroscience, 4*, 15–16.

Kay, T. (1993). Neuropsychological treatment of mild traumatic brain injury. *Journal of Head Trauma Rehabilitation, 8*, 74–85.

Kay, T. (1999). Interpreting apparent neuropsychological deficits: what is really wrong? In J. Sweet (Ed.), *Forensic neuropsychology: Fundamentals and practice. studies on neuropsychology, development and cognition* (pp. 145–183). Lisse, Netherlands: Swets & Zeitlinger.

Kay, T., Newman, B., Cavallo, M., Ezrachi, O., & Resnick, M. (1992). Toward a neuropsychological model of functional disability after mild traumatic brain injury. *Neuropsychology, 6*, 371–384.

Kay, T., Harrington, D.E., Adams, R., Anderson, T., Berrol, S., Cicerone, K., Dahlberg, C., Gerber, D., Goka, R., Harley, P., Hilt, J., Horn, L., Lehmkuhl, D., & Malec, J. (1993). Definition of mild traumatic brain injury. *Journal of Head Trauma Rehabilitation, 8(3)*, 86–87.

Keane, J., Calder, A.J., Hodges, J.R., & Young, A.W. (2002). Face and emotion processing in frontal variant frontotemporal dementia. *Neuropsychologia, 40*(6), 655–665.

Keck, P.E., McElroy, S.L., & Arnold, L.M. (2001). Bipolar disorder. *Medical Clinics of North America, 85*, 647–661.

Keidel, M., & Diener, H.C. (1997). Post-traumatic headache. *Nervenarzt, 68*(10), 769–77.

Kellehear, A. (1993). Culture, biology, and the near-death experience. A reappraisal. *Journal of Nervous and Mental Disease, 181*(3), 148–156.

Kelly, E.W. (2001). Near-death experiences with reports of meeting deceased people. *Death Studies, 25*(3), 229–249.

Kelly, M.P., Johnson, C.T., Knoller, N., Drubach, D.A., & Winslow, M.M. (1997). Substance abuse, traumatic brain injury and neuropsychological outcome. *Brain Injury, 11*(6), 391–402.

Kelly, R. (1975). The post-traumatic syndrome: An iatrogenic disease. *Forensic Science, 6*, 17–24.

Kelly, A.E., & Kahn, J.H. (1994). Effects of suppression of personal intrusive thoughts. *Journal of Personality and Social Psychology, 66*, 998–1006.

Kemp, S., Biswas, R., Neumann, V., & Coughlan, A. (2004). The value of melatonin for sleep disorders occurring post-head injury: A pilot RCT. *Brain Injury, 18*(9), 911–919.

Kendall, E., & Terry, D.J. (1996). Psychosocial adjustment following closed head injury: A model for understanding individual differences and predicting outcome. *Neuropsychological Rehabilitation, 6*(2), 101–132.

Kent, H. (1999). Letter to the editor (comment on Awareness Intervention: Who needs it? By Sohlberg, M.M., Mateer, C., Penkman, L., Glang, A., & Todis B. (1998). *Journal of Head Trauma Rehabilitation, 13*, 62–78). *Journal of Head Trauma Rehabilitation, 14(4),* vii–ix.

Keppel, C.C., & Crowe, S.F. (2000). Changes to body image and self-esteem following stroke in young adults. *Neuropsychological Rehabilitation, 10,* 15–31.

Kersel, D.A., Marsh, N.V., Havill, J.H., & Sleigh, J.W. (2001a). Neuropsychological functioning during the year following severe traumatic brain injury. *Brain Injury, 15*(4), 283–296.

Kersel, D.A., Marsh, N.V., Havill, J.H., & Sleigh, J.W. (2001b). Psychosocial functioning during the year following severe traumatic brain injury. *Brain Injury, 15*(8), 683–696.

Keshavan, M.S., Channabasavanna, S.M., & Reddy, G.N. (1981). Post-traumatic psychiatric disturbances: patterns and predictors of outcome. *British Journal of Psychiatry, 138,* 157–160.

Kesler, S.R., Adams, H.F., Blasey, C.M., & Bigler, E.D. (2003). Premorbid intellectual functioning, education, and brain size in traumatic brain injury: An investigation of the cognitive reserve hypothesis. *Applied Neuropsychology, 10*(3), 153–162.

Kessler, R.C., Berglund, P., Demler, O., Jin, R., & Walters, E.E. (2005). Lifetime prevalence and age of onset distributions of DSM–IV disorders in the National Comorbidity Survey Replication. *Archives of General Psychiatry, 62*, 593–602.

Kettl, P.A., & Marks, I.M. (1986). Neurological factors in obsessive compulsive disorder. Two case reports and a review of the literature. *British Journal of Psychiatry, 149,* 315–319.

Khan-Bourne, N., & Brown, R.G. (2003). Cognitive behaviour therapy for the treatment of depression in individuals with brain injury. *Neuropsychological Rehabilitation, 13 (1/2),* 89–107.

Khanna, S., Narayan, H.S., Sharma, S.D., & Mukundan, C.R. (1985). Posttraumatic obsessive compulsive disorder: A single case report. *Indian Journal of Psychiatry, 27*, 337–340.

Khouzam, H.R., & Donnelly, N.J. (1998). Remission of traumatic brain injury-induced compulsions during Venlafaxine treatment. *General Hospital Psychiatry, 20,* 62–63.

Killgore, W.D., & DellaPietra, L. (2000). Using the WMS-III to detect malingering: empirical validation of the rarely missed index (RMI). *Journal of Clinical and Experimental Neuropsychology, 22*(6), 761–771.

Kim, E. (2002). Agitation, aggression, and disinhibition syndromes after traumatic brain injury. *NeuroRehabilitation, 17*, 297–310.

Kim, S.H., Manes, F., Kosier, T., Baruah, S., & Robinson, R.G. (1999). Irritability following traumatic brain injury. *Journal of Nervous and Mental Disease, 187*(6), 327–335.

Kimberg, D.Y., & Farah, M.J. (1993). A unified account of cognitive impairments following frontal lobe damage: the role of working memory in complex, organized behavior. *Journal of Experimental Psychology, General, 122*(4), 411–428.

Kimble, M., Lyons, M., O'Donnell, B., Nestor, P., Niznikiewicz, M., & Toomey, R. (2000). The effect of family status and schizotypy on electrophysiological measures of attention and semantic processing. *Biological Psychiatry, 47*, 402–412.

King, N. (1997). Mild Head injury: Neuropathology, sequelae, measurement and recovery. *British Journal of Clinical Psychology, 36*, 161–184.

King, N. (2003). Post-concussive syndrome: Clarity amid the controversy? *British Journal of Psychiatry, 183*, 276–278 .

King, L.R., Knowles, H.C., McLaurin, R.L., Brielmaier, J., Perisutti, G., & Piziak, V.K. (1981). Pituitary hormone response to head injury. *Neurosurgery, 9*, 229–235.

Kinsella, G., Moran, C., Ford, B., & Ponsford, J. (1988). Emotional disorder and its assessment within the severe head injured population. *Psychological Medicine, 18*(1), 57–63.

Kleeman, F.J. (1970). The physiology of the internal urinary sphincter. *Journal of Urology, 104,* 549–554.

Kleppel, J.B., Lincoln, A.E., & Winston, F.K. (2002). Assessing head-injury survivors of motor vehicle crashes at discharge from trauma care. *American Journal of Physical Medicine and Rehabilitation, 81*(2), 114–122; quiz 123–115, 142.

Klonoff, H. (1971). Head injuries in children: predisposing factors accident conditions, accident proneness and sequelae. *American Journal of Public Health, 61*(12), 2405–2417.

Kluckhohn, C., & Murray, H.A. (1953). Personality formation: The determinants. In C. Kluckhohn, H.A. Murray, & D.M. Schneider (Eds.). *Personality in nature, society and culture* (2nd ed). New York: Knopf.

Kluver, H. (1958). The temporal lobe syndrome. In M. Baldwin, & P. Bailey (Eds.), *Temporal lobe epilepsy.* Springfield, IL: Thomas.

Kluver, H., & Bucy, P. (1937). "Psychic blindness" and other symptoms following bilateral temporal lobectomy in rhesus monkeys. *American Journal of Physiology, 119,* 352–353.

Kluver, H., & Bucy, P. (1938). An analysis of certain effects of bilateral temporal lobectomy in the rhesus monkey, with special reference to "psychic blindness". *The Journal of Physiology, 5,* 33–54.

Kluver, H., & Bucy, P.C. (1939). Preliminary analysis of functions of the temporal lobes in monkeys. *Archives of Neurology and Psychiatry, 42,* 979.

Kolakowsky-Hayner, S.A., Gourley, E.V., Kreutzer, J.S., Marwitz, J.H., Meade, M.A., & Cifu, D.X. (2002). Post-injury substance abuse among persons with brain injury and persons with spinal cord injury. *Brain Injury, 16*(7), 583–592.

Kolb, B., & Whishaw, I.Q. (1990). *Fundamentals of human neuropsychology.* New York: W.H. Freeman and Co.

Koponen, S., Taimen, T., Portin, R., Himanen, L., Isoniemi, H., Heinonen, H., Hinkka, S., & Tenuovo, O. (2002). Axis I and II psychiatric disorders after traumatic brain injury: A 30-year follow-up study. *American Journal of Psychiatry, 159,* 1315–1321.

Kornack, D.R., & Rakic, P. (1999). Continuation of neurogenesis in the hippocampus of the adult macaque monkey. *Proceedings of the National Academy of Science, USA, 96,* 5768–5773.

Kosteljanetz, M., Jensen, T.S., Norgard, B., Lunde, I., Jensen, P.B., & Johnsen, S.G. (1981). Sexual and hypothalamic dysfunction in the post-concussional syndrome. *Acta Neurologica Scandanavica, 63,* 169–180.

Koufen, H., & Hagel, K.H. (1987). Systematic EEG follow-up study of traumatic psychosis. *European Archives of Psychiatry and Neurological Sciences, 237*(1), 2–7.

Kraepelin, E. (1896). *Psychiatrie* (5th ed.). Barth: Leipzig.

Kraepelin, E. (1910). *Psychiatrie, Vol. 2: Klinische Psychiatrie.* Barth: Leipzig.

Kraus, J.F., & Chu, L.D. (2005). Epidemiology. In J.M. Silver, T.W. McAllister, & S.C. Yudofsky (Eds.), *Textbook of traumatic brain injury* (pp. 3–26). Washington, DC: American Psychiatric Publishing.

Kraus, J.F., & MacArthur, D.L. (1996). Epidemiologic aspects of brain injury. *Neurologic Clinics, 14,* 435–450.

Kraus, J.F., & Sorenson, S.B. (1994). Epidemiology. In J.M. Silver, S.C. Yudofsky, & R.E. Hales (Eds.), *Neuropsychiatry of traumatic brain injury.* Washington, DC: American Psychiatric Press.

Kraus, M.F., & Maki, P. (1997a). The combined use of amantadine and l–dopa/carbidopa in the treatment of chronic brain injury. *Brain Injury, 11*(6), 455–460.

Kraus, M.F., & Maki, P.M. (1997b). Effect of amantadine hydrochloride on symptoms of frontal lobe dysfunction in brain injury: Case studies and review. *Journal of Neuropsychiatry and Clinical Neuroscience, 9*(2), 222–230.

Krauthammer, C., & Klerman, G.L. (1978). Secondary mania: manic syndromes associated with antecedent physical illness or drugs. *Archives of General Psychiatry, 35*, 1333–1339.

Kreuter, M., Dallhof, A.G., Gudjonsson, G., Sullivan, M., & Siosteen, A. (1998). Sexual adjustment and its predictors after traumatic brain injury. *Brain Injury, 12*(5), 349–368.

Kreutzer, J.S., Marwitz, J.H., & Witol, A.D. (1995). Interrelationships between crime, substance abuse, and aggressive behaviours among persons with traumatic brain injury. *Brain Injury, 9*(8), 757–768.

Kreutzer, J.S., Seel, R.T., & Gourley, E. (2001). The prevalence and symptom rates of depression after traumatic brain injury: A comprehensive examination. *Brain Injury, 15*(7), 563–576.

Kreutzer, J.S., & Zasler, N.D. (1989). Psychosexual consequences of traumatic brain injury: Methodology and preliminary findings. *Brain Injury, 3*, 177–186.

Kreutzer, J.S., Wehman, P.H., Harris, J.A., Burns, C.T., & Young, H.F. (1991). Substance abuse and crime patterns among persons with traumatic brain injury referred for supported employment. *Brain Injury, 5*(2), 177–187.

Kreutzer, J.S., Witol, A.D., & Marwitz, J.H. (1996). Alcohol and drug use among young persons with traumatic brain injury. *Journal of Learning Disabilities, 29*(6), 643–651.

Kuhn, H.G., Dickinson-Anson, H., & Gage, F.H. (1996). Continuation of neurogenesis in the dentate gyrus of the adult rat: Age–related decrease of neuronal progenitor proliferation. *Journal of Neuroscience, 16*, 2027–2033.

Labbate, L.A., Warden, D., & Murray, G.B. (1997). Salutary change after frontal brain trauma. *Annals of Clinical Psychiatry, 9*(1), 27–30.

LaFuente, J.V., & Cervos-Navarro, J. (1999). Craniocerebral trauma induces hemorheological disturbances. *Journal of Neurotrauma, 16*, 425–430.

Lahz, S., & Bryant, R. A. (1996). Incidence of chronic pain following traumatic brain injury. *Archives of Physical Medicine and Rehabilitation, 77*(9), 889–891.

Lankford, A., Wellman, J.J., & O'Hara, C. (1994). Posttraumatic narcolepsy in mild to moderate closed head injury. *Sleep, 17*, S25–S28.

Lam, C.S., McMahon, B.T., Priddy, D.A., & Gehred-Schultz, A. (1988). Deficit awareness and treatment performance among traumatic head injury adults. *Brain Injury, 2*(3), 235–242.

Laplane, D., Boulliat, J., Baron, J.C., Pillon, B., & Baulac, M. (1988). Obsessive-compulsive behaviour caused by bilateral lesions of the lenticular nuclei. A new case. *L'Encéphale, 14*(1), 27–32.

Larrabee, G.J. (1992). On modifying recognition memory tests for detection of malingering. *Neuropsychology, 6*(1), 23–27.

Larrabee, G.J. (1998). Somatic malingering on the MMPI and MMPI-2 in personal injury litigants. *The Clinical Neuropsychologist, 12*(2), 179–188.

Larrabee, G.J. (2000). Association between IQ and neuropsychological test performance: commentary on Tremont, Hoffman, Scott, and Adams (1998). *Clinical Neuropsychology, 14*(1), 139–145.

Larrabee, G.J. (2001). *Assessment of malingering.* Paper presented at National Academy of Neuropsychology Conference (Nov. 3), San Francisco, CA.

Larrabee, G.J. (2005). *Forensic neuropsychology: A scientific approach.* New York; Oxford University Press.

Lavy, E.H., & van den Hout, M. (1990). Thought suppression induces intrusions. *Behavioural Psychotherapy, 18*, 251–258.

Layton, B.S., & Wardi-Zonna, K. (1995), Posttraumatic stress disorder with neurogenic amnesia for the traumatic event. *The Clinical Neuropsychologist, 9*, 2–10.

Lebrun, Y. (1987). Anosognosia in aphasics. *Cortex, 23*, 251–263.

Le Doux, J.E. (1996). *The emotional brain*. New York: Simon & Schuster.

Le Doux, J.E. (1998). *The emotional brain: The mysterious underpinnings of emotional life*. New York: Touchstone.

Lees-Haley, P.R. (1992). Efficacy of MMPI-2 validity scales and MCMI-II modifier scales for detecting spurious PTSD claims: F, F-K, Fake Bad Scale, ego strength, subtle-obvious subscales, DIS, and DEB. *Journal of Clinical Psychology, 48(5)*, 681–9.

Lees-Haley, P.R. (1997). MMPI-2 base rates for 492 personal injury plaintiffs: implications and challenges for forensic assessment. *Journal of Clinical Psychology, 53*(7), 745–755.

Lees-Haley, P.R., & Dunn, J.T. (1994). The ability of naive subjects to report symptoms of mild brain injury, post-traumatic stress disorder, major depression, and generalized anxiety disorder. *Journal of Clinical Psychology, 50*(2), 252–256.

Lees-Haley, P.R., English, L.T., & Glenn, W.J. (1991). A Fake Bad Scale on the MMPI-2 for personal injury claimants. *Psychological Reports, 68*(1), 203–210.

Lees-Haley, P.R., Williams, C.W., Zasler, N.D., Marguilies, S., English, L.T., & Stevens, K.B. (1997). Response bias in plaintiff's histories. *Brain Injury, 11*, 791–799.

Leger, D. (1994). The cost of sleep-related accidents: A report for the National Commission on Sleep Disorders Research. *Sleep, 17*, 84–93.

Lehne, G. (1986). Brain damage and paraphilia: treated with medroxy-progesterone acetate. *Sexuality Disability, 7*, 145–158.

Lenninger, B.E., Gramling, S.E., Farrell, A.D., Kreutzer, J.S. & Peck, E.A. (1990). Neuropsychological deficits in symptomatic minor head injury patients after concussion and mild concussion. *Journal of Neurology, Neurosurgery and Psychiatry, 53*, 293–296.

Levin, H.S. (1995). Prediction of recovery from traumatic brain injury. *Journal of Neurotrauma, 12*(5), 913–922.

Levin, H.S., Benavidez, D.A., Verger-Maestre, K., Perachio, N., Song, J., Mendelsohn, D.B., & Fletcher, J.M. (2000). Reduction of corpus callosum growth after severe traumatic brain injury in children. *Neurology, 54*, 647–653.

Levin, H.S., Benton, A.L., & Grossman, R.G. (1982). *Neurobehavioural consequences of closed head injury*. New York: Oxford University Press.

Levin, H.S., Brown, S.A., Song, J.X., McCauley, S.R., Boake, C., Contant, C.F., Goodman, H., & Kotrla, K.J. (2001). Depression and posttraumatic stress disorder at three months after mild to moderate traumatic brain injury. *Journal of Clinical and Experimental Neuropsychology, 23*, 754–769.

Levin, H.S., Gary, H.E., High, W.M., Mattis, S.M., Ruff, R.M., Eisenberg, H.M., Marshall, L.F., & Tabaddor, K. (1987). Minor head injury and the postconcussional syndrome: Methodological issues in outcome studies. *Neurobehavioral recovery from head injury* (pp. 262–275). New York: Oxford University Press.

Levin, H.S., & Grossman, R.G. (1978). Behavioral sequelae of closed head injury. A quantitative study. *Archives of Neurology, 35*(11), 720–727.

Levin, H.S., High, W.M., & Eisenberg, H.M. (1985). Impairment of olfactory recognition after closed head injury. *Brain, 108 (Pt 3)*, 579–591.

Levin, H.S., High, W.M., & Eisenberg, H.M. (1988). Learning and forgetting during posttraumatic amnesia in head injured patients. *Journal of Neurology, Neurosurgery and Psychiatry, 51*, 14–20.

Levin, H.S., High, W.M., Goethe, K.E., Sisson, R.A., Overall, J.E., Rhoades, H.M., Eisenberg, H.M., Kalisky, Z., & Gary, H.E. (1987). The neurobehavioural rating scale: Assessment of the behavioural sequelae of head injury by the clinician. *Journal of Neurology Neurosurgery and Psychiatry, 50*(2), 183–193.

Levin, H.S., & Kraus, M.F. (1994). The frontal lobes and traumatic brain injury. *Journal of Neuropsychiatry and Clinical Neuroscience, 6*(4), 443–454.

Levin, H.S., Mattis, S., Ruff, R.M., Eisenberg, H.M., Marshall, L.F., Tabaddor, K., High, W.M. Jr., & Frankowski, R.F. (1987). Neurobehavioral outcome following minor head injury: A three-center study. *Journal of Neurosurgery, 66(2),* 234–43.

Levin, H.S., O'Donnell, V.M., & Grossman, R.G. (1979). The Galveston Orientation and amnesia test. *Journal of Nervous and Mental Disease, 167*, 675–684.

Levin, H.S., Williams, D.H., Eisenberg, H.M., High, W.M., Jr., & Guinto, F.C. Jr. (1992). Serial MRI and neurobehavioural findings after mild to moderate closed head injury. *Journal of Neurology, Neurosurgery and Psychiatry, 55(4*), 255–262.

Levin, J., & Summers, D. (1992). Anorexia due to brain injury. *Brain Injury, 6*, 99–201.

Levine, D.N., & Finkelstein, S. (1982). Delayed Psychosis after right temporoparietal stroke or trauma: relation to epilepsy. *Neurology, 32*, 267–273.

Levy, M.L., Cummings, J.L., Fairbanks, L.A., Masterman, D., Miller, B.L., Craig, A.H., Paulsen, J.S., & Litvan, I. (1998). Apathy is not depression. *Journal of Neuropsychiatry and Clinical Neuroscience, 10*(3), 314–319.

Lewine, J.D., Davis, J.T., Sloan, J.H., Kodituwakku, P.W., & Orrison, W.W., Jr. (1999). Neuromagnetic assessment of pathophysiologic brain activity induced by minor head trauma. *American Journal of Neuroradiology, 20*, 857–66.

Lewis, A. (1942). Discussion on differential diagnosis and treatment of post-concussional states. *Proceedings of the Royal Society of Medicine, 35*, 607–614.

Lewis, L., & Rosenberg, S.J. (1990). Psychoanalytic psychotherapy with brain-injured adult psychiatric patients. *Journal of Nervous and Mental Disease, 178*(2), 69–77.

Lezak, M.D. (1978). Living with the characterologically altered brain injured patient. *Journal of Clinical Psychiatry, 39*(7), 592–598.

Lezak, M.D. (1995). *Neuropsychological assessment* (3rd ed.). New York: Oxford University Press.

Lezak, M.D., Howieson, D.B., & Loring, D.W. (Eds.). (2004). *Neuropsychological assessment* (4th ed.). New York: Oxford University Press.

Liberman, R.P., Musser, K.T., & Wallace, C.T. (1986). Social skill training for schizophrenic individuals at risk for relapse. *American Journal of Psychiatry, 147*, 523–526.

Liberzon, I., Krstov, M., & Young, E.A. (1997). Stress-restress: effects on ACTH and fast feedback. *Psychoneuroendocrinology, 22*(6), 443–453.

Liberzon, I., Taylor, S.F., Fig, L.M., & Koeppe, R.A. (1996). Alteration of corticothalamic perfusion ratios during a PTSD flashback. *Depress Anxiety, 4*(3), 146–150.

Lichter, D.G., & Cummings, J.L. (2001). *Frontal-subcortical circuits in psychiatric and neurological disorders.* New York: Guilford Press.

Liddle, P.F. (1987). The symptoms of chronic schizophrenia: A re-examination of the positive-negative dichotomy. *British Journal of Psychiatry, 151,* 145–151.

Liddle, P.F., Ngan, E.T.C., Caissie, S.L., Anderson, C.M., & Bates, A.T. (2002). Thought and language index: An instrument for assessing thought and language in schizophrenia. *British Journal of Psychiatry, 181*, 326–330.

Lilly, R., Cummings, J.L., Benson, D.F., & Frankel, M. (1983). The human Kluver–Bucy syndrome. *Neurology, 33,* 1141–1145.

Lishman, W.A. (1966). Psychiatric disability after head injury: the significance of brain damage. *Proceedings of the Royal Society of Medicine, 59*(3), 261–266.

Lishman, W.A. (1968). Brain damage in relation to psychiatric disability after head injury. *British Journal of Psychiatry, 114*(509), 373–410.

Lishman, W.A. (1973). The psychiatric sequelae of head injury: A review. *Psychological Medicine, 3,* 304–318.

Lishman, W.A. (1978). Psychiatric sequelae of head injuries: problems in diagnosis. *Irish Medical Journal, 71*(9), 306–314.

Lishman, W.A. (1987). *Organic psychiatry: The psychological consequences of cerebral disorder* (2nd ed.). Oxford: Blackwell Scientific.

Lishman, W.A. (1988). Physiogenesis and psychogenesis in the 'post-concussional syndrome'. *British Journal of Psychiatry, 153*, 460–9.

Lishman, W.A. (1997). *Organic psychiatry: The psychological consequences of cerebral disorder* (3rd ed.). Oxford: Blackwell Scientific.

Livingston, D.H., Loder, P.A., Koziol, J., & Hunt, C.D. (1991). The use of CT scanning to triage patients requiring admission following minimal head injury. *Journal of Trauma, 31(4),* 483–489.

Livingston, M.G., Brooks, D.N., & Bond, M.R. (1985a). Patient outcome in the year following severe head injury and relatives' psychiatric and social functioning. *Journal of Neurology Neurosurgery and Psychiatry, 48*(9), 876–881.

Livingston, M.G., Brooks, D.N., & Bond, M.R. (1985b). Three months after severe head injury: psychiatric and social impact on relatives. *Journal of Neurology Neurosurgery and Psychiatry, 48*(9), 870–875.

Loyd, D.W., & Tsuang, M.T. (1981). A snake lady: post-concussion syndrome manifesting visual hallucinations of snakes. *Journal of Clinical Psychiatry, 42*(6), 246–247.

Lundberg, P.O. (1992). Sexual dysfunction in patients with neurological disorders. *Annual Review of Sex Research, 3,* 121–150.

Lupien, S.J., & McEwen, B.S. (1997). The acute effects of corticosteroids on cognition: Integration of animal and human model studies. *Brain Research: Brain Research Reviews, 24*(1), 1–27.

Luria, A.R. (1969). Frontal lobe syndromes. In P.J. Vinken & G.W. Bruyn (Eds.), *Handbook of clinical neurology* (Vol. 2, pp. 725–757). Amsterdam: North-Holland.

Luria, A.R. (1973). *The working brain.* London: Penguin.

McAllister, T.W. (1992). Neuropsychiatric sequelae of head injuries. *Psychiatric Clinics of North America, 15*, 395–413.

McAllister, T.W. (1994). Mild traumatic brain injury and the post-concussive syndrome." In J. Silver, S. Yudofsky, & R. Hales (Eds.), *The neuropsychiatry of traumatic brain injury* (pp. 357–392), Washington D.C.: American Psychiatric Press.

McAllister, T.W. (1998). Traumatic brain injury and psychosis: What is the connection? *Seminars in Clinical Neuropsychiatry, 3*(3), 211–223.

McAllister, T.W., & Arciniegas, D. (2002). Evaluation and treatment of postconcussive symptoms. *NeuroRehabilitation, 17,* 265–283.

McAllister, T.W., & Ferrell, R.B. (2002). Evaluation and treatment of psychosis after traumatic brain injury. *NeuroRehabilitation, 17*(4), 357–368.

McAllister-Williams, R.H., Ferrier, I.N., & Young, A.H. (1998). Mood and neuropsychological function in depression: the role of corticosteroids and serotonin. *Psychological Medicine, 28*(3), 573–584.

McCarthy, K. (2001). Traumatic brain injury: The challenge of community management. *Medicine Today, March*, 57–64.

McCauley, S.R., Boake, C., Levin, H.S., Constant, C.F., & Song, J.X. (2001). Postconcussional disorder following mild to moderate traumatic brain injury: Anxiety, depression, and social support as risk factors and comorbidities. *Journal of Clinical and Experimental Neuropsychology, 23*(6), 792–808.

McCleary, C., Satz, P., Forney, D., Light, R., Zaucha, K., Asarnow, R., & Namerow, N. (1998). Depression after traumatic brain injury as a function of Glasgow Outcome Score. *Journal of Clinical and Experimental Neuropsychology, 20*(2), 270–279.

McClelland, R.J. (1996). The postconcussional syndrome: A rose by any other name. *Journal of Psychosomatic Research, 40(6)*, 563–8.

McClelland, R.J., Fenton, G.W., & Rutherford, W. (1994). The post-concussional syndrome revisited. *Journal of the Royal Society of Medicine, 87*, 508–510.

McCrory, P. (2002). Treatment of recurrent concussion. *Current Sports Medicine Reports, 1*, 28–32.

McDonald, S., Flanagan, S., Rollins, J., & Kinch, J. (2003). TASIT: A new clinical tool for assessing social perception after traumatic brain injury. *Journal of Head Trauma Rehabilitation, 18*(3), 219–238.

McDonald, S., Togher, L., & Code, C. (1999). Communication disorders following traumatic brain injury. Hove, East Sussex, UK: Psychology Press.

McFarlane, A.C. (1988). Posttraumatic stress disorder and blindness. *Comprehensive Psychiatry, 29*(6), 558–560.

McGuffin, P., & Katz, R. (1989a). The genetics of depression and manic-depressive disorder. *British Journal of Psychiatry, 155*, 294–304.

McGuffin, P., & Katz, R. (1989b). The genetics of depression: current approaches. *British Journal of Psychiatry,* (Suppl. 6), 18–26.

McIntosh, T.K., Smith, D.H., Meaney, D.F., Kotapka, M.J., Gennarelli, T.A., & Graham, D.I. (1996). Neuropathological sequelae of traumatic brain injury: relationship to neurochemical and biomechanical mechanisms. *Laboratory Investigation, 74*(2), 315–42.

MacKay, L.E., Morgan, A.S., & Bernstein, B.A. (1999). Swallowing disorders in severe brain injury: risk factors affecting return to oral intake. *Archives of Physical Medicine and Rehabilitation, 80*(4), 365–71.

McKenzie, E.J., Edelstein, S.L., & Flynn, J.P. (1989). Hospitalized head-injured patients in Maryland: Incidence and severity of injuries. *Maryland Medical Journal, 38*, 725–732.

McKenzie, T.B., Robiner, W.N., & Knopman, D.S. (1989). Differences between patient and family assessments of depression in Alzheimer's disease. *American Journal of Psychiatry, 146*, 1174–1178.

McKeon, J., McGuffin, P., & Robinson, P. (1984). Obsessive-compulsive neurosis following head injury: A report of four cases. *British Journal of Psychiatry, 144*, 190–192.

McKinlay, W.W., & Brooks, D.N. (1984). Methodological problems in assessing psychosocial recovery following severe head injury. *Journal of Clinical Neuropsychology, 6*(1), 87–99.

McKinlay, W.W., Brooks, D.N., Bond, M.R., Martinage, D.P., & Marshall, M.M. (1981). The short-term outcome of severe blunt head injury as reported by relatives of the injured persons. *Journal of Neurology Neurosurgery and Psychiatry, 44*(6), 527–533.

McLaren, S., & Crowe, S.F. (2003). The contribution of perceived control of stressful life events and thought suppression to the symptoms of obsessive-compulsive disorder in both non-clinical and clinical samples. *Journal of Anxiety Disorders, 17*(4), 389–403.

MacLean, P.D. (1975). Brain mechanisms of primal sexual functions and related behavior. In M. Sandler & G.L. Gessa (Eds.), *Sexual behavior: pharmacology and biochemistry* (pp.1–11). New York: Raven Press.

McLean, A., Dikmen, S.S., Temkin, N.R., Wyler, A.R., & Gale, J.L. (1984). Psychosocial functioning at one month after head injury. *Neurosurgery, 14*, 393–399.

McLean, A., Jr., Dikmen, S.S., & Temkin, N.R. (1993). Psychosocial recovery after head injury. *Archives of Physical Medicine and Rehabilitation, 74*(10), 1041–1046.

MacLean, P.D., Denniston, R.H., Dua, S., & Ploog, D.W. (1962). Hippocampal changes with brain stimulation eliciting penile erection. *Colloques Internationaux du Centre National de la Recherche Scientifique, 107,* 491–510.

MacLean, P.D., Dua, S., & Denniston, R.H. (1963). Cerebral localization for scratching and seminal discharge. *Archives of Neurology, 9,* 485–497.

MacLean, P.D., & Ploog, D.W. (1962). Cerebral representation of penile erection. *Journal of Neurophysiology, 25,* 29–55.

MacMillan, P.J., Martelli, M.F., Hart, R.P., & Zasler, N.D. (2002). Pre-injury status and adaptation following traumatic brain injury. *Brain Injury, 16*(1), 41–49.

McMillan, T.M. (1991). Post-traumatic stress disorder and severe head injury. *British Journal of Psychiatry, 159*, 431–433.

McMillan, T.M. (1996). Post-traumatic stress disorder following minor and severe closed head injury: 10 single cases. *Brain Injury, 10*(10), 749–758.

McMillan, T.M. (1997). Minor head injury. *Current Opinion in Neurology, 10*, 479–483.

McMillan, T.M. (2001). Errors in diagnosing post-traumatic stress disorder after traumatic brain injury. *Brain Injury, 15*(1), 39–46.

McMillan, T.M., & Jacobson, R.R. (1999). Traumatic brain injury and post-traumatic stress disorder. *British Journal of Psychiatry, 174*, 274–275.

McMillan, T.M., Jongen, E.L., & Greenwood, R.J. (1996). Assessment of post-traumatic amnesia after severe closed head injury: retrospective or prospective? *Journal of Neurology, Neurosurgery and Psychiatry, 60*, 422–427.

McMillan, T.M., Williams, W.H., & Bryant, R. (2003). Post-traumatic stress disorder and traumatic brain injury: A review of causal mechanisms, assessment, and treatment. *Neuropsychological Rehabilitation, 13*, 149–164.

McNeil, J.E., & Greenwood, R. (1996). Can PTSD occur with amnesia for the precipitating event? *Cognitive Neuropsychiatry, 1,* 239–46.

Malec, J., & Moessner, A. (2000). Self-awareness, distress, and postacute rehabilitation outcome. *Rehabilitation Psychology,* 45(3), 227–241.

Malloy, P., Bihrle, A., Duffy, J., & Cimino, C. (1993). The orbitomedial frontal syndrome. *Archives of Clinical Neuropsychology, 8*(3), 185–201.

Mandel S. (1989). Minor head injury may not be 'minor'. *Postgraduate Medicine, 85(6)*, 213–217, 220, 225.

Mandleberg, I.A. (1976). Cognitive recovery after severe head injury: 3. WAIS Verbal and Performance IQ's as a function of post-traumatic amnesia duration and time from injury. *Journal of Neurology, Neurosurgery and Psychiatry, 39*, 1001–1007.

Mann, N.R., Fichtenberg, N.L., Putnam, S., & DeSantis, N.M. (1997). Sleep disorders among TBI survivors: A comparative study. *Archives of Physical Medicine and Rehabilitation, 78*, 1055.

Mapou, R.L. (1990). Traumatic brain injury rehabilitation with gay and lesbian individuals. *Journal of Head Trauma Rehabilitation, 5,* 67–72.

Margulies, S. (2000). The post concussion syndrome after mild head trauma: Is brain damage over diagnosed? Part 1. *Journal of Clinical Neuroscience, 7(5)*, 400–408.

Marin, R.S. (1991). Apathy: A neuropsychiatric syndrome. *Journal of Neuropsychiatry and Clinical Neuroscience, 3*(3), 243–254.

Marin, R.S. (1997). Differential diagnosis of apathy and related disorders of diminished motivation. *Psychiatric Annals, 27,* 30–33.

Marin, R.S., Biedrzycki, R.C., & Firinciogullari, S. (1991). Reliability and validity of the Apathy Evaluation Scale. *Psychiatry Research, 38*(2), 143–162.

Marin, R.S., & Chakravorty, S. (2005). Disorders of diminished motivation. In J.M. Silver, T.W. McAllister, & S.C. Yudofsky (Eds.), *Textbook of traumatic brain injury* (pp. 337–352). Washington, DC: American Psychiatric Publishing.

Marin, R.S., Fogel, B.S., Hawkins, J., Duffy, J., & Krupp, B. (1995). Apathy: A treatable syndrome. *Journal of Neuropsychiatry and Clinical Neuroscience, 7*(1), 23–30.

Marshall, J.C., Halligan, P.W., & Wade, D.T. (1995). Reduplication of an event after head injury? A cautionary case report. *Cortex, 31*(1), 183–190.

Marshall, L.F., Gautille, T., Klauber, M.R., Eisenberg, H.M., Jane, J.A., Luerssen, T.G., Marmarou, A., & Foulkes, M.A. (1991). The outcome of severe head injury. *Journal of Neurosurgery, 75*, 528–536.

Martelli, M.E., Grayson, R.L., & Zasler, N.D. (1999). Posttraumatic headache: neuropsychological and psychological effects and treatment implications. *Journal of Head Trauma Rehabilitation, 14*, 49–69.

Martelli, M.E., & Zasler, N.D. (2001). Ethics and objectivity in medicolegal contexts: Recommendations for experts. In R.B. Weiner (Eds.), *Pain management: A practical guide for clinicians* (6th ed.). Boca Raton, FL: St. Lucie Press.

Martin, L.L., & Kleiber, D.A. (2005). Letting go of the negative: Psychological growth from a close brush with death. *Traumatology, 11*(4), 221–232.

Martzke, J.S., Swan, C.S., & Varney, N.R. (1991). Posttraumatic anosmia and orbital frontal damage: Neuropsychological and neuropsychiatric correlates. *Neuropsychology, 5*, 213–225.

Mason, O., Claridge, G., & Jackson, M. (1995). New scales for the assessment of schizotypy. *Personality and Individual Differences, 18(1)*, 7–13.

Masson, F., Maurette, P., & Salmi, L.R. (1996). Prevalence of impairments 5 years after a head injury, and their relationship with disabilities and outcome. *Brain Injury, 10*, 487–497.

Matser, E.J.T., Kessels, A.G., Lezak, M.D., Jordan, B.D., & Troost, J. (1999). Neuropsychological impairment in amateur soccer players. *Journal of the American Medical Association, 282(10)*, 971–973.

Matser, J.T., Kessels, A.G., Jordan, B.D., Lezak, M.D., & Troost, J. (1998). Chronic traumatic brain injury in professional soccer players. *Neurology, 51(3)*, 791–6.

Maudsley, C. & Ferguson, F. R. (1963). Neurological disease in boxers. *Lancet, 2*, 799–801.

Mauss-Clum, N. & Ryan, M. (1981). Brain injury and the family. *Journal of Neurological Nursing, 13*, 165–169.

Max, J.E., Smith, W.L., Jr., Lindgren, S.D., Robin, D.A., Mattheis, P., Stierwalt, J., & Morrisey, M. (1995). Case study: obsessive–compulsive disorder after severe traumatic brain injury in an adolescent. *Journal of the American Academy of Child and Adolescent Psychiatry, 34*(1), 45–49.

Max, W., McKenzie, E., & Rice, D. (1991). Head injuries: cost and consequences. *Journal of Head Trauma Rehabilitation, 6*, 76–91.

May, P.R.A., Fuster, J.M., Haber, J., & Hirschman, A. (1979). Woodpecker drilling behavior: An endorsement of the rotational theory of impact brain injury. *Archives of Neurology, 36*, 370–373.

Mayberg, H.S. (2006). Defining neurocircuits in depression: Strategies toward treatment selection based on neuroimaging phenotypes. *Psychiatric Annals, 36(4)*, 259–268.

Mayberg, H.S. (2001). Depression and frontal subcortical circuits. In D.G. Lichter, & J.L. Cummings (Eds.), *Frontal–subcortical circuits in psychiatric and neurological disorders* (pp. 177–206). New York, NY: Guilford Press.

Mayberg, H.S. (1997). Limbic–cortical dysregulation: A proposed model of depression. *Journal of Neuropsychiatry, 4*, 471–481.

Mayou, R., Bryant, B., & Duthie, R. (1993). Psychiatric consequences of road traffic accidents. *British Medical Journal, 307*(6905), 647–651.

Mazaux, J.M., Masson, F., & Levin, H.S. (1997). Long-term neuropsychological outcome and loss of social autonomy after traumatic brain injury. *Archives of Physical Medicine and Rehabilitation, 78*, 1316–1320.

Medlar, T.M. (1993). Sexual counseling and traumatic brain injury. *Sexuality and Disability, 11,* 57–71.

Medlar, T. and Medlar, J. (1990). Nursing management of sexuality issues. *Journal of Head Trauma Rehabilitation, 5,* 46–51.

Meehl, P.E. (1962). Schizotaxia, schizotypy, schizophrenia. *American Psychologist, 17,* 827–838.

Meehl, P.E. (1990). Toward an integrated theory of schizotaxia, schizotypy, and schizophrenia. *Journal of Personality Disorders, 4*, 1–199.

Mega, M.S., & Cohenour, R.C. (1997). Akinetic mutism: Disconnection of frontal-subcortical circuits. *Neuropsychiatry, Neuropsychology and Behavioral Neurology, 10*, 254–259.

Merskey, H. & Bogduk, N. (Eds.). *IASP Task Force on taxonomy.* Seattle, WA: IASP Press, pp. 209–214.

Merskey, H., & Woodforde, J.M. (1972). Psychiatric sequelae of minor head injury. *Brain, 95*(3), 521–8.

Mesulam, M.M. (1985). *Principles of behavioral neurology.* Philadelphia, PA: F. A. Davis.

Mesulam, M.M. (2000a). *Principles of behavioral and cognitive neurology.* New York: Oxford University Press.

Mesulam, M.M. (2000b). Brain, mind, and the evolution of connectivity. *Brain Cognition, 42*(1), 4–6.

Meyer, J.E. (1955). Die Sexuellen storungen der hirverlezten. *Archiv fur psychiatrie and Zeitschrift Neurolgic, 193,* 449–469.

Meyer, J.E. (1971). Sexual disturbances after cerebral injuries. *Journal of Neurovisceral Relations,* (Suppl. X), 519–523.

Mickeviüiene, D., Schrader, H., Nestvold, K., Surkiene, D., Kunickas, R., & Stovner, L.J., & Sand, T. (2002). A controlled historical cohort study on the post-concussion syndrome. *European Journal of Neurology, 9*, 581–587.

Mickeviüiene, D., Schrader, H., Obelieniene, D., Surkiene, D., Kunickas, R., Stovner, L.J., & Sand, T. (2004). A controlled prospective inception cohort study on the post-concussion syndrome outside the medicolegal context. *European Journal of Neurology, 11*, 411–419.

Middleboe, T., Anderson, H.S., & Birket-Smith, M. (1992). Minor head injury: Impact on general health after 1 year: A prospective follow-up study. *Acta Neurologica Scandinavica, 85*, 5–9.

Milders, M., Fuchs, S., & Crawford, J.R. (2003). Neuropsychological impairments and changes in emotional and social behaviour following severe traumatic brain injury. *Journal of Clinical and Experimental Neuropsychology, 25*(2), 157–172.

Miller, E. (1983). A note on the interpretation of data derived from neuropsychological tests. *Cortex, 19,* 131–132.

Miller, H. (1961). Accident neurosis. *British Medical Journal, 1*, 919–925.

Miller, L. (1994). Sex and the brain-injured patient: Regaining love, pleasure and intimacy. *Journal of Cognitive Rehabilitation, May/June*, 12–20.

Miller, L. (1996). Neuropsychology and pathophysiology of mild head injury and the post-concussion syndrome: Clinical and forensic considerations. *The Journal of Cognitive Rehabilitation, January/February, 1996,* 8–23.

Miller, L. (2001). Not just malingering: Syndrome diagnosis in traumatic brain injury litigation. *NeuroRehabilitation, 16,* 109–122.

Miller, B.L., Cummings, J.L., McIntyre, H., Ebers, G. & Grodes, M. (1986). Hypersexuality or altered sexual preference following brain injury. *Journal of Neurology, Neurosurgery and Psychiatry, 49,* 867–873.

Miller, B.L., Cummings, J.L., Villanueva-Meyer, J., Boone, K., Mehringer, C.M., Lesser, I.M., & Mena, I. (1991). Frontal lobe degeneration: clinical, neuropsychological, and SPECT characteristics. *Neurology, 41*(9), 1374–1382.

Miller, H., & Stern, G. (1965). The Long–Term Prognosis of Severe Head Injury. *Lancet, 191,* 225–229.

Millis, S.R. (1992). The Recogntiion Memory Test in the detection of malingered and exaggerated memory deficits. *The Clinical Neuropsychologist, 6,* 406–414.

Millis, S.R., & Kler, S. (1995). Limitations of the Rey Fifteen-Item Test in the detection of malingering. *The Clinical Neuropsychologist, 9,* 241–244.

Millis, S.R., Rosenthal, M., Novack, T.A., Sherer, M., Nick, T., Kreutzer, J.S., High, W.M., & Ricker, J.H. (2001). Long-term neuropsychological outcome after traumatic brain injury. *Journal of Head Trauma Rehabilitation, 16,* 343–355.

Millis, S.R., Ross, S.R., & Ricker, J.H. (1998). Detection of incomplete effort on the Wechsler Adult Intelligence Scale–Revised: A cross-validation. *Journal of Clinical and Experimental Neuropsychology, 20,* 167–173.

Millon, T., Green, C., & Meagher, R. (1979). The MBHI: A new inventory for the psychodiagnostician in medial settings. *Professional Psychology, 10,* 529–539.

Milner, B., & Petrides, M. (1984). Behavioural effects of frontal-lobe lesions in man. *Trends in Neurosciences, 7,* 403–407.

Mitchell, W., Falconer, M.A., & Hill, D. (1954). Epilepsy with fetishism relieved by temporal lobectomy. *Lancet, 2,* 626–630.

Mittenberg, W., Azrin, R., Millsaps, C., & Heilbronner, R. (1993). Identification of malingered head injury on the Wechsler Memory Scale–Revised. *Psychological Assessment, 5,* 34–40.

Mittenberg, W., Canyock, E.M., Condit, D., & Patton, C. (2001). Treatment of post-concussion syndrome following mild head injury. *Journal of Clinical and Experimental Neuropsychology, 23,* 829–836.

Mittenberg, W., DiGiulio, D.V., Perrin, S., & Bass, A.E. (1992). Symptoms following mild head injury: expectation as aetiology. *Journal of Neurology, Neurosurgery and Psychiatry, 55(3),* 200–4.

Mittenberg, W., Patton, C., Canyock, E.M., & Condit, D.C. (2002). Base rates of malingering and symptom exaggeration. *Journal of Clinical and Experimental Neuropsychology, 24*(8), 1094–1102.

Mittenberg, W., Rotholc, A., Russell, E., & Heilbronner, R. (1996). Identification of malingered head injury on the Halstead–Reitan battery. *Archives of Clinical Neuropsychology, 11*(4), 271–281.

Mittenberg, W., Theroux-Fichera, S., Zielinski, R., & Heilbronner, R.L. (1995). Identification of malingered head injury on the Wechsler Adult Intelligence Scale–Revised. *Professional Psychology: Research and Practice, 26,* 491–498.

Mittenberg, W., Tremont, G., Zielinski, R.E., Fichera, S., & Rayls, K.R. (1996). Cognitive–behavioral prevention of postconcussion syndrome. *Archives of Clinical Neuropsychology, 11(2),* 139–45.

Molitch, M.E. (1992). Pathologic hyperprolactinemia. *Endocrinology and Metabolism Clinics of North America, 21*, 877–901.

Money, J. (1990). Forensic sexology: Paraphillic serial rape (biastophilia) and lust murder (erotophonophilia). *American Journal of Psychotherapy, 94,* 26–36.

Mooney, G., & Speed, J. (1997). Differential diagnosis in mild brain injury: understanding the role of non–organic conditions. *Neurorehabilitation, 8*, 223–233.

Mooney, G., & Speed, J. (2001). The association between mild traumatic brain injury and psychiatric conditions. *Brain Injury, 15*(10), 865–877.

Moore, A.D., & Stambrook, M. (1995). Cognitive moderators of outcome following traumatic brain injury: A conceptual model and implications for rehabilitation. *Brain Injury, 9*(2), 109–130.

Moore, E.L., Terryberry-Spohr, L., & Hope, D.A. (2006). Mild traumatic brain injury and anxiety sequelae: A review of the literature. *Brain Injury, 20*(2), 117–132.

Morgan, A.B., & Lilenfield, S.O. (2000). A meta-analytic review of the relation between antisocial behaviour and neuropsychological measures of executive function. *Clinical Psychology Review, 20*, 113–136.

Morse, P.A. & Montgomery, C.E. (1992). Neuropsychological evaluation of traumatic brain injury. In R.F. White (Ed.), *Clinical syndromes in adult neuropsychology: the practitioner's handbook* (pp. 85–176). New York: Elsevier Science Publishers B.V.

Mortensen, P.B., Mors, O., Frydenberg, M., & Ewald, H. (2003). Head injury as a risk factor for bipolar affective disorder. *Journal of Affective Disorders, 76*, 79–83.

Mortimer, J.A., French, L.R., Hutton, J.T., & Schuman, L.M. (1985). Head injury as a risk factor for Alzheimer's disease. *Neurology, 35*(2), 264–267.

Morton, M.V., & Wehman, P. (1995). Psychosocial and emotional sequelae of individuals with traumatic brain injury: A literature review and recommendations. *Brain Injury, 9*, 81–92.

Moss, N.E., Crawford, S., & Wade, D.T. (1994). Post-concussion symptoms: is stress a mediating factor? *Clinical Rehabilitation, 8*(2), 149–156.

Murai, T., Toichi, M., Sengoku, A., Miyoshi, K., & Morimune, S. (1997). Reduplicative paramnesia in patients with focal brain damage. *Neuropsychiatry Neuropsychology and Behavioral Neurology, 10*(3), 190–196.

Murelius, O., & Haglund, Y. (1991). Does Swedish amateur boxing lead to chronic brain damage? 4. A retrospective neuropsychological study. *Acta Neurologica Scandinavica, 83*, 9–13.

Muris, P., Merckelbach, H., & Horselenberg, R. (1996). Individual differences in thought suppression. The White Bear Suppression Inventory: Factor structure, reliability, validity and correlates. *Behaviour Research and Therapy, 34*(5–6), 501–513.

Mysiw, W.J., Bogner, J.A., Arnett, J.A., Clinchot, D.M., & Corrigna, J.D. (1996). The Orientation Group Monitoring System for measuring duration of posttraumatic amnesia and assessing therapeutic interventions. *Journal of Head Trauma Rehabilitation, 11,* 1–8.

Mysiw, W.J., Corrigan, J.D., Carpenter, D., & Chock, S.K. (1990). Prospective assessment of posttraumatic amnesia: A Comparison of the GOAT and OGMS. *Journal of Head Trauma Rehabilitation, 5*, 65–72.

Nakase-Thompson, R., Sherer, M., Yablon, S., Nick, T., & Trzepacz, P. (2004). Acute confusion following traumatic brain injury. *Brain Injury, 18*(2), 131–142.

Narushima, K., Kosier, J.T., & Robinson, R.G. (2003). A reappraisal of post-stroke depression, intra- and inter-hemispheric lesion location using meta-analysis. *Journal of Neuropsychiatry and Clincial Neuroscience, 15,* 423–430.

Nasrallah, H.A., Fowler, R.C., & Judd, L.L. (1981). Schizophrenia-like illness following head injury. *Psychosomatics, 22*(4), 359–361.

National Head Injury Foundation. (1989) *National Head Injury Foundation Taskforce on Special Education: educator's manual: What educators need to know about students with traumatic brain injury.* Southborough, MA: National Head Injury Foundation.

National Institutes of Health (NIH) (1998). Rehabilitation of persons with traumatic brain injury. *National Institutes of Health Consensus Statement, 16*(1).

National Institutes of Health (NIH) Consensus Development Panel. (1999). Consensus conference. Rehabilitation of persons with traumatic brain injury. *Journal of American Medical Association, 282(10),* 974–83.

Ndetei, D.M., & Vadher, A. (1984). A cross-cultural study of the frequencies of Schneider's first rank symptoms of schizophrenia. *Acta Psychiatrica Scandinavica, 70,* 540–544.

Nelson, E., & Rice, J. (1997). Stability of diagnosis of obsessive-compulsive disorder in the Epidemiologic Catchment Area study. *American Journal of Psychiatry, 154*(6), 826–831.

Nelson, L.D., Drebing, C., Satz, P., & Uchiyama, C. (1998). Personality change in head trauma: A validity study of the Neuropsychology Behavior and Affect Profile. *Archives of Clinical Neuropsychology, 13*(6), 549–560.

Nelson, R. (1988). Nonoperative management of impotence. *Journal of Urology, 139,* 2–5.

Nemeroff, C.B. (1998). *Biological Psychiatry, 44,* 517–525.

Netter, P., Croes, S., Merz, P., & Müller, M. (1991). Emotional and cortisol response to uncontrollable stress. In C.D. Spielberger, J.G. Sarason, J. Strelau, & J. Brebner (Eds.), *Stress and anxiety* (Vol. 13, pp. 193–208). Washington, DC: Hemisphere.

Nevin, N.C. (1967). Neuropathological changes in the white matter following head injury. *Journal of Neuropathology and Experimental Neurology, 26*(1), 77–84.

Nicholson, K. (2000). Pain, cognition and traumatic brain injury. *NeuroRehabilitation, 4,* 95–103.

Nielsen, A.S., Mortensen, P.B., O'Callaghan, E., Mors, O., & Ewald, H. (2002). Is head injury a risk factor for schizophrenia? *Schizophrenia Research, 55*(1–2), 93–98.

Nies, K.J., & Sweet, J.J. (1994). Neuropsychological assessment and malingering: A critical review of past and present strategies. *Archives of Clinical Neuropsychology, 9*(6), 501–552.

Niznikiewicz, M.A., Shenton, M.E., Voglmaier, M., Nestor, P.G., Dickey, C.C., Frumin, M., Seidman, L.J., Allen, C.G., & McCarley, R.W. (2002). Semantic dysfunction in women with schizotypal personality disorder. *American Journal of Psychiatry, 159,* 1767–1774.

Norris, F.H. (1992). Epidemiology of trauma: Frequency and impact of different potentially traumatic events on different demographic groups. *Journal of Consulting and Clinical Psychology, 60,* 409–418.

Obrenovich, T.P., & Urenjak, J. (1997). Is high extracellular glutamate the key to excitotoxicity in traumatic brain injury? *Journal of Neurotrauma, 14,* 677–698.

O'Carroll, R.E., Woodrow, J., & Maroun, F. (1991). Psychosexual and psychosocial sequelae of closed head injury. *Brain Injury, 5,* 303–313.

O'Connor, P., & Cripps, R. (1999). *Needs and opportunities for improved surveillance of brain injury. A progress report.* Canberra: Australian Institute of Health and Welfare.

Oddy, M., Coughlan, T., Tyerman, A., & Jenkins, D. (1985). Social adjustment after closed head injury: A further follow-up seven years after injury. *Journal of Neurology Neurosurgery and Psychiatry, 48*(6), 564–568.

Oddy, M.J. & Humphrey, M.E. (1980). Social recovery during the year following severe head injury. *Journal of Neurology, Neurosurgery and Psychiatry, 43,* 798–802.

Oddy, M.J., Humphrey, M.E., & Utley, D. (1978). Subjective impairment and social recovery after closed head injury. *Journal of Neurology, Neurosurgery and Psychiatry, 4,* 611–616.

O'Donnell, J.P., Cooper, J.E., Gersner, J.E., Shehan, I., & Ashley, J. (1981). Alcohol, drugs, and spinal cord injury. *Alcohol, Health and Research World, 148*, 209–212.

O'Flynn, K., Gruzelier, J.H., Bergman, A., & Siever, L.J. (2003). The schizophrenia spectrum personality disorders. In S.R. Hirsch, & D. Weinberger (Eds.), *Schizophrenia* (2nd ed., pp. 80–100). Chichester, UK: Blackwell.

O'Hara, C., & Harrell, M. (1991). *Rehabilitation with brain injury survivors: An empowerment approach.* Aspen: Gaithersburg, MD.

Ohry, A., Rattock, J., & Solomon, Z. (1996). Post-traumatic stress disorder in brain injury patients. *Brain Injury, 10(9),* 687–695.

Olds, J., & Milner, P. (1954). Positive reinforcement produced by electrical stimulation of septal area and other regions of the rat brain. *Journal of Comparative and Physiological Psychology, 47,* 419–427.

Ommaya, A.K., Faas, F., & Yarnell, P.R. (1968). Whiplash injury and brain damage: An experimental study. *Journal of the American Medical Association, 204,* 285–289.

Ommaya, A.K., & Gennarelli, T.A. (1974). Cerebral concussion and traumatic unconsciousness: Correlation of experimental and clinical observations on blunt head injuries. *Brain, 97,* 633–654.

Ommaya, A.K., Goldsmith, W., & Thibault, L. (2001). Biomechanics and neuropathology of adult and paediatric head injury. *British Journal of Neurosurgery, 16(3)*, 220–242.

Oquendo, M.A., Friedman, J.H., Grunebaum, M.F., Burke, A., Silver, J.M., & Mann, J.J. (2004). Suicidal behavior and mild traumatic brain injury in major depression. *Journal of Nervous and Mental Diseases, 192,* 430–434.

O'Shanick, G.T., & O'Shanick, A.M. (1994). Personality and intellectual changes. In J. Silver, S. Yudofsky, & R. Hales (Eds.), *Neuropsychiatry of traumatic brain injury* (pp. 163–188). Washington, DC: American Psychiatric Press.

O'Shanick, G.T., & O'Shanick, A.M. (2005). Personality disorders. In J.M. Silver, T.W. McAllister, & S.C. Yudofsky (Eds.), *Textbook of traumatic brain injury* (pp. 245–258). Washington, DC: American Psychiatric Publishing Inc.

Ota, Y. (1969). Head trauma––from the viewpoint of psychiatry. *Nippon Rinsho, 27*(9), 2239–2241.

Ouellet, M.C., & Morin, C.M. (2004). Cognitive behavioral therapy for insomnia associated with traumatic brain injury: A single-case study. *Archives of Physical Medicine and Rehabilitation, 85*, 1298–1302.

Overby, L.A. (1992). Perceptual asymmetry in psychosis-prone college students: Evidence for left-hemisphere overactivation. *Journal of Abnormal Psychology, 101*, 96–103.

Overholser, J.C., Norman, W.H., & Miller, I.W. (1990). Life stress and social supports in depressed inpatients. *Behav Med, 16*(3), 125–132.

Owens, J.E., Cook, E.W., & Stevenson, I. (1990). Features of "near-death experience" in relation to whether or not patients were near death. *Lancet, 336*(8724), 1175–1177.

Ownsworth, T. (2005). The impact of defensive denial upon adjustment following traumatic brain injury. *Neuro-Psychoanalysis, 7*, 83–94.

Ownsworth, T.L., & Oei, T.P. (1998). Depression after traumatic brain injury: conceptualization and treatment considerations. *Brain Injury, 12*(9), 735–751.

Packan, D.R., & Sapolsky, R.M. (1990). Glucocorticoid endangerment of the hippocampus: tissue, steroid and receptor specificity. *Neuroendocrinology, 51*(6), 613–618.

Pankratz, L. (1979). Symptom validity testing and symptom retraining: Procedures for the assessment and treatment of functional sensory deficits. *Journal of Consulting and Clinical Psychology, 47*, 409–410.

Pankratz, L., Fausti, S.A., & Peed, S. (1975). A forced-choice technique to evaluate deafness in the hysterical or malingering patient. *Journal of Consulting & Clinical Psychology, 43*(3), 421–422.

Parker, N. (1957). Manic-depressive psychosis following head injury. *Medical Journal of Australia, 44*(1), 20–22.

Parnas, J., Korsgaard, S., Krautwald, O., & Jensen, P.S. (1982). Chronic psychosis in epilepsy. A clinical investigation of 29 patients. *Acta Psychiatrica Scandinavica, 66*(4), 282–293.

Parnia, S., Waller, D.G., Yeates, R., & Fenwick, P. (2001). A qualitative and quantitative study of the incidence, features and aetiology of near-death experiences in cardiac arrest survivors. *Resuscitation, 48*(2), 149–156.

Patel, M. & Bontke, C.F. (1990). Impact of traumatic brain injury on pregnancy. *Journal of Head Trauma Rehabilitation, 5,* 60–66.

Patten, S.B., & Lauderdale, W.M. (1992). Delayed sleep phase disorder after traumatic brain injury. *Journal of the American Academy of Child and Adolescent Psychiatry, 31*(1), 100–102.

Pauls, D.L., & Alsobrook, J.P. 2nd. (1999). The inheritance of obsessive-compulsive disorder. *Child Adolescent Psychiatric Clinics of North America, 8*(3), 481–496, viii.

Pauls, D.L., Towbin, K.E., Leckman, J.F., Zahner, G.E.P., & Cohen, D.J. (1986). Gilles de la Tourette syndrome and obsessive-compulsive disorder: evidence supporting a genetic relationship. *Archives of General Psychiatry, 43*, 1180–2.

Paykel, E.S., & Dowlatshahi, D. (1988). Life events and mental disorder. In: S. Fisher, & J. Reason (Eds.), *Handbook of life stress, cognition and health.* Chichester (UK): John Wiley.

Paykel, E.S. (1974). Recent life events and clinical depression. In E.K. Gunderson, & R.H. Rahe (Eds.), *Life stress and illness.* Springfield, IL: Charles C. Thomas.

Paykel, E.S., Myers, J., Dienelt, M., Klerman, G., Lindenthal, J., & Pepper, M. (1969). Life events and depression. *Archives of General Psychiatry, 21*, 753–760.

Pelco, L., Sawyer, M., Duffield, G., Prior, M., & Kinsella, G. (1992). Premorbid emotional and behavioural adjustment in children with mild head injuries. *Brain Injury, 6*, 29–37.

Pellman, E.J., Lovell, M.R., Viano, D.C., Casson, I.R., & Tucker, A. (2004). Concussion in professional football: Neuropsychological testing—Part 6. *Neurosurgery, 55(6),* 1290–1305.

Pellman, E.J., Lovell, M.R., Viano, D.C., & Casson, I.R. (2006). Concussion in professional football: Recovery of NFL and high school athletes assessed by computerized neuropsychological testing—Part 12. *Neurosurgery, 58(2),* 263–274.

Penfield, W., & Jasper, H. (1954). *Epilepsy and the functional anatomy of the human brain.* Boston: Little Brown.

Penfield, W., & Rasmussen, T. (1950). *The cerebral cortex of man.* New York: MacMillan.

Perino, C., Rago, R., Cicolini, A., Torta, R., & Monaco, F. (2001). Mood and behavioural disorders following traumatic brain injury: clinical evaluation and pharmacological management. *Brain Injury, 15*(2), 139–148.

Perlesz, A., Kinsella, G., & Crowe, S. (2000). Psychological distress and family satisfaction following traumatic brain injury: injured individuals and their primary, secondary, and tertiary carers. *Journal of Head Trauma Rehabilitation, 15*(3), 909–929.

Pick, A. (1903). On reduplicative paramnesia. *Brain, 26*, 242–267.

Plum, F., & Posner, J.B. (1972). Diagnosis of stupor and coma. *Contemporary neurology series* (2nd ed.). Philadelphia, PA: F.A. Davis & Co.

Poeck, K. (1985). The Klüver–Bucy syndrome in man. In P.J. Vinken, G.W. Bruyn, & H.L. Klawans (Eds.), *Handbook of clinical neurology, Vol. 1(45):* Clinical neuropsychology (pp. 257–263). Amsterdam: Elsevier Science.

Pollens, R.D., McBrantie, B.P., & Burton, P.L. (1988). Beyond cognition: Executive functions in closed head injury. *Cognitive Rehabilitation, September/October*, 26–30.

Pollock, R.A., & Carter, A.S. (1999). The familial and developmental context of obsessive–compulsive disorder. *Child and Adolescent Psychiatry Clinics of North America, 8*(3), 461–479, vii–viii.

Ponsford, J. (2004). *Cognitive and behavioral rehabilitation: From neurobiology to clinical practice.* New York: Guilford Press.

Ponsford, J. (2003). Sexual changes associated with traumatic brain injury. *Neuropsychological Rehabilitation, 13*, (1–2), 275–289.

Ponsford, J., Facem, P.C., Willmott, C., Rothwell, A., Kelly, A., Nelms, R., & Ng, K.T. (2004). Use of the Westmead PTA scale to monitor recovery of memory after mild traumatic head injury. *Brain Injury, 18,* 603–614.

Ponsford, J., Sloan, S., & Snow, P. (1995). *Traumatic brain injury: Rehabilitation for everyday adaptive living.* Hove, UK: Lawrence Erlbaum Associates.

Ponsford, J., Willmott, C., Rothwell, A., Cameron, P., Kelly, A.M., Nelms, R., & Curran, C. (2002). Impact of early intervention on outcome following mild head injury in adults. *Journal of Neurology, Neurosurgery and Psychiatry, 73*, 330–332.

Ponsford, J., Willmott, C., Rothwell, A., Cameron, P., Kelly, A.M., Nelms, R., Curran, C., & Ng, K.T. (2000). Factors influencing outcome following mild traumatic brain injury in adults. *Journal of the International Neuropsychological Society, 6*, 568–579.

Pope, H.G., McElroy, S.L., & Satlin, A. (1988). Head injury, bipolar disorder, and response to valproate. *Comprehensive Psychiatry, 29(*1), 34–8.

Post, R.M. (2000). Neural substrates of psychiatric syndromes. In M. Mesulam (Ed.), *Principles of behavioral and cognitive neurology* (2nd ed.) (pp. 406–438). New York, NY: Oxford University Press.

Povlishock, J.T., & Christman, C.W. (1995). The pathobiology of traumatically induced axonal injury in animals and humans: A review of current thoughts. *Journal of Neurotrauma, 12*, 555–564.

Price, K.P. (1994). Post-traumatic stress disorder and concussion: Are they incompatible? Defense Law Journal, 43, 113–120.

Price, J.R., & Stevens, K.B. (1997). Psycholegal implications of malingered head trauma. *Applied Neuropsychology, 4*(1), 75–83.

Prigatano, G.P. (1991). Disturbances of self-awareness of deficit after traumatic brain injury. In G.P. Prigatano & D.L. Schacter (Eds.), *Awareness of deficit after brain injury: Clinical and theoretical issues* (pp. 111–126). New York: Oxford University Press.

Prigatano, G.P. (1992). Personality disturbances associated with traumatic brain injury. *Journal of Consulting and Clinical Psychology, 60*(3), 360–368.

Prigatano, G.P. (1996). Behavioral limitations TBI patients tend to underestimate: A replication and extension to patients with lateralized cerebral dysfunction. *Clinical Neuropsychologist, 10*, 191–201.

Prigatano, G.P., & Altman, I.M. (1990). Impaired awareness of behavioral limitations after traumatic brain injury. *Archives of Physical Medicine Rehabilitation, 71*(13), 1058–1064.

Prigatano, G.P., Altman, I.M., & O'Brien, K.P. (1990). Behavioral limitations that brain injured patients tend to underestimate. *Clinical Neuropsychologist, 4*, 163–176.

Prigatano, G.P., Bruna, O., Mataro, M., Munoz, J.M., Fernandez, S., & Junque, C. (1998). Initial disturbances of consciousness and resultant impaired awareness in Spanish patients with traumatic brain injury. *Journal of Head Trauma Rehabilitation, 13*(5), 29–38.

Prigatano, G.P., Fordyce, D., Zeiner, H.K., Roueche, J.R., Pepping, M., & Wood, B.C. (1986). *Neuropsychological rehabilitation after brain injury.* Baltimore: The Johns Hopkins University Press.

Prigatano, G.P., & Johnson, S.C. (2003). The three vectors of consciousness and their disturbances after brain injury. *Neuropsychological Rehabilitation, 13*(1/2), 13–29.

Prigatano, G.P., & Klonoff, P.S. (1997). A clinician's rating scale for evaluating impaired self awareness and denial of disability after brain injury. *The Clinical Neuropsychologist, 11*(1), 1–12.

Prigatano, G.P., & Leathem, J.M. (1993). Awareness of behavioural limitations after traumatic brain injury: A cross-cultural study of New Zealand Maoris and non-Maoris. *Clinical Neuropsychologist, 7,* 123–143.

Prigatano, G.P., O'Brien, K.P., & Klonoff, P.S. (1988). The clinical management of paranoid delusions in postacute traumatic brain-injured patients. *Journal of Head Trauma Rehabilitation, 3,* 23–32.

Prigatano, G.P., Ogano, M., & Amakusa, B. (1997). A cross-cultural study on impaired self-awareness in Japanese patients with brain dysfunction. *Neuropsychiatry, Neuropsychology and Behavioral Neurology, 10*(2), 135–143.

Prigatano, G.P., & Pribram, K.H. (1982). Perception and memory of facial affect following brain injury. *Percept Mot Skills, 54*(3), 859–869.

Prigatano, G.P., Stahl, M.L., Orr, W.C., & Zeiner, H.K. (1982). Sleep and dreaming disturbances in closed head injury patients. *Journal of Neurology, Neurosurgery and Psychiatry, 45,* 78–80.

Proctor, A., Wilson, B., Sanchez, C., & Wesley, E. (2000). Executive function and verbal working memory in adolescents with closed head injury (CHI). *Brain Injury,* 14(7), 633–647.

Pudenz, R.H., & Sheldon, L.H. (1946). The lucite calvarium: A method for direct observation of the brain. II. Cranial trauma and brain movement. *Journal of Neurosurgery, 3,* 487–505.

Quinto, C., Gellido, C., & Chokroverty, S. (2000). Posttraumatic delayed sleep phase syndrome. *Neurology, 54,* 250–252.

Radanov, B.P., Di Stefano, G.D., Schnidrig, A., & Ballinari, P. (1991). Role of psychological stress in recovery from common whiplash. *Lancet, 338,* 712–715.

Rao, V., & Lyketsos, C. (2000). Neuropsychiatric sequelae of traumatic brain injury. *Psychosomatics, 41,* 95–103.

Rao, V., & Lyketsos, C.G. (2002). Psychiatric aspects of traumatic brain injury. *The Psychiatric Clinics of North America, 25*(1), 43–69.

Rao, V., & Rollings, P. (2002). Sleep disturbances following traumatic brain injury. *Current Treatment Options in Neurology, 4*(1), 77–87.

Rapoport, M.J., & Feinstein, A. (2000). Outcome following traumatic brain injury in the elderly: A critical review. *Brain Injury, 14*(8), 749–761.

Rapoport, M., McCauley, S., Levin, H., Song, J., & Feinstein, A. (2002). The role of injury severity in neurobehavioral outcome three months after traumatic brain injury. *Neuropsychiatry, Neuropsychology and Behavioral Neurology, 15(2),* 123–132.

Rapoport, M.J., McCullagh, S., Streiner, D., & Feinstein, A. (2003). The clinical significance of major depression following mild traumatic brain injury. *Psychosomatics: Journal of Consultation Liaison Psychiatry, 44(1),* 31–37.

Rapport, L.J., Farchione, T.J., Coleman, R.D., & Axelrod, B.N. (1998). Effects of coaching on malingered motor function profiles. *Journal of Clinical and Experimental Neuropsychology, 20*(1), 89–97.

Rasmussen, S., & Eisen, J.L. (1991). Phenomenology of OCD: Clinical subtypes, heterogeneity and coexistence. In J. Zohar, T. Insel, & S. Rasmussen (Eds.), *The psychobiology of obsessive-compulsive disorder* (pp. 13–43). New York: Springer.

Raspe, R.E. (1859). The surprising adventures of Baron Munchausen. United Kingdom: Meridian.

Ratanalert, S., Chompikul, J., & Hirunpat, S. (2002). Talked and deteriorated head injury patients: how many poor outcomes can be avoided? *Journal of Clinical Neuroscience, 9*, 640–643.

Rattock, J., & Ross, B. (1993). Post traumatic stress disorder in the traumatically head injured. *Journal of Clinical and Experimental Neuropsychology, 15*, 403.

Rauch, S.L., Jenike, M.A., Alpert, N.M., Baer, L., Breiter, H.C., & Savage, C.R. (1994). Regional cerebral blood flow measured during symptom provocation in obsessive-compulsive disorder using oxygen 15-labeled carbon dioxide and positron emission tomography. *Archives of General Psychiatry, 51*(1), 62–70.

Rauch, S.L., van der Kolk, B.A., Fisler, R.E., Alpert, N.M., Orr, S.P., Savage, C.R., Fischman, A.J., Jenike, M.A., & Pitman, R. (1996). A symptom provocation study of posttraumatic stress disorder using positron emission tomography and script driven imagery. *Archives of General Psychiatry, 53*, 380–387.

Rauch, S.L., Whalen, P.J., Shin, L.M., McInerney, S.C., Macklin, M.L., Lasko, N.B., Orr, S.P., & Pitman, R.K. (2000). Exaggerated amygdala response to masked fearful vs. happy facial stimuli in posttraumatic stress disorder: A functional MRI study. *Biological Psychiatry, 47*, 769–776.

Rawling, P., & Brooks, N. (1990). Simulation Index: A method for detecting factitious errors on the WAIS-R and WMS. Special Section: Forensic-legal medical issues of neuropsychology. *Neuropsychology, 4*, 223–238.

Reading, P. (1991). Frontal lobe dysfunction in schizophrenia and Parkinson's disease–Meeting point for neurology, psychology and psychiatry. *Journal of the Royal Society of Medicine, 84*(6), 349–353.

Regestein, Q.R., & Reich, P. (1978). Pedophilia occurring after onset of cognitive impairment. *Journal of Nervous and Mental Disease, 166*, 794–8.

Reilly, P.L. (2001). Brain injury: the pathophysiology of the first hours. "Talk and die revisited". *Journal of Clinical Neuroscience, 8*, 398–403.

Reilly, P.L., Adams, J.H., Graham, D.I., & Jennett, B. (1975). Patients with head injury who talk and die. *Lancet, 11*, 375–377.

Reitan, R.M., & Wolfson, D. (1997). Emotional disturbances and their intention with neuropsychological deficits. *Neuropsychology Review, 7(1)*, 3–19.

Remillard, G. M., Andermann, F., & Testa, G. (1983). Sexual ictal manifestations predominate in women with temporal lobe epilepsy: A finding suggesting sexual dimorphism in the human brain. *Neurology, 33*, 323–330.

Resick, P.A. (2001a). *Stress and trauma*. London, England: Psychology Press Ltd.

Resick, P.A. (2001b). Cognitive therapy for posttraumatic stress disorder. *Journal of Cognitive Psychotherapy, 15*, 321–329.

Rey, A. (1964). *L-examen clinique en psychologie*. Paris: Universitaires de France.

Ribot, T. (1882). *Diseases of memory: An essay in the positive psychology*. New York: Appleton.

Richardson, A. (1969). *Mental imagery*. New York: Springer.

Richelson, E. (1993). Treatment of acute depression. *Psychiatry Clinics of North America, 16*(3), 461–478.

Rieger, M., & Gauggel, S. (2002). Inhibition of ongoing responses in patients with traumatic brain injury. *Neuropsychologia, 40*(1), 76–85.

Riggs, D.S., Rothbaum, B.O., & Foa, E.B. (1995). A prospective examination of symptoms of posttraumatic stress disorder in victims of nonsexual assault. *Journal of Interpersonal Violence, 10*, 201–214.

Rimel, R.W., Giordani, B., Barth, J.T., Boll, T.J., & Jane, J.A. (1981). Disability caused by minor head injury. *Neurosurgery, 9*, 221–228.

Rimel, R.W., Giordani, B.G., Barth, J.T., & Jane, J.A. (1982). Moderate head injury: Completing the clinical spectrum of brain trauma. *Neurosurgery, 2*(3), 344–351.

Rimel, R.W., Jane, J.A., & Bond, M.R. (1990). Characteristics of the head injured patient. In M. Rosenthal, E.R. Griffith, M.R. Bond, & J.D. Miller (Eds.), *Rehabilitation of the adult and child with traumatic brain injury*. Philadelphia: E A. Davis.

Ringman, J., & Cummings, J.L. (2000). Alterations in sexual behavior following focal brain injury. In J. Bogousslavsky, & J.L. Cummings (Eds.), *Behavior and mood disorders in focal brain lesions* (pp. 437–464). Cambridge: Cambridge University Press.

Roberts, G.W., Allsop, D., & Bruton, C. (1990). The occult aftermath of boxing. *Journal of Neurology, Neurosurgery and Psychiatry, 53*, 373–378.

Robertson, E., Rath, B., & Fournet, G. (1994). Assessment of mild brain trauma: A preliminary study of the influence of premorbid factors. *The Clinical Neuropsychologist, 8*, 69–74.

Robinson, R.G. (2000). Depression and lesion location in stroke. In J. Bogousslavsky, & J.L. Cummings (Eds.), *Behavior and mood disorders in focal brain lesions* (pp. 95–121). Cambridge: Cambridge University Press.

Robinson, R.G., & Jorge, R. (1994). Mood disorders. In J.M. Silver, S.C. Yudofsky, & R.E. Hales (Eds.), *Neuropsychiatry of traumatic brain injury* (pp. 219–250). Washington, DC: American Psychiatric Press.

Robinson, R.G., & Jorge, R. (2005). Mood disorders. In J.M. Silver, T.W. McAllister, & S.C. Yudofsky (Eds.), *Textbook of traumatic brain injury* (pp. 201–212). Washington, DC: American Psychiatric Publishing Inc.

Robinson, R.G., Boston, J.D., Starkstein, S.E., & Price, T.R. (1988). Comparison of mania and depression after brain injury: causal factors. *American Journal of Psychiatry, 145*, 172–178.

Roemer, L., & Borkovec, T.D. (1994). Effects of suppressing thoughts about emotional material. *Journal of Abnormal Psychology, 103*(3), 467–474.

Rogers, M.J., & Franzen, M.D. (1992). Delusional reduplication following closed-head injury. *Brain Injury, 6*(5), 469–476.

Rogers, R. (1988). *Clinical assessment of malingering and deception*. New York: Guilford Press.

Rogers, R. (1997). *Clinical assessment of malingering and deception*. New York: Guilford Press.

Rogers, R.D., Owen, A.M., Middleton, H.C., Williams, E.J., Pickard, J.D., Sahakian, B.J., & Robbins, T.W. (1999). Choosing between small, likely rewards and large, unlikely rewards activates inferior and orbital prefrontal cortex. *The Journal of Neuroscience, 19*(20), 9029–9038.

Rogers, R., Sewell, K.W., & Salekin, R.J. (1994). A meta-analysis of malingering on the MMPI-2. *Assessment, 1*, 227–237.

Rogers, R., Sewell, K.W., & Ustad, K.L. (1995). Feigning among chronic outpatients on the MMPI–2: A systematic examination of Fake-Bad indicators. *Assessment, 2*, 81–89.

Rohling, M.L., Green, P., Allen, L.M., & Iverson, G.L. (2002). Depressive symptoms and neurocognitive test scores in patients passing symptom validity tests. *Archives of Clinical Neuropsychology, 17*(3), 205–222.

Rojas, L. (1947). Impotencia sexual post traumatica. *Acta Espanola Neurologica y Psiquiatrica, 6,* 43–45.

Rolls, E.T. (1999). *The brain and emotion.* Oxford: Oxford University Press.

Rolls, E.T. (2000). The orbitofrontal cortex and reward. *Cerebral Cortex, 10,* 284–294.

Rolls, E.T., Hornak, J., Wade, D., & McGrath, J. (1994). Emotion-related learning in patients with social and emotional changes associated with frontal lobe damage. *Journal of Neurology Neurosurgery and Psychiatry, 57*(12), 1518–1524.

Ron, S., Algom, D., Hary, D., & Cohen, M. (1980). Time related changes in the distribution of sleep stages in brain injured patients. *Electroencephalography and Clinical Neurophysiology, 48,* 432–441.

Rosenbaum, A., & Hoggs, S.K. (1989). Head injury and marital aggression. *American Journal of Psychiatry, 146,* 8–15.

Rosenbaum, M., & Najenson, T. (1976). Changes in life patterns and symptoms of low mood as reported by wives of severely brain-injured soldiers. *Journal of Consulting and Clinical Psychology, 44,* 881–888.

Rosenstein, L.D. (1998). Differential diagnosis of the major progressive dementias and depression in middle and late adulthood: A summary of the literature of the early 1990s. Neuropsychology Review, 8(3), 109–67.

Rosenthal, M., Griffith, E.R., Bond, M.R., & Miller, J.D. (1990). Rehabilitation of the adult and child with traumatic brain injury. Philadelphia, PA: Davis.

Roth, M. (1955). The natural history of mental disorders in old age. *Journal of Mental Science, 101,* 281–301.

Ruff, R.M. (1996). *Ruff Figural Fluency Test (RFFT) professional manual.* Odessa, FL: Psychological Assessment Resources.

Ruff, R.M., Camenzuli, L., & Mueller, J. (1996). Miserable minority: emotional risk factors that influence the outcome of a mild traumatic brain injury. *Brain Injury, 10*(8), 551–65.

Ruff, R.M., Crouch, J.A., Tröster, A.I., Marshall, L.F., Buchsbaum, M.S., Lottenberg, S., & Somers, L.M. (1994). Selected cases of poor outcome following a minor brain trauma: Comparing neuropsychological and positron emission tomography assessment. *Brain Injury, 8(4),* 297–308.

Ruff, R.M., & Grant, I. (1999). Postconcussional disorder: background to DSV-IV and future considerations. In N. Varney & R. Roberts (Eds.), *The evaluation and treatment of mild traumatic brain injury.* Mahwah, NJ: Lawrence Erlbaum Associates.

Ruff, R.M., & Jurica, P. (1999). In search of a unified definition for mild traumatic brain injury. *Brain Injury, 13*(12), 943–952.

Ruff, R.M., Marshall, L.F., Klauber, M.R., Blunt, B.A., Grant, I., Foulkes, M.A., Eisenberg, H., Jane, J., & Marmarou, A. (1990). Alcohol abuse and neurological outcome of the severely head injured. *Journal of Head Trauma Rehabilitation, 5,* 21–31.

Ruff, R.M., & Richardson, A.M. (1999). Mild traumatic brain injury. In J. Sweet (Ed.), *Forensic neuropsychology: fundamentals and practice. Studies on neuropsychology, development and cognition* (pp. 315–358). Lisse, Netherlands: Swets & Zeitlinger.

Russell, J.D., & Roxanas, M.G. (1990). Psychiatry and the frontal lobes. *Australia and New Zealand Journal of Psychiatry, 24*(1), 113–132.

Russell, R., & Smith, A. (1961). Post-traumatic amnesia in closed head injury. *Archives of Neurology, 5,* 16–29.

Russell, W.R. (1932). Cerebral involvement in head injury. *Brain, 55,* 549–603.

Russell, W.R. (1960). Injury to the cranial nerves and optic chiasm. In S. Brock (Ed), *Injuries of the brain and spinal cord and their coverings* (4th ed) (pp. 118–126). New York: Springer Verlag.

Rutherford, W.H. (1989). Postconcussion symptoms: relationship to acute neurological indices, individual differences, and circumstances of injury. In H.S. Levin, H.M. Eisenberg, & A.L Benton (Eds.), *Mild head injury*. Oxford: Oxford University Press.

Rutherford, W.H., Merritt, J.D., & McDonald, J.R. (1977). Sequelae of concussion caused by minor head injuries. *Lancet, 1*, 1–4.

Rutherford, W.H., Merrett, J.D., & McDonald, J.R. (1978). Symptoms at 1 year following concussion from minor head injuries. *Injury, 10*, 225–30.

Rutherford, W.H., Merrett, J.D., & McDonald, J.R. (1979). Symptoms at one year following concussion from minor head injuries. *Injury, 10*(3), 225–230.

Ryan, A.J. (1998). Intracranial injuries resulting from boxing. *Clinical Sports Medicine, 17(1)*, 155–168.

Sabhesan, S., Arumugham, R., Ramasany, P., & Natarajan, M. (1987). Persistent alcohol abuse and late outcome in head injury. *Indian Journal of Psychological Medicine, 10*, 61–65.

Sabhesan, S., & Natarajan, M. (1989). Sexual behaviour after head injury in Indian men and women. *Archives of Sexual Behavior, 18*, 349–356.

Sachdev, P., Smith, J.S., & Cathcart, S. (2001). Schizophrenia-like psychosis following traumatic brain injury: A chart-based descriptive and case-control study. *Psychological Medicine, 31*(2), 231–239.

Sadock, B.J., & Sadock, V.A. (Eds.). (2004). *The comprehensive textbook of psychiatry* (8th ed.). Baltimore, MD: Williams & Wilkins.

Salim, A., Kim, K.A., Kimbrell, B.J., Petrone, P., Roldan, G., & Asensio, J.A. (2002). Kluver-Bucy syndrome as a result of minor head trauma. *Southern Medical Journal, 95*(8), 929–31.

Salkovskis, P.M. (1985). Obsessional-compulsive problems: A cognitive-behavioural analysis. *Behaviour Research and Therapy, 23*(5), 571–583.

Salkovskis, P.M., & Campbell, P. (1994). Thought suppression induces intrusion in naturally occurring negative intrusive thoughts. *Behaviour Research and Therapy, 32*(1), 1–8.

Sanderson, W.C., Rapee, R.M., & Barlow, D.H. (1989). The influence of an illusion of control on panic attacks induced via inhalation of 5.5% carbon dioxide-enriched air. *Archives of General Psychiatry, 46*(2), 157–162.

Sandel, M.E., Williams, K.S., Dellapietra, L. & Derogatis, L.R. (1996). Sexual functioning following traumatic brain injury. *Brain Injury, 10*, 719–728.

Sapolsky, R.M. (1990). Glucocorticoids, hippocampal damage and the glutamatergic synapse. *Progressive Brain Research, 86*, 13–23.

Sapolsky, R.M. (1994). Glucocorticoids, stress and exacerbation of excitotoxic neuron death. *Seminars in Neuroscience, 6*, 323–331.

Sapolsky, R.M. (2000). Glucocorticoids and hippocampal atrophy in neuropsychiatric disorders. *Archives of General Psychiatry, 57*, 925–935.

Sarapata, M., Herrmann, D., Johnson, T., & Aycock, R. (1998). The role of head injury in cognitive functioning, emotional adjustment and criminal behaviour. *Brain Injury, 12*(10), 821–42.

Satish, U., Streufert, S., & Eslinger, P.J. (1999). Complex decision making after orbitofrontal damage: neuropsychological and strategic management simulation assessment. *Neurocase, 5*, 355–364.

Satz, P., Forney, D.L., Zaucha, K., Asarnow, R.R., Light, R., McCleary, C., Levin, H., Kelly, D., Bergsneider, M., Hovda, D., Martin, N., Namerow, N., & Becker, D. (1998). Depression, cognition, and functional correlates of recovery outcome after traumatic brain injury. *Brain Injury, 12(7)*, 537–553.

Saver, J.L., & Damasio, A.R. (1991). Preserved access and processing of social knowledge in a patient with acquired sociopathy due to ventromedial frontal damage. *Neuropsychologia, 29*(12), 1241–1249.

Savola, O., & Hillbom, M. (2003). Early predictors of post-concussion symptoms in patients with mild head injury. *European Journal of Neurology, 10*, 175–181.

Sbordone, R.J. (1991). Overcoming obstacles in cognitive rehabilitation of persons with severe traumatic brain injury. In J.S. Kreutzer, & P.H. Wehman (Eds.), *Cognitive rehabilitation for persons with traumatic brain injury*. Bisbee, Arizona: Imaginart Press.

Sbordone, R.J., & Guilmette, T.J. (1999). Ecological validity: prediction of everyday and vocational functioning from neuropsychological test data. In J.J. Sweet (Ed.), *Forensic neuropsychology* (pp. 227–254). Lisse: Swets & Zeitlinger.

Sbordone, R.J., & Liter, J.C. (1995). Mild traumatic brain injury does not produce post-traumatic stress disorder. *Brain Injury, 9 (4)*, 405–412.

Sbordone, R.J., Seyranian, G.D., & Ruff, R.M. (1998). Are the subjective complaints of traumatically brain injured patients reliable? *Brain Injury, 12*(6), 505–515.

Schacter, D.L. (1992). Implicit knowledge: new perspectives on unconscious processes. *Procedings of the National Academy of Science USA, 89*(23), 11113–11117.

Schacter, D.L., & Crovitz, H.F. (1977). Memory function after closed head injury: A review of the quantitative research. *Cortex, 13*, 150–176.

Schachter, S., & Singer, J.E. (1962). Cognitive, social and physiological determinants of emotional state. *Psychological Review, 69*, 379–399.

Schechter, P.J., & Henkins, R.I. (1974). Abnormalities of taste and smell after head trauma. *Journal of Neurology, Neurosurgery and Psychiatry, 37*, 802–810.

Scheutzow, M.H., & Wiercisiewski, D.R. (1999). Panic disorder in a patient with traumatic brain injury: A case report and discussion. *Brain Injury, 9*, 705–714.

Schneider, K. (1959). *Clinical psychopathology*. New York: Grune and Stratton.

Schoenhuber, R., & Gentilini, M. (1988). Anxiety and depression after mild head injury: A case control study. *Journal of Neurology Neurosurgery and Psychiatry, 51*(5), 722–724.

Schreiber, S., Klag, E., Gross, Y., Segman, R.H., & Pick, C.G. (1998). Beneficial effect of risperidone on sleep disturbance and psychosis following traumatic brain injury. *International Clinical Psychopharmacology, 13*(6), 273–5.

Schretlen, D., Brandt, J., Krafft, L., & Van Gorp, W. (1991). Some caveats in using the Rey 15-Item memory test to detect malingered amnesia. *Psychological Assessment, 3*, 667–672.

Schretlen, D., & Shapiro, A.M. (2003). A quantitative review of the effects of traumatic brain injury on cognitive functioning. *International Review of Psychiatry, 15*, 341–349.

Schwartz, M.L., Carruth, F., Binns, M.A., Brandys, C., Moulton, R., Snow, W.G., & Stuss, D.T. (1998). The course of post-traumatic amnesia: three little words. *Canadian Journal of Neurological Sciences, 25*, 108–116.

Schwartz, O., & Sisler, G.C. (1971). A clinical study of post-traumatic amnesia. *Canadian Psychiatric Association Journal, 16*, 341–346.

Scoville, W.B., & Milner, B. (1957). Loss of recent memory after bilateral hippocampal lesions. *Journal of Neurology, Neurosurgery and Psychiatry, 20*, 11–21.

Segraves, R.T. (1988). Hormones and libido. In S.R. Leiblum & R.C. Rosen (Eds.), *Sexual desire disorders* (pp. 271–312). London: Guildford.

Segraves, R.T. (1996). Neuropsychiatric aspects of sexual dysfunction. In B.S. Fogel, R.B. Schiffer & S.M. Rao (Eds.), *Neuropsychiatry* (pp. 757–770). Baltimore: Williams and Wilkins.

Sem-Jacobsen, C.W. (1968). *Depth-electrographic stimulation of the human brain and behaviour*. Springfield, Ill.: C. C. Thomas.

Semple, W.E., Goyer, P., McCormick, R., Compton-Toth, B., Morris, E., Donovan, B., Muswick, G., Nelson, D., Garnett, M.L., Sharkoff, J., Leisure, G., Miraldi, F., & Schulz, S.C. (1996). Attention and regional cerebral blood flow in posttraumatic stress disorder patients with substance abuse histories. *Psychiatry Research, 67,* 17–28.

Shallice, T. (1988). *From neuropsychology to mental structure.* New York: Cambridge.

Shaw, N.A. (2002). The neurophysiology of concussion. *Progress in Neurobiology, 67,* 281–344.

Sheehan, P.W. (1967). A shortened form of Bett's questionnaire upon mental imagery. *Journal of Clinical Psychology, 23,* 386–389.

Sherer, M., Bergloff, P., Levin, E., High, W.M., Jr., Oden, K.E., & Nick, T.G. (1998). Impaired awareness and employment outcome after traumatic brain injury. *Journal of Head Trauma Rehabilitation, 13*(5), 52–61.

Sherer, M., Hart, T., Nick, T.G., Whyte, J., Thompson, R.N., & Yablon, S.A. (2003). Early impaired self-awareness after traumatic brain injury. *Archives of Physical Medicine Rehabilitation, 84*(2), 168–176.

Sherer, M., & Struchen, M. (2004, November 17). *Course 7: Outcome after traumatic brain injury: A review of factors that affect long-term functional status.* Workshop presented at the National Academy of Neuropsychology 24th Annual Conference, Seattle, Washington.

Shin, L.M. (1997). Visual imagery and perception in posttraumatic stress disorder. *Archives of General Psychiatry, 54,* 233–241.

Shores, A.E., & Carstairs, J.R. (1998). Accuracy of the MMPI-2 Computerized Minnesota Report in identifying fake-good and fake-bad response sets. *The Clinical Neuropsychologist, 12*(1), 101–106.

Shores, E.A., Marosszeky, J.E., Sandanam, J., & Batchelor, J. (1986). Preliminary validation of a scale fro measuring the duration of post-traumatic amnesia. *Medical Journal of Australia, 144,* 569–572.

Shores, T.J., Seib, T.B., Levine, S., & Rose, G.M. (1989). Inescapable versus escapable shock modulates long-term potentiation in the rat hippocampus. *Science, 244,* 224–226.

Shukla, S., Cook, B.L., Mukherjee, S., Godwin, C., & Miller, M.G. (1987). Mania following head trauma. *American Journal of Psychiatry, 144,* 93–96.

Signer, S.F., & Cummings, J.L. (1987). De Clerambault's syndrome in organic affective disorder. *British Journal of Psychiatry, 151,* 404–407.

Silva, J.A., Leong, G.B., & Luong, M.T. (1989). Split body and self: An unusual case of misidentification. *Canadian Journal of Psychiatry, 34*(7), 728–730.

Silver, J., Kramer, R., Greenwald, S., & Weissman, M. (2001). The association between head injuries and psychiatric disorders: Findings from the New Haven NIMH Epidemiologic Catchment Area Study. *Brain Injury, 15,* 935–945.

Silver, J., & McAllister, T. (1997). Forensic issues in the neuropsychiatric evaluation of the patient with mild traumatic brain injury. *Neuropsychiatric Practice and Opinion, 9,* 102 –113.

Simpson, G.K., Blaszczynski, A., & Hodgkinson, A. (1999). Sex offending as a psychosocial sequela of traumatic brain injury. *The Journal of Head Trauma Rehabilitation, 14,* 567–580.

Simpson, G.K, Tate, R., Ferry, K., Hodgkinson, A., & Blaszczynski, A. (2001). Social, neuroradiologic, medical and neuropsychologic correlates of sexually aberrant behaviour after traumatic brain injury: A controlled study. *The Journal of Head Trauma Rehabilitation, 16*(6), 556–572.

Sinanan, K. (1984). Mania as a sequel to a road traffic accident. *British Journal of Psychiatry, 144,* 330–331.

Slater, E., Beard, A.W., & Glithero, E. (1963). The schizophrenia-like psychoses of epilepsy. *British Journal of Psychiatry, 109*, 95–105.

Slaughter, J., Bobo, W., & Childers, M.K. (1999). Selective serotonin reuptake inhibitor treatment of post-traumatic Kluver-Bucy syndrome. *Brain Injury, 13*(1), 59–62.

Slick, D.J., Hopp, G., Strauss, E., Hunter, M., & Pinch, D. (1994). Detecting dissimulation: profiles of simulated malingerers, traumatic brain-injury patients, and normal controls on a revised version of Hiscock and Hiscock's Forced-Choice Memory Test. *Journal of Clinical and Experimental Neuropsychology, 16*(3), 472–481.

Slick, D.J., Sherman, E.M., & Iverson, G.L. (1999). Diagnostic criteria for malingered neurocognitive dysfunction: proposed standards for clinical practice and research. *Clinical Neuropsychology, 13*(4), 545–561.

Slick, D.J., Tan, J.E., Strauss, E.H., & Hultsch, D.F. (2004). Detecting malingering: A survey of experts' practices. *Archives of Clinical Neuropsychology, 19*(4), 465–473.

Smeltzer, D.J., Nasrallah, H.A., & Miller, S.C. (1994). Psychotic disorders. In J.M. Silver, S.C. Yudofsky, & R.E. Hales (Eds.), *Neuropsychiatry of traumatic brain injury* (pp. 251–283). Washington, DC: American Psychiatric Press.

Smith, B.H. & Khatri, A.M. (1979). Cortical localization of sexual feeling. *Psychosomatics, 20*, 771–776.

Smith, D., & Over, R. (1987). Correlates of fantasy-induced and film-induced male sexual arousal. *Archives of Sexual Behavior, 16*, 395–409.

Smith, D. & Over, R. (1990). Enhancement of fantasy-induced sexual arousal in men through training in sexual imagery. *Archives of Sexual Behavior, 19*, 477–489.

Smith, M.E. (2005). Bilateral hippocampal volume reduction in adults with post-traumatic stress disorder: A meta-analysis of structural MRI studies. *Hippocampus, 15*(6): 798–807.

Sohlberg, M.M., Mateer, C., Penkman, L., Glang, A., & Todis, B. (1998). Awareness intervention: Who needs it? *Journal of Head Trauma Rehabilitation, 13*, 62–78.

Solomon, D.A., & Malloy, P.E. (1992). Alcohol, head injury and neuropsychological function. *Neuropsychology Review, 3*(3), 249–280.

Sparadeo, F.R., & Gill, D. (1989). Effects of prior alcohol use on head injury recovery. *Journal of Head Trauma Rehabilitation, 4*(1), 75–82.

Sparadeo, F.R., Strauss, D., & Barth, J.T. (1990). The incidence, impact and treatment of substance abuse in head trauma rehabilitation. *Journal of Head Trauma Rehabilitation, 5*, 1–8.

Spell, L.A., & Frank, E.M. (2000). Recognition of nonverbal communication of affect following traumatic brain injury, *Journal of Nonverbal Behavior, 24*(4), 285–300.

Spielberger, C.D. (1983). *State-Trait Anxiety Inventory (Form Y)*. California: Mind Culture.

Spielberger, C.D., Lushene, R.E., & McAdoo, W.G. (1977). Theory and measurement of anxiety states. In R.B. Cattell & R.M. Dreger (Eds.) *Handbook of modern personality theory* (pp. 253–293). New York: Hemisphere/Wiley.

Spreen, O., & Strauss, E. (1998). *A Compendium of Neuropsychological Tests: Administration, Norms and Commentary* (2nd edition). New York: Oxford University Press.

Starkman, M.N., Gebarski, S.S., Berent, S., & Schteingart, D.E. (1992). Hippocampal formation volume, memory dysfunction, and cortisol levels in patients with Cushing's syndrome. *Biological Psychiatry, 32*(9), 756–765.

Starkstein, S.E., Pearlson, G.D., Boston, J., & Robinson, R.G. (1987). Mania after brain injury: A controlled study of causative factors. *Archives of Neurology, 44*, 1069–1073.

Starkstein, S.E., & Robinson, R.G. (1991). Dementia of depression in Parkinson's disease and stroke. *Journal of Nervous and Mental Disease, 179*(10), 593–601.

Starkstein, S.E., & Robinson, R.G. (1997). Mechanism of disinhibition after brain lesions. *Journal of Nervous and Mental Disease, 185*(2), 108–114.

Stavrakaki, C., & Vargo, B. (1986). The relationship of anxiety and depression: A review of the literature. *The British Journal of Psychiatry, 149*, 7–16.

Stein, M.B., Koverola, C., Hanna, C., Torchia, M.G., & McClarty, B. (1997). Hippocampal volume in women victimized by childhood sexual abuse. *Psychological Medicine, 27*(4), 951–959.

Stein, M.B., Forde, D.R., Anderson, G., & Walker, J.R. (1997). Obsessive–compulsive disorder in the community: An epidemiologic survey with clinical reappraisal. *American Journal of Psychiatry, 154*(8), 1120–1126.

Stern, R.S. (1978). Obsessive thoughts: the problem of therapy. *The British Journal of Psychiatry,* 133, 200–205.

Sterr, A., Herron, K.A., Hayward, C., & Montaldi, D. (2006). Are mild head injuries as mild as we think? Neurobehavioral concomitants of chronic post-concussion syndrome. *BMC Neurology, 6*, 7.

Stevenson, I., Williams-Cook, E., & McClean-Rice, N. (1989). Are persons reporting "near death experiences" really near death? A study of medical records. *Omega, 20*, 45–54.

Stevenson, I., & Greyson, B. (1979). Near-death experiences. Relevance to the question of survival after death. *Journal of the American Medical Association, 242*(3), 265–267.

Stewart, J.T., & Hemsath, R.H. (1988). Bipolar illness following traumatic brain injury: treatment with lithium and carbamazepine. *Journal of Clinical Psychiatry, 49(2)*, 74–75.

Stier, E. (1938). The visiting doctor. *TBI Challenge, Spring,* 44.

Stone, L.R., & Keenan, M.A. (1992). Deep-vein thrombosis of the upper extremity after traumatic brain injury. *Archives of Physical Medicine Rehabilitation, 73*, 486–489.

Strich, S.J. (1956). Diffuse degeneration of the cerebral white matter in severe dementia following head injury. *Journal of Neurology, Neurosurgery and Psychiatry, 19*, 893–895.

Strauss, E., & Moscovitch, M. (1981). Perception of facial expressions. *Brain Lang, 13*(2), 308–332.

Streeter, C.C., van Reekum, R., Shorr, R.L., & Bachman, D.L. (1995). Prior head injury in male veterans with borderline personality disorder. *The Journal of Nervous and Mental Disease, 183*(9), 577–581.

Stuss, D.T., & Benson, D.F. (1986). *The frontal lobes.* New York: Raven Press.

Stuss, D.T., Binns, M.A., Carruth, F.G., Levine, B., Brandys, C.E., Moulton, R.J., Snow, W.G., & Schwartz, M.L. (1999). The acute period of recovery from traumatic brain injury: posttraumatic amnesia or posttraumatic confusional state? *Journal of Neurosurgery, 90*, 635–643.

Stuss, D.T., & Gow, A.D. (1992). Frontal dysfunction after traumatic brain injury. *Neuropsychiatry, Neuropsychology and Behaviour Neurology, 5*, 272–282.

Suhr, J.A., & Boyer, D. (1999). Use of the Wisconsin Card Sorting Test in the detection of malingering in student simulator and patient samples. *Journal of Clinical and Experimental Neuropsychology, 21*(5), 701–708.

Suhr, J.A., & Gunstad, J. (2002). Postconcussive symptom report: the relative influence of head injury and depression. *Journal of Clinical and Experimental Neuropsychology, 24(8)*, 981–93.

Sweeney, J.E. (1992). Non-impact brain injury: Grounds for clinical study of the neuropsychological effects of acceleration forces. *Clinical Neuropsychologist, 6(4),* 443–457.

Sweet, J.J., Wolfe, P., Sattlberger, E., Numan, B., Rosenfeld, J.P., Clingerman, S., & Nies, K.J. (2000). Further investigation of traumatic brain injury versus insufficient effort with the California Verbal Learning Test. *Archives of Clinical Neuropsychology, 15,* 105–113.

Symonds, C.P., & Russell, W.R. (1943). Accidental head injuries. *Lancet, 1,* 7–10.

Szasz, G. (1983). Sexual health care. In C.P. Zejdlik (Ed.), *Management of spinal cord injury.* Monterey, CA: Wadsworth Health Sciences Division.

Szekeres, S.F., Ylvisaker, M., & Cohen, S.B. (1987). A framework for cognitive rehabilitation therapy. In M. Ylvisaker & E.M.R. Gobble (Eds.), *Community re-entry for head injured adults* (pp. 87–136). Boston, MA: College-Hill Press.

Tamminga, C.A., Thaker, G.K., Buchanan, R., Kirkpatrick, B., Alphs, L.D., Chase, T.N., & Carpenter, W.T. (1992). Limbic system abnormalities identified in schizophrenia using positron emission tomography with fluorodeoxyglucose and neocortical alterations with deficit syndrome. *Archives of General Psychiatry, 49,* 522–530.

Tate, R.L. (1987). Issues in the management of behaviour disturbance as a consequence of severe head injury. *Scandinavian Journal of Rehabilitation Medicine, 19*(1), 13–18.

Tate, R.L. (1999). Executive dysfunction and characterological changes after traumatic brain injury: two sides of the same coin? *Cortex, 35*(1), 39–55.

Tate, R.L. (2003). Impact of pre-injury factors on outcome after severe traumatic brain injury: Does post-traumatic personality change represent an exacerbation of pre-morbid traits? *Neuropsychological Rehabilitation, 13*(1–2), 43–64.

Tate, R.L., & Pfaff, A. (2000). Problems and pitfalls in the assessment of posttraumatic amnesia. *Brain Impairment, 1,* 116–129.

Tate, R.L., Pfaff, A., & Jurjevic, L. (2000). Resolution of disorientation and amnesia during post-traumatic amnesia. *Journal of Neurology, Neurosurgery and Psychiatry, 68,* 178–185.

Tate, R.L., Pfaff, A., Hodgkinson, A.E., Baguley, I.J., Gurka, J.A., Marosszeky, J.E., & King, C. (2005). *Post-Traumatic Amnesia: An Investigation into the Validity of Measuring Instruments.* New South Wales: Motor Accidents Authority of New South Wales.

Tate, R.L., Simpson, G.K., Flanagan, S., & Coffey, M. (1997). Completed suicide after traumatic brain injury. *Journal of Head Trauma Rehabilitation, 12*(6), 16–28.

Taylor, L.A., Kreutzer, J.S., Demm, S.R., & Meade, M.A. (2003). Traumatic brain injury and substance abuse: A review and analysis of the literature. *Neuropsychological Rehabilitation, 13*(1), 165–188.

Teasdale, J. (1993). Emotion and two kinds of meaning: Cognitive therapy and applied cognitive science. *Behavior Research and Therapy, 31(4),* 339–354.

Teasdale, J., & Barnard, P. (1993). *Affect cognition and change: Remodelling depressive thought.* Hove, UK: Lawrence Erlbaum.

Teasdale, G., & Jennett, B. (1974). Assessment of coma and impaired consciousness: A practical scale. *The Lancet, July 13,* 81–84.

Teasdale, G., & Jennett, B. (1976). Assessment of prognosis of coma after head injury. *Acta Neurochirurgica, 34,* 45–55.

Teasdale, T.W., & Engberg, A.W. (2001). Suicide after traumatic brain injury: A population study. *Journal of Neurology Neurosurgery and Psychiatry, 71*(4), 436–440.

Tellegen, A., & Atkinson, G. (1974). Openness to absorbing and self-altering experiences ("absorption"), a trait related to hypnotic suggestibility. *Journal of Abnormal Psychology, 83,* 268–277.

Tenhula, W.N., & Sweet, J.J. (1996). Double cross-validation of the Booklet Category Test in detecting malingered traumatic brain injury. *The Clinical Neuropsychologist, 10,* 104–116.

Teuber, H.L. (1964). Speech as a motor skill with special reference to nonaphasic disorders: formal discussion. *Monograms in Social Research of Child Development, 29,* 131–138.

Thatcher, R.W., Camacho, M., Salazar, A., Lindern, C., Biver, C., & Clare, E. (1997). Quantitative MRI of the gray-white matter distribution in traumatic brain injury. *Journal of Neurotrauma, 12,* 1–14.

Thompson, H.J., Pinto-Martin, J., & Bullock, M.R. (2003). Neurogenic fever after traumatic brain injury: An epidemiological study. *Journal of Neurology, Neurosurgery and Psychiatry, 74*(5), 614–619.

Thomsen, I.V. (1984). Late outcome of very severe blunt head trauma: A 10–15 year second follow-up. *Journal of Neurology, Neurosurgery, and Psychiatry, 47,* 260–268.

Thomsen, I.V. (1987). Late psychosocial outcome in severe blunt head trauma. *Brain Injury, 1*(2), 131–143.

Thurman, D.L, Alverson, C., Browne, D., Dunn, K.A., Guerrero, L., Johnson, R., Johnson, V., Langlois, L., Pilkey, D., Sniezek, J.E., & Toel, S. (1999). *Traumatic brain injury in the United States: A report to Congress.*

Tiihonen, J., Kuikka, J., Kupila, J., Partanen, K., Vainio, P., Airaksinen, J., Eronen, M., Hallikainen, T., Paanila, J., Kinnunen, I., & Huttunen, J. (1994). Increase in cerebral blood flow of right prefrontal cortex in man during orgasm. *Neuroscience Letters, 170*(2), 241–243.

Tobe, E.H., Schneider, J.S., Mrozik, T., & Lidsky, T.I. (1999). Persisting insomnia following traumatic brain injury. *The Journal of Neuropsychiatry and Clinical Neuroscience, 11*(4), 504–6.

Tokuda, T., Ikeda, S., Yanagisawa, N., Ihara, Y., & Glenner, G.G. (1991). Re-examination of ex-boxers brains using immunohistochemistry with antibodies to amyloid beta-protein and tau protein. *Acta Neuropathologica, 82,* 280–285.

Tombaugh, T.N. (1996). *Test of Memory Malingering.* North Tonawanda, NY: Multi-Health Systems.

Tombaugh, T.N. (1997). The Test of Memory Malingering (TOMM): Normative data from cognitively intact and cognitively impaired individuals. *Psychological Assessment, 9,* 260–268.

Torgersen, S. (1985a). Developmental differentiation of anxiety and affective neuroses. *Acta Psychiatrica Scandinavica, 71*(3), 304–310.

Torgersen, S. (1985b). Hereditary differentiation of anxiety and affective neuroses. *British Journal of Psychiatry, 146,* 530–534.

Tranel, D., Bechara, A., & Damasio, A.R. (2000). Decision-making and the somatic marker hypothesis. In M. Gazzaniga (Ed.), *The cognitive neurosciences* (pp. 1047–1061). Cambridge, MA: MIT Press.

Tranel, D., Bechara, A., & Denburg, N.L. (2002). Asymmetric functional roles of right and left ventromedial prefrontal cortices in social conduct, decision-making, and emotional processing. *Cortex, 38*(4), 589–612.

Trivedi, M.H. (1996). Functional neuroanatomy of obsessive-compulsive disorder. *Journal of Clinical Psychiatry, 57*(Suppl. 8), 26–35; discussion 36.

Tsushima, W.T., & Tsushima, V.G. (2001). Comparison of the Fake Bad Scale and other MMPI-2 validity scales with personal injury litigants. *Assessment, 8*(2), 205–212.

Turnbull, S.J., Campbell, E.A., & Swann, I.A. (2001). Post-traumatic stress disorder symptoms following a head injury: does amnesia for the event influence the development of symptoms? *Brain Injury, 15*(9), 775–85.

Tyerman, A., & Humphrey, M. (1984). Changes in self-concept following severe head injury. *International Journal of Rehabilitation Research, 7*(1), 11–23.

Tyrer, S.P. (1986). Learned pain behaviour. *British Medical Journal (Clinical Research Edition), 292*, 1–2.

Tyrer, S.P., & Lievesley, A. (2003). Pain following traumatic brain injury: Assessment and management. *Neuropsychological Rehabilitation, 13*, 189–210.

Tysvaer, A.T., & Storli, O.V. (1989). Soccer injuries to the brain: A neurological and electroencephalographic study of active football players. *American Journal of Sports Medicine, 17(4)*, 573–578.

Umile, E.M., Sandel, M.E, Alavi, A., Terry, C.M., & Plotkin, R.C. (2002). Dynamic imaging in mild traumatic brain injury: Support for the theory of medial temporal vulnerability. *Archives of Physical Medicine and Rehabilitation, 83(11)*, 1506–1513.

Uno, H., Tarara, R., Else, J.G., Suleman, M.A., & Sapolsky, R.M. (1989). Hippocampal damage associated with prolonged and fatal stress in primates. *Journal of Neuroscience, 9*(5), 1705–1711.

Uomoto, J.M., & Essleman, P.C. (1993). Traumatic brain injury and chronic pain: differential types and rates of head injury severity. *Archives of Physical Medicine Rehabilitation, 74*, 61–4.

Valenstein, E.S. (1986). *Great and desperate cures: the rise and decline of psychosurgery and other radical treatments for mental illness.* London: H.K. Lewis.

Valenta, L.J., & De Feo, D.R. (1980). Post-traumatic hypopituitarism due to a hypothalamic lesion. *American Journal of Medicine, 68*, 614–617.

Vallabhajosula, B., & van Gorp, W.G. (2001). Post-Daubert admissibility of scientific evidence on malingering of cognitive deficits. *Journal of the American Academy of Psychiatry and Law, 29*(2), 207–215.

van der Naalt, J., van Zomeren, A.H., Sluiter, W.J., & Minderhoud, J.M. (1999). One year outcome in mild to moderate head injury: the predictive value of acute injury characteristics related to complaints and return to work. *Journal of Neurology Neurosurgery and Psychiatry, 66*(2), 207–213.

Van Praag, H., Schinder, A.F., Christie, B.R., Toni, N., Palmer, T.D., & Gage, F.H. (2002). Functional neurogenesis in the adult hippocampus. *Nature, 415*, 1030–1034.

Van Reekum, R., Bolago, I., Finlayson, M.A.J., Garner, S., & Links, P.S. (1996). Psychiatric disorders after traumatic brain injury. *Brain Injury, 10(5)*, 319–327.

van Reekum, R., Cohen, T., & Wong, J. (2000). Can traumatic brain injury cause psychiatric disorders? *Journal of Neuro-psychiatry and Clinical Neuroscience, 12*, 316–327.

van Woerkom, T.C., Minderhoud, J.M., Gottschalk, T., & Nicolai, G. (1982). Neurotransmitters in the treatment of patients with severe head injuries. *European Neurology, 21*(4), 227–234.

Van Zomeren, A., & Van Den Berg, W. (1985). Residual complaints of patients two years after severe head injury. *Journal of Neurology, Neurosurgery, and Psychiatry, 48*, 21–28.

Varney, N.R. (1988). Prognostic significance of anosmia in patients with closed-head trauma. *Journal of Clinical and Experimental Neuropsychology, 10*(2), 250–254.

Varney, N.R. (2002). Wishing doesn't make it so: A reply to Greiffenstein, Baker and Gola. *Journal of Clinical and Experimental Neuropsychology, 24*(6), 852–853.

Varney, N.R., Martzke, J.S., & Roberts, R.J. (1987). Major depression in patients with closed head injury. *Neuropsychology, 1(1)*, 7–9.

Varney, N.R., & Menefee, L. (1993). Psychosocial and executive deficits following closed head injury: implications for orbital frontal cortex. *Journal of Head Trauma Rehabilitation, 8*, 32–41.

Vataja, R., Leppävuori, A., Pohjasvaara, T., Mäntylä, R., Aronen, H.J., Salonen, O., Kaste, M., & Erkinjuntti T. (2004). Poststroke depression and lesion location revisited. *Journal of Neuropsychiatry and Clinical Neuroscience, 16*, 156–162.

Vaukhonen, K. (1959). Suicide among the male disabled with war injuries to the brain. *Acta Psychiatrica Neurologica Scandinavica, 137*(Suppl.), 90–91.

Veiel, H.O. (1997). A preliminary profile of neuropsychological deficits associated with major depression. *Journal of Clinical and Experimental Neuropsychology, 19*(4), 587–603.

Velakoulis, D., Wood, S.J., Wong, M.T.H., McGorry, P.D., Yung, A., Phillips, L., Smith, D., Brewer, W., Proffitt, T., Desmond, P., & Pantelis, C. (2006). Hippocampal and amygdala volumes according to psychosis stage and diagnosis: A magnetic resonance imaging study of chronic schizophrenia, first-episode psychosis, and ultra-high-risk individuals. Archives of General Psychiatry, 63(2), 139–149.

Vespa, P., Prins, M., Ronne-Engstrom, E., Caron, M., Shalmon, E., Hovda, D.A., Martin, N.A., & Becker, D.P. (1998). Increase in extracellular glutamate caused by reduced cerebral perfusion pressure and seizures after traumatic brain injury: A microdialysis study. *Journal of Neurosurgery, 89*, 971–982.

Villki, J., Ahola, K., Holst, P., Ohman, J., Sevo, A., & Heiskanen, O. (1994). Prediction of psychosocial recovery after head injury with cognitive tests and neurobehavioral ratings. *Journal of Clinical and Experimental Neuropsychology, 16*(3), 325–38.

Violon, A., & De Mol, J. (1987). Psychological sequelae after head traumas in adults. *Acta Neurochirurgica (Wien), 85*(3–4), 96–102.

Volkow, N.D., & Fowler, J.S. (2000). Addiction, a disease of compulsion and drive: involvement of the orbitofrontal cortex. *Cerebral Cortex, 10*(3), 318–325.

Waddell, P.A., & Gronwall, D.M. (1984). Sensitivity to light and sound following minor head injury. *Acta Neurologica Scandinavica, 69(5)*, 270–6.

Walker, A.E. (1972). Long-term evaluation of the social and family adjustment to head injury. *Scandinavian Journal of Rehabilitation Medicine, 4,* 5–8.

Walker, A.E. (1976). The neurological basis of sex. *Neurology India, 24,* 1–13.

Walker, A.E., & Jablon, S. (1961). *A follow-up study of head wounds in World War II.* Washington DC: Veteran's Administration Medical Monograph.

Wall, S.E., Williams, W.H., Cartwright-Hatton, S., Kelly, T.P., Murray, J., Murray, M., Owen, A., & Turner, M. (2006). Neuropsychological dysfunction following repeat concussions in jockeys. *Journal of Neurology, Neurosurgery, and Psychiatry*, 77, 518–520.

Wallace, C.A. (2000). Unawareness of deficits: Emotional implications for patients and significant others. *Dissertation Abstracts International: Section B: the Sciences & Engineering, 60,* 4257.

Walsh, K.W. (1991). *Understanding brain damage: A primer of neuropsychological evaluation* (2nd ed.). Edinburgh: Churchill Livingstone.

Warden, D.L., Gordon, B., McAllister, T.W., Silver, J.M., Barth, J.T., Bruns, J., Drake, A., Gentry, T., Jagoda, A., Katz, D.I., Kraus, J., Labbate, L.A., Ryan, L.M., Sparling, M.B., Walters, B., Whyte, J., Zapata, A., & Zitnay, G. (2006). Guidelines for the pharmacologic treatment of neurobehavioral sequelae of traumatic brain injury. *Journal of Neurotrauma, 23*(10), 1468–1501.

Warden, D.L., Labbate, L.A., Salazar, A.M., Nelson, R., Sheley, E., Staudenmeier, J., & Martin, E. (1997). Posttraumatic stress disorder in patients with traumatic brain injury and amnesia for the event? *Journal of Neuropsychiatry and Clinical Neurosciences, 9*, 18–22.

Warren, R., & Zgourides, G.D. (1991). *Anxiety disorders: A rational-emotive perspective.* Elmsford, NY: Pergamon.

Warrington, E.K. (1984). *Recognition Memory Test.* Windsor, UK: NFER-Nelson.

Weber, J.B., Coverdale, J.H., & Kunik, M.E. (2004). Delirium: current trends in prevention and treatment. *International Medical Journal, 34(*3),115–121.

Webster, J.B., Bell, K.R., Hussey, J.D., Natale, T.K., & Lakshminarayan, S. (2001). Sleep apnea in adults with traumatic brain injury: A preliminary investigation. *Archives of Physical Medicine and Rehabilitation, 82, 316–321.*

Wechsler, D. (1997). *Wechsler Adult Intelligence Scale-III.* New York: Psychological Corporation.

Weddell, R., Oddy, M., & Jenkins, D. (1980). Social adjustment after rehabilitation: A two year follow-up of patients with severe head injury. *Psychological Medicine, 10,* 257–263.

Wegner, D.M., & Zanakos, S. (1994). Chronic thought suppression. *J Pers, 62*(4), 616–640.

Weinberger, D.R., Berman, K.S., & Zec, R.F. (1986). Physiological dysfunction of dorsolateral prefrontal cortex in schizophrenia: 1. Regional cerebral blood flow evidence. *Archives of General Psychiatry, 43,* 1114–1124.

Weissman, M.M., Bland, R.C., Canino, G.J., Greenwald, S., Hwu, H.G., Lee, C.K., Newman, S.C., Oakley-Browne, M.A., Rubio-Stipec, M., & Wickramaratne, P.J. (1994). The cross national epidemiology of obsessive compulsive disorder. The Cross National Collaborative Group. *Journal of Clinical Psychiatry, 55*(Suppl.), 5–10.

Wenzlaff, R.M., Wegner, D.M., & Klein, S.B. (1991). The role of thought suppression in the bonding of thought and mood. *Journal of Personality and Social Psychology, 60,* 500–508.

Wesolowski, M.D., & Burke, W.H. (1988). Behaviour management techniques. In P.M. Deutsch, & K. Fralish (Eds.), *Innovations in head injury rehabilitation* (pp. 27–58). New York: Matthew Bender.

Weston, M.J., & Whitlock, F.A. (1971). The Capgras syndrome following head injury. *British Journal of Psychiatry, 119*(548), 25–31.

Wetter, M.W., Baer, R.A., Berry, D.T.R., Smith, G.T., & Larsen, L.H. (1992). Sensitivity of MMPI–2 validity scales to random responding and malingering. *Psychological Assessment, A Journal of Consulting and Clinical Psychology, 4,* 369–374.

Whalen, R.E., & Luttge, W.G. (1970). Para-chlorophenylalanine methylester: An aphrodisiac. *Science, 169,* 1000–1001.

Whitman, S., Coonley-Hoganson, R., & Desai, B.T. (1984). Comparative head trauma experiences in two socioeconomically different Chicago-area communities: A population study. *American Journal of Epidemiology, 119,* 570–580.

Wilcox, J.A., & Nasrallah, H.A. (1987a). Childhood head trauma and psychosis. *Psychiatry Research, 21*(4), 303–306.

Wilcox, J.A., & Nasrallah, H.A. (1987b). Perinatal distress and prognosis of psychotic illness. *Neuropsychobiology, 17*(4), 173–175.

Wilcox, J.A., & Nasrallah, H.A. (1987c). Perinatal insult as a risk factor in paranoid and nonparanoid schizophrenia. *Psychopathology, 20*(5–6), 285–287.

Wilde, E.A., Bigler, E.D., Gandhi, P.V., Lowry, C.M., Blatter, D.D., Brooks, J., & Ryser, D.K. (2004). Alcohol abuse and traumatic brain injury: Quantitative magnetic resonance imaging and neuropsychological outcome. *Journal of Neurotrauma, 21(2),* 137–147.

Williams, D.H., Levin, H.S., & Eisenberg, H.M. (1990). Mild head injury classification. *Neurosurgery, 27*(3), 422–428.

Williams, W.H. & Evans, J.J. (2003). Brain injury and emotion: An overview to a special issue on biopsychosocial approaches in neurorehabilitation. *Neuropsychological Rehabilitation, 13,* 1–11.

Williams, W.H., Evans, J.J., & Fleminger, S. (2003). Neurorehabilitation and cognitive-behaviour therapy of anxiety disorders after brain injury: An overview and a case illustration of obsessive-compulsive disorder. *Neuropsychological Rehabilitation, 13,* 133–148.

Williams, W.H., Evans, J.J., Wilson, B.A., & Needham, P. (2002). Brief report: prevalence of post-traumatic stress disorder symptoms after severe traumatic brain injury in a representative community sample. *Brain Injury, 16*(8), 673–679.

Williams, W.H., Williams, J.M.G., & Ghadiali, E.J. (1998). Autobiographical memory in traumatic brain injury: Neuropsychological and mood predictors of recall. *Neuropsychological Rehabilitation, 8(1)*, 43–60.

Wilson, B.A. (2003). *Neuropsychological rehabilitation: Theory and practice.* Hove, UK: Lawrence Erlbaum Associates.

Wilson, J.T.L., Teasdale, G.M., Hadley, D.M., Wiedmann, K.D., & Lang, D. (1993). Post-traumatic amnesia: still a valuable yardstick. *Journal of Neurology, Neurosurgery and Psychiatry, 56*, 198–201.

Wise, M.G., & Rundell, J.R. (1999). Anxiety and neurological disorders. *Seminars in Clinical Neuropsychiatry, 4*(2), 98–102.

Woessner, R., & Caplan, B. (1995). Affective disorders following mild to moderate brain injury: Interpretive hazards of the SCL-90-R. *Journal of Head Trauma Rehabilitation, 10(2)*, 78–89.

Wood, R.L. (1987). *Brain injury rehabilitation: A neurobehavioural approach.* London: Croom Helm.

Wood, R.L. (1990). Towards a model of cognitive rehabilitation. In R.L. Wood & I. Fussey (eds). *Cognitive rehabilitation in perspective* (pp. 3–25). Hove, UK: Lawrence Erlbaum Associates.

Woolf, P.D., Hamill, R.W., Lee, A.L., Cox, C., & McDonald, J. (1987). The predictive value of catecholamines in assessing outcome in traumatic brain injury. *Journal of Neurosurgery, 66*, 875–882.

World Health Organisation. (1992). *The ICD-10 classification of mental and behavioural disorders.* Geneva: WHO.

Worthington, A.D., & Melia, Y. (2006). Rehabilitation is compromised by arousal and sleep disorders: Results of a survey of rehabilitation centres. *Brain Injury, 20*(3), 327–332.

Wrightson, P. (1989). Management of disability and rehabilitation services after mild head injury. In H.S. Levin, H.M. Eisenberg, & A.L. Benton, *Mild head injury.* New York: Oxford.

Wrightson, P. (2000). The development of the concept of mild head injury. *Journal of Clinical Neuroscience, 7(5)*, 384–388.

Wrightson, P., & Gronwall, D. (1981). Time off work and symptoms after minor head injury. *Injury, 12*(6), 445–54.

Xiong, Y., Gu, Q., Peterson, P.L., Muizelaar, J.P., & Lee, C.P. (1997). Mitochondrial dysfunction and calcium perturbation induced by traumatic brain injury. *Journal of Neurotrauma, 14*, 23–34.

Yalla, S.V. (1994). Sexual dysfunction in the paraplegic and quadriplegic. In A.H. Bennett (Ed.), *Management of male impotence* (pp.181–191). Baltimore: Williams & Wilkins.

Yamaguchi, M. (1992). Incidence of headache and severity of head injury. *Headache, 32*, 427–431.

Yarnell, P.R., & Lynch, S. (1970). Retrograde memory immediately after concussion. *Lancet, 1*, 863–865.

Young, A.W., Robertson, I.H., Hellawell, D.J., de Pauw, K.W., & Pentland, B. (1992). Cotard delusion after brain injury. *Psychological Medicine, 22*(3), 799–804.

Young, H., Olin, M., & Schmidek, H. (1980). Fractures of the sella turcica. *Neurosurgery, 7*, 23–29.

Young, M.E., Rintala, D.H., Rossi, C.D., Hart, K.A., & Fuhrer, M.J. (1995). Alcohol and marijuana use in a community-based sample of persons with spinal cord injury. *Archives of Physical Medicine and Rehabilitation, 76*(6), 525–532.

Young, M.A., Scheftner, W.A., Fawcett, J., & Klerman, G.L. (1990). Gender differences in the clinical features of unipolar major depressive disorder. *Journal of Nervous and Mental Disease, 178*(3), 200–203.

Young, T., Evans, L., Finn, L., & Palta, M. (1997). Estimation of clinically diagnosed proportion of sleep apnea syndrome in middle-aged men and women. *Sleep, 20*, 705–706.

Yücel, M., Pantelis, C., Stuart, G.W., Wood, S.J., Maruff, P., Velakoulis, D., Pipingas, A., Crowe, S.F., Tochon-Danguy, H.J., & Egan, G.F. (2002). Anterior cingulate activation during Stroop task performance: A PET to MRI co registration study of individual patients with schizophrenia *American Journal of Psychiatry, 159*(2), 251–254.

Yücel, M., Stuart, G.W., Maruff, P., Velakoulis, D., Crowe, S.F., Savage, G., & Pantelis, C. (2001). Hemispheric and gender-related differences in gross morphology of the anterior cingulate/paracingulate cortex in normal volunteers: An IRM morphometric study. *Cerebral Cortex, 11,* 17–25.

Zasler, N.D. (1991). Sexuality in neurological disability: An overview. *Sexuality and Disability, 9,* 11–27.

Zasler, N.D. (1998). Sexuality issues after traumatic brain injury. *Sexuality Update, 1,* 1–3.

Zasler, N.D., & Horn, L. (1990). Rehabilitative management of sexual dysfunction. *Journal of Head Trauma Rehabilitation, 5,* 14–24.

Zeman, A. (2001). Invited review: Consciousness. *Brain, 124,* 1263–1289.

Zencius, A., Wesolowski, M.D., Bourke, W.H., & Hough, S. (1990). Managing hypersexual disorders in brain-injured clients. *Brain Injury, 4,* 175–181.

Zhang, Q., & Sachdev, P.S. (2003). Psychotic disorder and traumatic brain injury. *Current Psychiatry Reports, 5*(3), 197–201.

Ziskin, J., & Faust, D. (1988). *Coping with psychiatric and psychological testimony* (Vols. 1–3, 4th ed.). Marina Del Ray, CA: Law & Psychology Press.

Zubkov, A.Y., Pilkington, A.S., Bernanke, D.H., Parent, A.D., & Zhang, J. (1999). Posttraumatic cerebral vasospasm: Clinical and morphological presentations. *Journal of Neurotrauma, 9*, 763–770.

Zuckerman, J.D., Mirabello, S.C., Newman, D., Gallagher, M., & Cuomo, F. (1991). The painful shoulder: Part II. Intrinsic disorders and impingement syndrome. *American Family Physician, 43*(2), 497–512.

Index

Page references given in **boldface** type refer to tables.

B

E

G

H

I

M

N

R

S

T

U

V

W

Y

Z